CLINICAL EDUCATION FOR THE ALLIED HEALTH PROFESSIONS

CLINICAL EDUCATION FOR THE ALLIED HEALTH PROFESSIONS

Edited by

CHARLES W. FORD, Ph.D.

THE C. V. MOSBY COMPANY

Saint Louis   1978

The C. V. Mosby Company
11830 Westline Industrial Drive, St. Louis, Missouri 63141

Library of Congress Cataloging in Publication Data

Main entry under title:

Clinical education for the allied health professions.

   Bibliography: p.
   Includes index.
   1. Paramedical education.   I. Ford, Charles W.
[DNLM: 1. Allied health personnel—Education.
2. Health occupations—Education. W18 C641]
R847.C54   610   78-3620
ISBN 0-8016-1623-9

TS/CB/B 9 8 7 6 5 4 3 2 1

CONTRIBUTORS

Clair Agriesti-Johnson, Ph.D., is Assistant Professor of Medical Dietetics, School of Allied Medical Professions (SAMP), the Ohio State University. As Curriculum Coordinator for the Division of Medical Dietetics, she conducts research in the area of curriculum evaluation. She has authored papers in journals relative to the delivery of both educational and health care services, and has served as a consultant on curriculum and evaluation to a variety of programs preparing clinical dietitians. She is active in teacher preparation for health professionals and has served on the staff of the Competency Based Curriculum Project, SAMP.

Jo Ivey Boufford, M.D., is Co-Director of the Institute for Health Team Development and Director of the Residency Program in Social Medicine at Montefiore Hospital and Medical Center in New York. She is also Assistant Professor in the Department of Community Health and Clinical Instructor in Pediatrics at the Albert Einstein College of Medicine. Her activities are largely in the fields of primary care residency training and interdisciplinary health team development. She is currently serving as a member of the National Advisory Council on Health Professions Education.

John P. Casbergue, Ph.D., is an Associate Professor, Office of Medical Education Research and Development, Michigan State University. He was previously at the School of Allied Medical Professions, the Ohio State University. As an educational consultant in faculty and educational development, he assists faculty in identifying educational needs, and designing and conducting workshops or other educational programs to meet those needs. His consulting role has also included working with professional educational program faculty in medicine, law, nursing, dietetics, and other allied health professions in the United States, Canada, and other countries.

Phyllis Drennan, R.N., Ph.D., is Dean and Professor of the School of Nursing, University of Northern Colorado, Greeley, Colorado. She has been active in nursing education and service for over twenty-five years. Membership includes: AERA Special Interest Group—Educational Research and Development Evaluators, Western Society for Research in Nursing, Pi Lambda Theta, Sigma Theta Tau, National League for Nursing, American Nurses Association, and Colorado Public Health Association. She has been a site visitor on accreditation for the National League for Nursing, North Central Commission, and is currently serving on the Veterans Administration Health Manpower Training Assistance Review Committee.

Shirley A. Eichenwald, B.S., RRA, is the Clinical Coordinator and Assistant Director of the Program in Health Information Administration at the College of St. Scholastica in Duluth, Minnesota. From 1974 to 1976 she coordinated a total curriculum revision project for the program. She is currently engaged in graduate study at the University of Minnesota, Duluth, and is President of the Minnesota Medical Record Association.

J. Kay Felt, J.D., is a partner in a Detroit law firm. She is also Adjunct Assistant Professor in the Department of Community Medicine, Wayne State University. A major portion of her practice is directed toward the health care delivery system. She

v

is an active member in several national associations relating to health law.

Charles W. Ford, Ph.D., is Associate Dean (Acting) at the School of Health Related Professions, State University of New York at Buffalo. Dr. Ford was previously on the staff of an allied health clinical education research project working with a consortium in Grand Rapids, Michigan. He also spent two years as an administrator in Ghana, West Africa. He is on the Medical Technology Review Committee for the National Accrediting Agency for Clinical Laboratory Sciences. He has served in over 60 projects and institutions as a consultant in the health professions. He and Margaret K. Morgan have edited *Teaching in the Health Professions*.

Leonard E. Heller, Ed.D., is Assistant Dean and Director of Educational Development, University of Kentucky College of Medicine. He was formerly Assistant Director with the Office of Educational Resources and Research at the University of Michigan College of Medicine and Coordinator of Evaluation at Baylor College of Medicine. Dr. Heller has served as an educational consultant for curriculum design and program evaluation to various programs in the health professions, especially those related to primary care.

J. Dennis Hoban, Ed.D., is Associate Professor of Biomedical Communications, College of Medicine, University of Cincinnati. He was formerly with the Office of Medical Education Research and Development at Michigan State University (MSU) where he directed a simulation laboratory. He was also a member of a research team studying the state of the art of simulation in medical education in a project funded by the National Library of Medicine. He has been actively involved in instructional and faculty development at both MSU and the University of Cincinnati.

Alan L. Hull, M.S.B.A., is a Research Associate, Office of Educational Resources and Research, The University of Michigan College of Medicine. He is a Ph.D. candidate in the Center for the Study of Higher Education at The University of Michigan, studying institutional characteristics that affect medical school success in sponsored research activity. He has evaluated several medical and nursing educational programs and conducted cost studies related to medical education in the state of Michigan.

David M. Irby, Ph.D., is Director, Training Program, Office of Research in Medical Education, University of Washington. He has been actively involved in curriculum and faculty development in allied health and medicine on the regional and national levels through workshops and consultation. He and Margaret K. Morgan have edited *Evaluating Clinical Competence in the Health Professions*.

Richard D. Kingston, D.D.S., is Associate Professor and Director, Center for Learning Resources, School of Allied Health Professions, University of Kentucky. Previously he was Vice-President and Director of Education for Comprenetics, Inc., Los Angeles, California. He also held positions in allied health with the Allied Health Professions Projects, UCLA, and with Weber State College, Ogden, Utah. Dr. Kingston writes in the media field, in allied health, and in fiction.

Anthony LaDuca, Ph.D., is Associate Professor of Health Professions Education, Center for Educational Development, University of Illinois at the Medical Center in Chicago. His recent work has focused on extensive analysis of selected allied health fields, development and validation of a new methodology for competence definition, construction of prototype evaluation instruments, and design of related curriculum revisions. In addition, Dr. LaDuca has been consultant to numerous professional organizations and has conducted workshops on criterion-referenced test development and evaluation of clinical performance.

M. Jeanne Madigan, M.A., OTR, is Associate Professor and Curriculum Coordinator, Curriculum in Occupational Therapy, School of Associated Medical Sciences, University of Illinois at the Medical Center in Chicago. For two years she was full-time consultant with the proficiency test development project of the University of Illinois Area Health Education System. More recently, she serves as Coordinator of Appraisal for the School of Associated Medical Sciences and holds appointment as Adjunct Associate Professor of Medical Education in the Center for Educational Development. She has chaired the Certification Committee of the American Occupational Therapy Association for four years.

Margaret K. Morgan, Ph.D., is Director, Center for Allied Health Instructional Personnel; Associate Professor, Curriculum and Instruction, and Adjunct Associate Professor, Health Related Professions, University of Florida. She was formerly Assistant Director of the University of Kentucky Center for Learning Resources for Allied Health. She has written or edited many publications, including *Teaching in the Health Professions, Evaluating Clinical Competence in the Health Professions, The Health Professions,* and *Cognitive and Affective Dimensions in Health Related Education.*

J. Warren Perry, Ph.D., is Professor of Health Sciences Administration at the State University of New York at Buffalo. From 1966 to 1977 he was the Dean of the School of Health Related Professions, where he was presented with the Chancellor's Award for Excellence in Administration in 1977. Dr. Perry was the second president of the American Society of Allied Health Professions and presented the Mary E. Switzer Memorial Lecture at the tenth annual meeting of ASAHP. He is well known for his extensive and visionary writing in allied health education. Among his many firsts was his responsibility as the first editor of the *Journal of Allied Health.*

Patricia J. Pierce, M.S., RRA, is Chairperson of the Department of Health Information Administration at the College of St. Scholastica in Duluth, Minnesota, and has also served as Chairperson of the Division of Health Sciences. She is a past president of the American Medical Record Association and has served on the Education and Registration Committee, as well as many other committees for that organization. She is on the Advisory Board of the *Journal of Clinical Computing* and has published a programmed instruction manual on computation of hospital statistics.

Craig L. Scanlan, M.Ed., RRT, is Assistant Professor and Educational Director of the Respiratory Therapy Program at Brookdale Community College, Lincroft, New Jersey. He is active professionally in state and national affairs, having chaired several committees on education and learning resources. He is presently a member of the Joint Review Committee on Respiratory Therapy Education of the American Medical Association. He

also serves as an assistant editor for *Respiratory Care,* Journal of the American Association for Respiratory Therapy, and has published several articles on allied health education.

Jennie D. Seaton, Ed.D., is an Associate Professor of Allied Health Education, School of Allied Health Professions, Health Sciences Division of Virginia Commonwealth University and Coordinator of the Veterans Administration/Medical College of Virginia Center for Allied Health Education at the McGuire Veterans Administration Hospital in Richmond. Her previous experiences include teaching clinical chemistry at the University of Kentucky and participating in the Administrative Internship Program of the School of Health Related Professions, State University of New York at Buffalo as a Kellogg Fellow.

Harold G. Smith, M.Ed., RPT, is Chief Physical Therapist, Eugene Talmadge Memorial Hospital. He was formerly Associate Professor in the Departments of Physical and Occupational Therapy, Medical College of Georgia, as well as the coordinator of Clinical Experiences, Department of Physical Therapy. He served as a task force member on evaluation of clinical education—Section for Education, American Physical Therapy Association. He has been on the faculty of several workshops in clinical education and evaluation, and is presently on a Veterans Administration Task Force developing guidelines for clinical affiliation for physical therapy students.

Shirley A. Weaver, M.A., MT(ASCP), is coordinating the Grand Rapids Cooperative In-service Program. She is also a Ph.D. candidate at Michigan State University in Medical Sociology. She was previously on the staff at a consortium for health professionals, Grand Rapids, Michigan. As a medical technology educator she has been involved in efforts to plan and coordinate medical technology education and clinical laboratory continuing education on a statewide basis. She presently serves as the chairperson of the Education Committee for the American Society for Medical Technology.

FOREWORD

From the perspective of time, the literature for allied health education can trace its expansion and growth to the passage of the Allied Health Education Act of 1966. The development of new colleges, schools, and divisions for these health professions, defined as "allied" by that legislation, became one of the most important educational administrative innovations in academic health centers, universities, and community colleges throughout the United States. Although many speakers were expounding on allied health philosophy and potential, educators in the departments and administrative offices of these new programs found a void in written communication concerning some of the real challenges in allied health education. Thus, it is encouraging to note that within the past few years this literature is beginning to develop through both texts and a quarterly journal; the "ballpark" for such educational literature for these health professions is now responding to some of the problems and issues in education in these fields.

I believe that this book should prove to be a hallmark among the new writings for these health professions, for it speaks directly to the area of clinical education, one of the most complex and important components of allied health education programs. This text also removes the stigma of on-the-job training in hospital settings and adds the responsibility of improving the clinical experience, supervised by the personnel in the educational settings working in harmony with clinical practitioners.

With major emphasis being placed on a more refined curricula for many of these fields and with new thrusts in clinical education based upon changes in health care delivery patterns, it is propitious to have this new text that will assist allied health educators learn how to plan, develop, and evaluate clinical education programs.

Historically, allied health education has made the transition from total emphasis on hospital-based settings to emphasis on academic settings—sometimes without regard to the health care settings. We now realize that one cannot separate didactic instruction from clinical instruction as though they were two distinct entities. We must concentrate on partnership program development with integration of components as the key. Although this book focuses on the issues of clinical education, it is in the context of total program improvement.

The editor of this text has had rich experience in participating in a unique allied health clinical education consortium; this gave him a breadth of practical experience with many fields at various educational levels. His former experience in an allied health instructional program has helped him develop the conceptual framework to clinical education. That is evident in both *Teaching in the Health Professions* and this text. It is little wonder, then, that he has become a sought-after educational

ix

consultant for allied health educational pursuits.

Faculty and administrative personnel who have had clinical education responsibilities and those who are now taking on new clinical education assignments will appreciate the comprehensive Table of Contents of this text. Here one finds a large number of competent, experienced educators who share their specialized expertise in discussing the various components of clinical education. Although some of the individual health fields have a rich history of experience in clinical education, this new text presents a special approach to the problems involved in the selection, development, and evaluation of clinical education programs. In fact, perhaps the most significant contribution of this text may be found in the fact that each chapter deals with an aspect of clinical education in such a way that faculty members and others now have an opportunity to evaluate existing programs in line with the ideas and concepts presented.

Hopefully, this author and others will focus their attention on other important aspects of allied health education and treat each topic in the comprehensive nature of this text. As activities such as these occur we will move further away from those days when we stressed manpower development and magnitude of programs to this imminently superior time when the quality aspects of each curriculum can now be given priority attention.

J. Warren Perry

PREFACE

To study the phenomenon of disease without books
is to sail an uncharted sea, while to study books without patients
is not to go to sea at all.

SIR WILLIAM OSLER

In a review of the book *Teaching in the Health Professions*, edited by Margaret K. Morgan of the University of Florida and myself, Bella J. May suggested that the book provided a needed tool for the health professions. She further suggested that the editors "might try to expand each of the sections into a book of its own." Dr. Morgan and Dr. Irby of the University of Washington have produced a textbook that explores assessment more fully: *Evaluating Clinical Competence in the Health Professions*. During the same period of time I have busied myself developing a book dealing with another aspect of *Teaching in the Health Professions*, namely clinical education.

This book on clinical education has evolved out of my work on a Division of Associated Health Professions contract. The contract called for the development of an allied health clinical education consortium model. In developing this model, I was forced to look and look again at the characteristics of clinical education in nearly twenty allied health professions.

The diversity of these clinical experiences ranged from hospital-based experiences controlled almost entirely by the health care facility to those set in the offices of private dentists and physicians as well as to clinical experiences occurring almost wholly on the campus of an educational facility. The extremes of these experiences suggested that commonalities would be scarce. However, as I continued to examine the clinical experiences, and methods to improve them, I soon discovered that there in fact were common problems and common solutions—if not in the specific, at least in the general.

Furthermore, I realized that many of the points that Dr. Morgan and I were trying to make in *Teaching in the Health Professions* were relevant to the clinical experience. This idea was crystallized when I attended a workshop on clinical education models at the University of Connecticut. After general workshop sessions with the faculty and participants, I discussed my hypothesis with Polly Fitz, workshop leader and Dean of the College of Allied Health. She agreed with some of my premises and gave me further suggestions, particularly from her experiences as a registered dietitian. With these ideas beginning to make sense, I worked up an outline embodying many of the concepts of a systems approach to clinical education. During this time, Shirley Weaver, my colleague in the consortium, provided some thoughtful input. The remainder is unimportant history.

What *is* important is for the reader to understand that there is a design to the book. In accord with a systems approach to instruction, this book states the belief that establishing goals, objectives, and policies must be the first decision point. The go–no–go decision should result from information at this early stage. The first position that needs assessment holds in this book reinforces this belief. If the needs cannot be clearly established, then what is the point of clinical experience?

The remainder of the chapters in Part I emphasize some of the important issues concerning the establishment of policies and procedures. As is the case with the entire book *some* of the issues, not *all* of them, are explored. The choice of content was a matter of setting content priorities and identifying persons capable of addressing each issue.

Part II parallels the second part of the suggested system, identifying student characteristics by focusing on identification of the kind of plans needed to match program intent.

Part III of the textbook parallels the idea that the instructor must facilitate learning by choosing among several alternatives. So, too, in clinical education must the faculty, both clinical and academic, choose the most cost efficient and effective means of reaching the objectives established for the program.

Part IV of this text directly parallels the evaluation stage of the systems model. A system is not complete until suggestions are made to help determine whether the objectives have been met. In this section I suggest the clinical education guide, which I have found to make a considerable difference in student and faculty attitudes and experiences during clinical education. Although not an assessment tool in itself, it is a tool for improving the assessment process. Other chapters in this section provide additional concrete suggestions.

This book neither addresses all the issues of clinical education nor attempts to deal with highly specialized and sophisticated issues that are more unusual than common. It does, however, address the issues that are most relevant and common for the greatest number of allied health practitioners and educators, particularly those new to allied health education.

My thanks go to a number of persons. I have already suggested two: Polly Fitz for helping me to see the problem of clinical education in a Gestalt, and Shirley Weaver for her constant, sometimes irritating questions that I had to answer—at least to my own satisfaction if not to hers.

I also owe thanks:

To Aaron Andrews and John Brady for allowing me to pursue a personal goal in the context of an assignment that dovetailed and integrated with it.

To Dolores Filson for serving as my second pair of eyes in the editing process as she made sure that all manuscripts were consistent and complete.

To Chris Clark and Helen Shively for typing the correspondence with the contributors.

To Sandy McCoy for typing the final copy that was ultimately set in type.

To Carol Elkins and Donna Watson for arranging for my participation in "practice" workshops.

And finally to many workshop participants who sat through sessions listening to ideas that germinated into this effort.

Charles W. Ford

CONTENTS

CLINICAL EDUCATION FOR THE ALLIED HEALTH PROFESSIONS

prologue **A PLACE TO BEGIN**
A SYSTEMS APPROACH TO
CLINICAL EDUCATION

Charles W. Ford

Show a child a toy pyramid tower made of various sized, doughnut-shaped plastic rings and a center post. Take the tower apart, give it to the child, and what results? The child will soon place the rings on the upright post to begin to form the tower. Initially, the child will not always place the largest rings at the base and proceed to construct the pyramid tower with a series of smaller rings; the child will make mistakes. With some guidance and a period of trial and error, the child will soon learn to construct the tower quickly, efficiently, and correctly. In simple terms, the child can be said to have become competent in building the pyramid tower.

This prologue addresses issues of competency in the context of a systems approach to instruction. The reasons are many. First, introduction of competency-based education requires an institutional commitment that demands a departure from traditional education. Clinical education for the allied health professions requires articulation among several institutions, with heavy dependence on health care institutions. Radical educational change might be possible within one educational institution, but it is less likely to be coordinated among several institutions, especially those that have a secondary commitment to education, a primary one to health care. Second, the present state of clinical education can benefit from focusing on a systems approach to instruction and from moving from a traditional approach toward competency-based education, particularly in the didactic portion of curricula. Third, the clinical portion of curricula can be improved by utilizing concepts and principles of a systems approach to instruction. Since the most difficult task in clinical education is evaluation, utilizing a system based upon competency will ensure improved instruction and evaluation.

There is little question that in the health professions competency has always been a central focus for the preparation of practitioners. I believe that a systems approach to instruction can provide a foundation that will enable faculty to introduce competency-based education into their own programs in an incremental fashion.

1

TERMINOLOGY

The English language provides an array of synonyms, while it preserves subtle distinctions among them that suggest specific nuances. The specialized language of education, on the other hand, often uses one word that is differently defined by each author. This chapter defines each word in a manner consistent with those definitions generally accepted by educators. New terminology is not introduced, for the language of education is already sufficiently complete. For example, *competency* is defined in this chapter as it is in the literature—as the ability to carry out a specific task within given parameters of control. Thus competency-based education is the designing of a course, program, or curriculum on the basis of what the student is supposed to learn to do.

Another term that frequently appears in the literature is *performance-based education*. Other authors attempt to differentiate the terms *competency* and *performance:*

Objectives describing a behavior, but without additional criteria, lead to performance-based education, while behavioral objectives with performance criteria lead to competency-based education (p. 89).[3]

Although some authors differentiate between the terms, this text concurs with Houston and Howsam:

Some see this [competency] as the more comprehensive of the alternative terms and hence as the more capable of including the wide range of types of objectives and of abilities to perform. At best, however, the choice must be recognized as an arbitrary one made in the interests of uniformity. The two terms remain synonymous and hence subject to personal choice (p. viii).[7]

Roueche, in the companion chapter to this one in *Teaching in the Health Professions*, also equates the terms:

In all definitions of learning, a basic condition associated with learning is changed behavior. *Competency-* or *performance-based* instruction implies that learning produces a change in the learner's behavior (p. 2).[11]

A straightforward comparison of a competency-based and a conventional educational system seems in order. Young and Van Mondfrans[15] have developed a table (see Table 1) that provides insight into the *pure* attributes of competency-based education in comparison with conventional education. The word *pure* is italicized with purpose. Broski and his colleagues at Ohio State University began their first published report on competency-based curriculum design with these words:

A competency-based curriculum, like a core curriculum, is often discussed, rarely defined, and seldom operationalized. In its pure, theoretical form, it probably has not been implemented anywhere—ever.[2]

The description of the competency-based system in Table 1 is approximated in application; perhaps it has not been implemented anywhere in a pure form. The reader must determine to what extent the principles in Table 1 can be applied to the clinical setting.

Fig. 1 is a model for systematic instruction. It includes concepts introduced by Tyler[14] and is integrated with the teaching model of DeCecco[4] (as adapted by Ford and Morgan). This eclectic systems model can be put into practice in a variety of ways. In this book, it is applied to clinical education.

Table 1

A comparison of competency-based and conventional systems of instruction

Issues	Competency-based	Conventional
1. Who sets the goals and objectives of instruction?	Both the teacher and student are usually involved. When the teacher sets the goals and objectives, the student is told what they are and often is allowed some choice of objective or goal.	The teacher usually sets the goals and objectives. Often they are not clearly defined. Students are usually not told what they are. Students usually do not have a choice.
2. Who decides on the means and procedures of instruction?	Students often have a choice of alternative routes, experiences, and materials to use in pursuing a given goal or objective. The student controls the amount of time spent on the goal or objective.	The teacher usually controls the situation and presents all students with the same materials and experiences for the same amount of time.
3. What is learned?	Students usually learn how to do something.	Students may learn about something.
4. Who decides on the evaluation procedures?	The teacher ensures that the evaluation procedures are consistent with the objectives. Often students have a choice of ways to demonstrate that they can perform as expected.	The teacher usually gives a test of his or her own design. Students often don't know what is expected of them. Testing procedures tend to be paper-and-pencil tests.
5. When does evaluation take place?	When the student indicates readiness.	When the teacher is through teaching a unit of instruction.
6. When does the student move on to the next set of learning goals and objectives?	When the student has mastered the last set of objectives and goals. The student continues working on a set of goals or objectives until mastery is achieved.	When the last unit has been taught and the evaluation of students is completed. Students may have "failed" or "passed" the last unit at various levels of proficiency. Nevertheless, all students move on to new content.

Adapted from Young, J. I., and Von Mondfroms, A. P.: Psychological implications of competency-based education. In Burns, R. W., and Klingstedt, J. L., editors: Competency-based education, Englewood Cliffs, N.J., 1973, Educational Technology Publications, Inc.

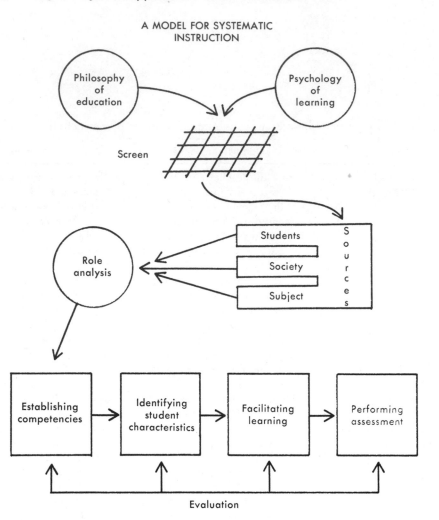

Fig. 1

A paradigm of the basic steps in a systems approach to instruction.

Although clinical education in most cases occurs within a wider context that includes both didactic and clinical education, the issues of clinical education are specific enough to demand individual attention. Neither this chapter nor any other chapter in this book presents an argument for this premise; it is an assumption that is accepted as a given.

THE MODEL

Fig. 1 is a simplified paradigm of the basic steps in a systematic approach to clinical education. The graphic is linear; other models exist in the literature that are circular. Whether the model is linear or circular, the *process* is the focus of attention. And the process is always in a state of becoming more than it already is; always developing; always being reconsidered; stable but not inflexible; flexible but not without form. To make sense out of some of the more prominent characteristics, the reader must examine the model in closer detail.

Philosophy of education

Curriculum designing occurs within the context of what the designer believes about education. *For whom?* and *for what?* are central questions. "Everyone should have the same opportunity" is not congruent with "only those with exceptional ability should have the opportunity." The former is democratic; the latter, elitist. These statements deal with the *for whom* of education.

The *for what* answer depends on the designer's view of man. Do human beings control the environment or does the environment control humans? Answers to these questions will lead to various emphases in the design of a curriculum and in the subsequent design of clinical experiences.

Any philosophical position of education for the health professions must define the relationship of education to patient care or, more appropriately, within the context of patient care. Is education mainly for preparing to live a life or preparing for a career? Is education to be technical or theoretical? What constraints or compromises must exist within the health professions if patients are to receive first priority?

Psychology of learning

What one believes about *how* students learn also has implications for curriculum design. For example, modeling is important in the health professions. Where is modeling most effective? To what extent should it be utilized? Is learning by social imitation really useful in preparing practitioners for new roles in a changing health care delivery system? Or is it more important to provide students with the thought processes necessary to put content and experience into an organized whole (Gestalt field theory)? Or is learning a result of providing the right stimulus in order to generate the correct response?[5]

Whether or not these questions are considered, the impact of learning theory on curriculum design is apparent as clinical experiences are designed. Several chapters in this book address the design of clinical experiences from different vantage points. Each reflects a theory of learning: Agriesti-Johnson, as she addresses early exposure and its limitations and implications; Kingston, as he discusses various approaches to graduate level experiences; Hoban and Casbergue, as they suggest ways to use simulation. These chapters and other emphasize that what one believes about learning should be reflected in the structures of the learning experiences.

Screen

The ideal should always be considered when dealing with the level of abstraction demanded in examining a philosophy of education and a psychology of learning. If the ideal is not considered at this juncture, it most likely will never be considered. Too often the ideal is prematurely dismissed as being unworkable. Once the ideal is considered and developed, then and only then should restraints and constraints serve to screen out the portion of the ideal that is unworkable.*

Sources

How does one determine what is to be taught? The answer is by examining the three major sources of available information. *Students* can provide a great deal of

---

*The original Tyler model suggests that screens should follow the generation of tentative general objectives. Popham and Baker[10] report that Tyler has more recently suggested using screens earlier.

insight into the teaching/learning process in terms of both content and methodology. In conventional programs, students are often disregarded as not possessing the "keys to the academic kingdom"; their suggestions are neither welcomed nor solicited. As indicated in Table 1, a competency-based program encourages student input into the goal-setting process.

Since *society* is both supplying funds and employing program graduates, it has a role in defining what is to be taught. This fact has been recognized for many years in the allied health professions. Community advisory committees provide this input, as do periodic follow-up questionnaires sent to employers.

The third source is the most widely used and accepted input for content: the *subject* itself. The historical development of curricula has centered on the content dictated by "what a health professional should know." Subject experts are epitomized by the professional organizations, which play a strong role in what a given professional will learn for the present and where the profession should go in the future. Of course, society does control some professions by licensure laws, which in most instances describe the bounds of practice.

Meeth,[9] rather than dividing sources into three broad categories, identifies seven authority bases that can be used to decide which competencies will be included in a program:

1. Individual students
2. Patients and clients of service
3. Practitioners
4. Faculty
5. Employers
6. Experts
7. Government (legislation)

Whether three broad categories or seven authority bases are cited, the point remains the same: the definition of the tasks the graduates will perform (be competent to do) must come from a variety of sources.

Role

The sources provide the information to be collated and categorized into role analysis. These tasks are identified at a given time, but they still undergo the constant reexamination that is necessary to maintain standards and they respond to the allied health professions that continue to become more sophisticated. Whether it be expanded duties for the dental hygienist or the inclusion of computer instruction for the medical records administrator, the process is always in a state of becoming. Thus the role analysis is not only what *is;* the analysis should also project the needs for the future.

Establishing competencies

The task lists are used for identification of the specific competencies needed within the profession. Competency-based education arises out of the development, teaching, and evaluation of these competencies. At this point, performance objectives must also be developed to help specify the competencies. Burns[3] contends that objectives are at the heart of performance- and competency-based learning. Since the issue is so important, it is addressed more extensively later in this prologue.

Identifying student characteristics

Another major component of the instructional model is the identification of who the students are and what ability they bring to the program. Again, general learning principles can be aptly applied to the clinical experience (that is, curriculum designers should determine the students' level of knowledge and what experiences, academic and/or experiential, the students have already had).

Facilitating learning

Once the competencies are known and the strengths and weaknesses of the students are known, the instructor must answer the question that is central to the teaching profession: what means are available to help the student learn in the most efficient manner? The diagnosis begins to occur as the instructor identifies student characteristics. The treatment and/or prescription can begin to occur as soon as the instructor selects some methods to help students achieve the desired competency.

Performing assessment

A final major component of the instructional model is the determination of results. Assessment data relating to the competencies delineated must be collected and analyzed. However, this process should not end with the assessment of *what is;* it must extend to *what could be*. The model's feedback loop provides for sending back messages for improving various components of the model in order to improve the system. Assessment becomes *evaluation* when the results of analysis are utilized.

Summary of the model

In a cursory way, the description of the steps in the instructional model provide an overview of the approach to the content of this book. The application is to clinical education, but the principles remain the same.

Establishing competencies in the instructional model has a counterpart in Part one: Formulating Goals, Policies, and Objectives. Identifying student characteristics has a counterpart in Part two: Designing Learning and Organizational Strategies. Facilitating learning has a counterpart in Part three: Developing and Implementing Programs. Performing assessment has a counterpart in Part four: Assessing Outcomes. The point of drawing attention to the parallel is that the systems approach to clinical education is the application of systems theory to a particular setting. Systems theory application leads to a planning and implementation model. Thus the concepts of a systems approach are repeated by different authors throughout this book, starting with Weaver, who in Chapter 1 discusses needs assessment.

IMPLEMENTATION OF THE MODEL

To implement a systems approach to clinical education, curriculum designers must state competencies in performance terms. This often requires a translation step. For example, the American Society of Medical Technology[1] has listed over 200 statements of competence of clinical laboratory practitioners. Four of these statements follow:

Evaluate the systems and procedures for receiving, controlling, and verifying laboratory performance for optimum efficiency and minimum cost to the patient and laboratory (p. 5).

Create an effective working relationship with lines of authority above and below management position and with peers (p. 5).

Consult with physicians on additional tests which may be necessary to illustrate any problem (p. 19).

Integrate the principles of host-parasite relationships, pathogenesis of infectious diseases, and epidemiology of infectious diseases in the establishment of protocols for investigating and reporting findings on microbial organisms and therapeutic indications (p. 20).

These four statements of competence help to define the tasks of a medical technologist, but they must be translated into behavioral or performance objectives, the key to competency-based education.

TAXONOMY OF OBJECTIVES

A taxonomic system is helpful in writing precise objectives:

1. It helps in determining the relative difficulty of achieving objectives.
2. It aids in determining the sequence of learning experiences.

This makes sense, because *taxonomy* literally means the department of knowledge that embodies the laws and principles of classification. The word derives from the Greek *taxis*, meaning arrangement, and *nomos*, meaning law.

When taxonomy is mentioned, Bloom invariably comes to mind. He and his associates set the stage for determining the levels of a cognitive taxonomy.* The work of Krathwohl, one of Bloom's associates, who developed a classification for affective levels, is less well known.* Several efforts to classify psychomotor skills have been undertaken. They are even less well known.[6,13] In order to reveal the Gestalt of taxonomies, this section outlines the three taxonomies and their application.

Table 2 indicates the cognitive levels, starting with the lowest and proceeding to the highest; definitions of each follow the terms.

Cognitive domain

Fig. 2 is a graphic illustration of the heirarchical steps in the cognitive domain. Under each level is a list of verbs that are useful in writing performance objectives.

---

*See bibliography at end of book.

Table 2
Classification of behavioral objectives: Cognitive domain

Level	Description
Knowledge	Remembering by recognition or recall facts, ideas, material, or phenomena
Comprehension	Understanding the literal message contained in a communication by translation, interpretation, or extrapolation
Application	Selecting and using technical principles, ideas, or theories in a problem-solving situation
Analysis	Breaking down material into constituent parts and relating how the parts are organized
Synthesis	Putting together elements and parts to form a whole that constitutes a new structure or pattern
Evaluation	Making qualitative and quantitative judgments in terms of meeting criteria

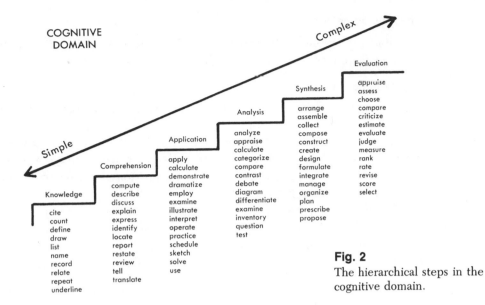

Fig. 2
The hierarchical steps in the cognitive domain.

Table 3
Classification of behavioral objectives: Affective domain

Level	Description
Receiving	Being aware of phenomena and stimuli and willing to control and direct attention
Responding	Complying with a suggestion, being willing to respond, and responding with satisfaction
Valuing	Accepting a value as a belief, preferring the value, and pursuing the value
Organizing	Conceptualizing a value and organizing a value system into an ordered relationship
Characterizing an internally consistent value system	Acting with consistency in accordance with values that are integrated into a total philosophy or world view

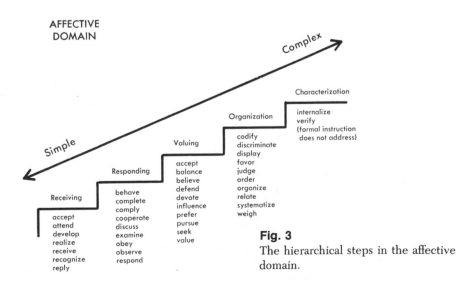

Fig. 3
The hierarchical steps in the affective domain.

Affective domain

Table 3 shows the affective domain in an analogous way. Fig. 3 suggests verbs for affective objectives.

Psychomotor domain

The psychomotor domain, as developed by Simpson,[13] is presented as a useful classification of levels of motor skills.

Simpson's work has not had the widespread publication of that of Bloom and Krathwohl. Just as their classification has provided some insight into the instructional process so can her taxonomy. As in the case of the previous domains, suggested verbs for writing objectives are listed in Fig. 4.

This prologue does not provide instructions on the writing of objectives, for others have done this quite well. Lynch and Holloway[8] have addressed this issue with sufficient clarity and depth for the health professions that it need not be repeated here. Segall and coworkers[12] have detailed the steps for examining the components of

Table 4
Classification of behavioral objectives: Psychomotor domain

Level	Description
Perception	Being aware of objects, qualities, or relations through the senses, selecting relevant cues, and relating the cues to motor act
Set	Being ready for response through a mental, physical and/or emotional set
Guided response	Imitating the performance of another person and/or repeating performance until correct (trial and error)
Mechanism	Responding to the demands of a situation with confidence and a degree of proficiency
Complex overt response	Performing without hesitating and with coordinated muscle control
Adaptation	Altering basic motor responses to inact demands of new situations
Origination	Creating new motor acts or ways of manipulating materials

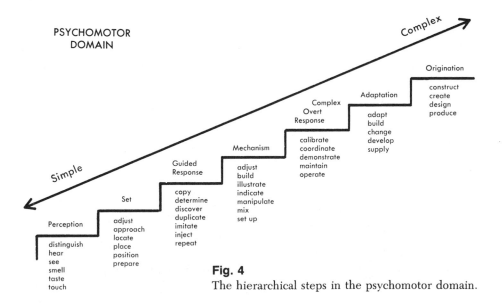

Fig. 4
The hierarchical steps in the psychomotor domain.

performance objectives and placing them in the context of audience, behavior, conditions, and degree. Information on the taxonomies is included here to point out the state of the art.

Health professionals have largely struggled with the classification of objectives in the cognitive domain. Particularly for clinical education, the focus of this book, there is an additional need to work through the classification systems in the affective and psychomotor domains. Clinical education purports to utilize cognitive knowledge in patient care. While it is true that much of the cognitive knowledge involves levels of a higher order, much of it is also intertwined with the application of psychomotor and affective skills. These skills need to be identified with as much precision as the taxonomy will allow.

Writing objectives is done neither for fun nor for accreditation; it needs to be done to improve the teaching/learning process in the clinical setting. It is not the only task within the systems approach to instruction, but it is one that is necessary to implement a systems approach to instruction.

Competency-based education in the pure form outlined in Table 1 cannot be implemented in all situations. However, it is possible to move the educational process toward that end. A systems approach can provide the framework.

REFERENCES

1. *ASMT News, 12,* (August) 1976.
   A regular publication of the American Society For Technology. This issue includes a list of over 200 competencies developed by the Competency Deliberation Committee.
2. Broski, D.; Alexander, D.; Brunner, M.; and others. Competency-based curriculum development: A pragmatic approach. *Journal of Allied Health, 6,* (Winter) 1977, 38-44.
   Examines the concepts of competency-based education, describes a model for its development, and applies the model to allied health education.
3. Burns, R. W., and Klingstedt, J. L. (Eds.). *Competency-Based Education,* Englewood Cliffs, N.J.: Educational Technology Publications, 1973.
   Nineteen chapters covering an array of topics that focus on competency-based education: philosophy, psychology, curriculum, certification, accreditation. The emphasis is on teacher education. The text was originally printed in the November 1972 issue of Educational Technology.
4. DeCecco, J. P. *The Psychology of learning and instruction: Educational Psychology.* Englewood Cliffs, N.J.: Prentice-Hall, 1968.
   Focuses on a systems approach to instruction. The author provides concrete suggestions for implementation.
5. Ford, C. W. Learning environment. In C. W. Ford and M. K. Morgan (Eds.), *Teaching in the Health Professions.* St. Louis: The C. V. Mosby Co., 1976.
   Examines three major theories of educational psychology: social imitation learning, Gestalt field theory, and stimulus-response.
6. Harrow, A. J. *A Taxonomy of the Psychomotor Domain.* New York: David McKay, 1972.
   A model for classifying movement behavior of children, based on theories of child growth and development. The book is an excellent reference for developing objectives in the psychomotor domain.
7. Houston, W. R., and Howsam, R. B. (Eds.). *Competency-Based Teacher Education.* Chicago: Science Research Associates, 1972.
   Eight chapters detailing CBTE: objectives, curriculum design, evaluation, consortia, and certification. The book provides a valuable review of the issues of CBTE.
8. Lynch, B. L., and Holloway, L. D. *Writing Objectives for Health Related Instruction.* Gainesville, Fla.: University of Florida, The Center for Allied Health Instructional Personnel, 1974.
   A self-directed manual of 43 pages for learning how to write objectives. Preassessment and postassessment evaluation forms are included, as are 12 checkpoints.
9. Meeth, R. L. The characteristics of competency-based curricula. *Regional Spotlight, 9,* (September) 1974, 2-3.
   Adapted from a speech on competency-based curricula in undergraduate programs. Southern Regional Education Board, June 1974.
10. Popham, W. S., and Baker, E. L. *Establishing Instructional Goals.* Englewood Cliffs, N.J.: Prentice-Hall, 1970.
    A self-instructional book with companion audiovisual materials. Emphasis is on using systematic instructional decision making.
11. Roueche, J. R. A place to begin: A systems approach

to instruction. In C. W. Ford and M. K. Morgan (Eds.), *Teaching in the Health Professions*. St. Louis: The C. V. Mosby Co., 1976.

A review of the key issues of a systems approach to instruction.

12. Segall, A. J.; Vanderschmidt, H.; Burglass, R.; and Frostman, T. *Systematic Course Design for the Health Fields*. New York: John Wiley and Sons, 1975.

A useful guide for curriculum design in the health fields. It is structured to enable teachers to work by themselves or as a team.

13. Simpson, E. J. The classification of educational objectives in the psychomotor domain. In *The Psychomotor Domain*. Washington, D.C.: Gryphon House, 1972.

Developed from a home economics curriculum, this taxonomy does not attempt to classify specific motor acts; the emphasis is on classifying objectives. It is clearly written with many examples.

14. Tyler, R. W. *Basic Principles of Curriculum and Instruction*. Chicago: University of Chicago Press, 1950.

A classic text presenting fundamental concepts. The author suggests four fundamental questions to be answered during program development.

15. Young, J. I., and Van Mondfrans, A. P. Psychological implications of competency-based education. In R. W. Burns and J. L. Klingstedt (Eds.), *Competency-Based Education*. Englewood Cliffs, N.J.: Educational Technology Publications, Inc., 1973.

Compares the procedures of competency-based and conventional education systems. Topics include interest, motivation, frustration, anxiety, and self-concept.

part one **FORMULATING GOALS, POLICIES, AND OBJECTIVES**

1

NEEDS ASSESSMENTS

Shirley A. Weaver

As Robert Kinsinger stressed in his foreword to *Teaching in the Health Professions*,[7] we are surfacing from a revolution in allied health education—a revolution characterized more by explosions in number and kinds of educational programs than by systematic responses to health manpower demands. Whereas urgent cries of manpower shortages were the motivating force for the revolution of the 1960s and early 1970s, more tempered voices now call for *quality* and *accountability*.[9] Systematic, comprehensive planning is essential to developing educational programs that satisfy those new, reasonable demands.

Planning is now a ubiquitous phenomenon in our society. In health care administration, for example, comprehensive planning has become the key to federal funds for expansion and improvement of health care facilities. The level of comprehensive health planning described in Public Law 93-641, the National Health Planning and Resources Development Act, has yet to be applied to health manpower planning. Allied health education administrators are, however, well advised that such comprehensive manpower planning may be their next administrative mandate. Thoughtful, effective planning can minimize the impact on individual allied health educational programs of any future governmental planning acts and, more importantly, can obviate the need for costly corrective action.

This text focuses on those aspects of allied health education programs that offer students an opportunity to test professional skills in the clinic. Comprehensive planning is integral to the efficient use of clinical sites. This chapter offers a general approach to planning educational programs, including a clinical component, by suggesting specific models and methodologies for the crucial first step in planning for change—needs assessment.

PERSPECTIVES IN PLANNING

Whether the educator is concerned with initiating a program or modifying an existing one, knowledge of legislation as well as educational and manpower trends is essential to innovative and effective planning.[5] In brief, legislation that the educator must consider includes: PL 93-641, the 1974 Amendment to the Taft-Hartley Act, affirmative action legislation (Title IX of the Higher Education Act), Social Security Act amendments related to health manpower, and current health professionals manpower training assistance legislation. Such legislation may suggest modifications to existing programs (such as accommodation of extended professional duties and different recruitment procedures) or may suggest new programs (such as credited continuing education, laddered programs, and totally new careers). Educators must also maintain current files on accreditation, certification, and licensure guidelines and be knowledgeable about educational trends endorsed by professional organizations and manpower utilization trends within the delivery systems.

Not only is knowledge of these influences on allied health educational programs a significant factor in the nature and quality of the planning, the planner's perspective is an equally significant variable. One typology of planner attitudes, credited to Ackoff,[12] delineates four attitudes (perspectives) exhibited by administrators when faced with a need for creative problem solving (planning):

1. *Reactive*—planning is retrospective. The administrator identifies individual problems and then removes the cause (e.g., the haphazard proliferation of allied health professions in response to advances in medical research and increased use of technology).

2. *Inactive*—planning is conservative, and as few changes as possible are made. This is the general mode in hospitals and universities.

3. *Preactive*—planning is forecast-oriented. Future predictions form the basis of planning, and the overall philosophy is that change is good.

4. *Interactive/proactive*—planning is directed toward achieving an ideal state. The planner/administrator tries to design a viable future and then works toward it (p. 19).

Ackoff further suggests that the first three perspectives advocate corrective surgery on isolated portions of the larger problem; only the last, interactive, approach to planning attempts to deal innovatively with the entire issue.

The perspective of the planner is a determinant in both *what* problem is selected and *how* the problem is solved. A hypothetical example would be a situation in which preliminary indications suggest that a college needs to institute a medical technology program. A *reactive planner* would perhaps state the problem in the following manner: "Do we have or can we get the resources necessary to initiate a medical technology program?" The *interactive/proactive planner,* on the other hand, might ask, "What kind of laboratory personnel will be needed to meet the future health care needs of this community/region/state?" The secondary questions and the respective data collection processes implicit in these two very different perspectives on the same initial problem should be apparent.

There is great risk in advocating a single problem-solving methodology. Perhaps the single commonality in the four planning perspectives is the general process: definition of the problem, collection of data (for identification of alternatives and selection of the most appropriate one), implementation of the selected alternative, evaluation of the outcome, and modification of the process.

Whatever the planning perspective, central to sound decision making is appropriate data. For education programs, data collection starts with a needs assessment; whether academic and clincial resources are available is a moot point if there is no need for the program or clinical experience.

NEEDS ASSESSMENT IN THE PLANNING PROCESS

Needs assessment is a process for collecting data from which administrators can determine whether a program and/or what program should exist. That is, a needs assessment should assist in answering such questions as: Should this program continue to exist? What skills does this practitioner need in that role? What clinical experiences will be most effective in developing a competent practitioner? The needs assessment is, in effect, a research project which, when carefully designed and effectively conducted, results in valid and reliable data on the need for a program and the definition of the program or experience.

Needs assessment programs are intended to provide data on the basis of which educators can: (1) identify the extent and kinds of needs there are in the community, (2) evaluate systematically their existing program, and (3) plan new ones in the light of the community's needs and educational programs.

In the limited definition of the process, a needs assessment does not provide data on the feasibility of actualizing the program. The feasibility study begins with the definition provided by the needs assessment and proceeds to determine whether there are sufficient resources to meet the needs. To complete the planning process, of course, the planners must design a program by which resources are directed to meet the need. A case in point: if a needs assessment shows that a sufficient number of inactive laboratory personnel are seeking reentry into a job market to justify initiating a retraining program in a given locale, if the assessment defines the retraining needs of those individuals, and if a feasibility study indicates that there are sufficient resources (faculty and facilities) to make the program a reality, there remains the task of designing the educational program to meet the originally described need.

APPROACHES TO NEEDS ASSESSMENT

Allied health educators currently face a perplexing paradox: increased demands for inclusion of valid needs assessments in program proposals coupled with a dearth of literature on needs assessment methodology. Federal grant proposals, with increasing frequency, have not been approved because of insufficient (or at least unconvincing) documentation of need. Yet, with the exception of nursing education literature and a single allied health article, a review of the limited texts on allied health education and health professions educational periodicals reveals no discussion of needs assessment methodology. The most pertinent literature is, unfortunately, in the form of government monographs of limited distribution.

Some literature from the human services delivery systems has recently appeared in health related periodicals.[14] While not specifically related to educational planning, the needs assessment models and methodology described for the delivery systems should be considered by conscientious educational planners. In the absence of tools for comprehensive planning, needs assessment has been limited to quantitative manpower estimates and projections.

Allied health manpower estimates

Lack of realistic allied health data on manpower needs and supply has plagued governmental efforts to project future manpower needs and to develop manpower training legislation. Review of federal health manpower laws and the methodology used to assess needs reveals a predominantly retrospective and status quo perspective. One comprehensive study concludes:

Any discussion of requirements for allied health manpower must recognize that the assumptions underlying an analysis of supply versus demand are not agreed upon, and that much essential data are not available. The most important lack is an objective against which our present ability to provide health services can be measured. These difficulties are especially apparent in attempting to determine or forecast requirements for medical and dental allied manpower, since requirements are related more to rising standards and demands for health care than to simple growth in population (p. 84).[4]

The designers of federal manpower needs estimates acknowledge that their projections of the number of workers are based on the following assumption: there will be no major changes in the health care system, in manpower utilization patterns, or in the economics of health. The estimates use data collection methodology from a *ratio model* of manpower assessment, which includes such approaches as:

Enumerating budgeted vacancies, e.g., determining the number of cytotechnologists needed in the service area by the number of unfilled, budgeted positions

Using established ratios of practitioners to total population, e.g., using the Public Health Service ratio of physicians to population to determine the number needed in the service area

Determining professional judgment of need, e.g., seeking the advice of the local medical society to determine the number of physician's assistants needed

Using established ratios of practitioners to patient population, e.g., using a ratio of medical records technicians to number of patient files to establish manpower needs

Determining requirements per unit of service, e.g., determining the number of radiologic technologists needed based on the total number of patients processed per year

Analyzing staffing patterns, e.g., determining the number of dental assistants needed in the service area based on the national ratio of dentists to dental assistants

Allied health educators attempting to use such federal manpower projections should understand that the estimates do not consider: (1) the extent to which increasing specialization will be efficient or desirable; (2) the extent to which duties (particularly primary care) will be delegated to lower level personnel; (3) the extent to which technological and sociological changes will alter personal service requirements; (4) the effect of new specialties on old ones; or (5) the effect of economics on the health care industry. The Committee for Economic Development in its 1973 study addressed the fallacies of past manpower planning efforts:

> Poor distribution, together with inadequate utilization, training and organization have aggravated the shortages of manpower in some areas while causing surpluses in others. Beyond some crude and increasingly doubtful ratios of professionals to population, it is not even known how many people are now needed, let alone how many would be needed under a better organized system (p. 33).[3]

Recent research has produced at least one model that addresses the multidimensional nature of manpower analysis. The *econometric model* is a sophisticated statistical tool that promises to give national and regional planners more realistic manpower projections. For example, the macroeconometric model posed by Yett and coworkers[15] provides for testing the impact of such variables as national health insurance alternatives on health service demand and manpower needs. In addition, the econometric approach makes possible simulation of the impact of various national policies on the health care delivery system. Planning tools made possible by such approaches have yet to be made available at the regional level, but, if and when available, they should be of considerable value in regional comprehensive manpower planning.

Such methods have yet to become routine tools for the planning process,* and it is un-

---

*A project funded by DHEW, Division of Associated Health Professions, for the examination of allied health manpower in California has attempted to utilize some of these methods (California State University and Colleges, unpublished, 1976).

likely that they will assist educators in defining new programs and determining the quantity and quality of clinical experiences within existing programs. The necessity for program planning requires models and guidelines for individual needs assessments. A review of the studies recently conducted suggests several needs assessment models.

Models for needs assessment

Four models for needs assessments seem applicable to clinical education in allied health. The first, a consumer model, has been extrapolated from a model developed for health service needs assessment. The second, a professional-expert model, reflects the method used in several allied health education studies. The third, a systematic educational needs assessment model, is a theoretical construct designed specifically for allied health education. The fourth, a continuing education needs assessment model, is currently being tested in a Michigan statewide cooperative continuing education project.

Consumer model for assessing professional service needs. The consumer model presents the planner with a method of assessing professional service needs by using consumers as the major source of input.[14] The consumer is defined as any community member who resides within the given geographic study area. The model supplies information on the priorities of need for additional service by target problem, population group, and geographic area. This model is most applicable to planning for a new career program or modifying an existing program to include expanded professional duties.

Study population. Within the model, four consumer groups are surveyed:

1. Health related agencies—agencies and individuals that use the services of the professional
2. Patients/clients—individuals who are using or have used the professional services in question
3. Community and civic groups—groups within the study area that are organized around a common goal or for specific purposes that relate directly to the profession under study

4. Community-at-large—a sample of area residents selected at random who may or may not be associated with the other three groups

Study methodology. The following are aspects of the study methodology:

1. The study is conducted within the service area or within a study area that approximates the sociodemographic characteristics of the overall service area population.

2. The study uses questionnaires and interviews designed to collect the types of data best provided by the specific consumer group. Specifically, health-related agencies provide current service and projected service data and identify and prioritize service problem areas; patients/clients provide data regarding service needs and the quality and quantity of services received; and community groups advocate services and their priorities and identify potential service consumers.

3. Statistical analysis of the data results in a frequency distribution and ranking of needed services for each consumer study group and for specific population groups according to such factors as age and sex.

Professional-expert model for assessing skill needs. The professional-expert model presents the planner with a method of assessing professional skill needs by using the professional practitioner as the major source of input.[11] The professional practitioner is defined as any person certified or licensed to provide any or all services ascribed to that occupation. This model is most applicable to identifying the need and planning for modification of an educational program.

Study population. Within the model, practitioners are identified according to:

1. Type of service agency—outpatient service, public school, acute care facility, rehabilitation center, etc.

2. Levels of certification or licensure—professional, technician, aide, specialist, etc.

3. Job title or position—administrator, chief technician, staff therapist, educator, etc.

4. Geographic location—urban, rural, regional, etc.

Study methodology. Within the model, the study methodology includes:

1. A study area that provides the most valid data for the problem at hand

2. Group techniques that focus expertise on a particular aspect of the problem, using such methods as brainstorming, nominal group process, and the Delphi technique

3. Survey and interview techniques to obtain the broadest base of input on specific issues

4. Identification of professional services provided, skills used, skill deficiencies, and priorities for problem resolution

5. Statistical interpretation of the data, to provide a profile of skill needs that can be translated into program proposals

Systematic educational needs assessment model. The systematic educational needs assessment model presents the planner with a method of identifying competencies that should be taught and identifying why, what, and for whom the instructional system is needed.[16] The model, as described, can be divided into eleven discrete steps; the first five can be considered as needs assessment according to the definition established within the chapter:

1. Develop a performance model that represents the knowledge, skills, and/or attitudes needed by the prospective target audience

2. Identify current levels of performance—discover what competencies the target audience has that are congruent with the performance model

3. Specify the desirable levels of performance—what is needed to raise the level of competency from the real (step 2) to the ideal (step 1)

4. Differentiate instructional from administrative needs—separate those discrepancies between the real and ideal that can be resolved through instruction from those that are outside the realm of competency development

5. Designate priorities—translate educa-

tional needs into instructional objectives and rank in an order of priority

Continuing education needs assessment model. The continuing education needs assessment model presents the planner with a method of assessing practitioner preferences and correlating them with objective indicators of need.[6] The model assumes a categorical service (i.e., medical laboratory service) rather than a categorical profession.

Study population. This model is intended for small laboratory service agencies. Within the model, two laboratory practitioner groups are surveyed:

1. Employees of hospitals of 100 beds or fewer—including all personnel, other than physicians, regardless of academic and certification level
2. Employees of small private laboratories and physicians' offices—including all personnel who perform laboratory procedures, regardless of professional preparation and quality and type of procedures performed

Study methodology. The study methodology includes:

1. A study that is conducted on a regionalized, statewide basis
2. Survey techniques, including questionnaires and interviews, that identify practitioner preferences
3. Analysis of state-level proficiency tests to identify practitioner needs
4. Preferences and needs are collated on a regional basis

These four models have a number of limitations: They are theoretical; as such, they are not necessarily pragmatic or validated; and, typical of models, they tend to be specifically focused on a limited number of variables.

Needs assessment is a research project, the breadth (or narrowness) of which depends on the perspective of the planners, and the outcome of which depends on the planners' research competence.

THE RESEARCH PROCESS AND METHODOLOGY

The design and implementation of a needs assessment require a vast array of educational and social research techniques. The unique nature of professional education, and particularly clinical education, requires methodology that borrows not only from social research, but also from systems analysis. Professional competency studies (task analyses), for example, fall under the latter research genre.

Fundamental to good research, of course, is familiarity with the *research process*. As Lawler and Hedl[7] note, research is a process of systematic investigation undertaken to provide answers to questions. The major steps of this process (scientific approach) are:

Problem identification. This is the crucial first step in research and the one for which authorities give the least guidance. In clinical education needs assessment studies, the initial question is often presented by an external agent, such as the college administration or a community group, or generated as an outcome of the educational program.

Formulation of research hypotheses. The initial question must be analyzed and restated as research objectives. For novices it may be easier to state the hypothesis as a question (for example, What clinical competencies are essential to physical therapists in pediatric practice?) Such a question may then provoke auxiliary questions (Which of those competencies are unique to pediatric practice? Which competencies require clinical versus simulated practice?) The series of questions then becomes the basis of the study objectives and the framework for the research project.

Development of techniques and measuring instruments. Techniques and measuring instruments must be developed that will provide objective data pertinent to the hypotheses. The researcher describes the methodological procedures to be used, including a specification of the sample, experimental design, and data collection instruments and procedures and develops instruments such as "opinionnaires" to be used in the collection process.

Collection of data. Once the experimental procedures, including the timetable for the process, have been described and instruments developed, data collection begins.

Analysis of data. The data must be evaluated to determine whether they permit an adequate investigation of the problem. Typically in scientific research, statistical analysis of the data is employed. In needs assessment studies, however, statistical procedures are often greatly simplified.

Drawing of conclusions relative to the hypotheses and based on the data. The final task of research is to answer the original questions, thereby establishing the direction for future action. In needs assessment studies, the conclusions provide the broad definitions for the new program or determine that no program is needed.

Definitions and concepts

A variety of *research methods* can be used in needs assessment studies. In clinical education needs assessments, social research methods are extensively used. Frequently, however, allied health educators are unfamiliar with research methods. That is why allied health practitioners, well aware of the competencies and tasks associated with their professions, often are more comfortable with job analyses. Since they may never have conducted field research, constructed a survey instrument, or led problem-solving group processes, a brief review of some important aspects of survey research follows.

Population versus sample. While a population is a total collection of persons that conform to a specific criterion or set of criteria, a sample is a portion of the population that is representative of the whole. Sampling design should be guided by at least four criteria: (1) *goal orientation,* the design and conditions of the study survey; (2) *measurability,* the kind of computations possible for determining the validity of the sample; (3) *practicality,* the reasonableness of fit with the model, even though the ideal is not possible; and (4) *economy,* the achievement of precision and accuracy within the budget limitations.

The sampling accuracy depends on such matters as: (1) the characteristics of the population, its homogeneity; (2) the nature of the information required, its complexity; (3) the procedures used in drawing the sample, its bias; and (4) the degree of confidence, its reliability.

Data-gathering techniques

Regardless of the type of survey used to gather needs assessment information, the principal tasks of the investigator are related to the securing of information from the survey population. Efforts must be made to ensure *validity* and *reliability* of the data, and the results must be recorded in a way that permits easy and economical retrieval and analysis. There are three major techniques used to gather information during a survey research: interviews, mailed questionnaires, and group processes. The differences among them are in the types of data that can be collected and the cost of conducting the research.

Interviews. Person-to-person interviews and telephone interviews involve a personal encounter between an interviewer and respondent. If guided by a structured list of questions (an interview schedule), this method has definite advantages over the mailed questionnaire. More importantly, the interview involves a dialogue that maximizes the likelihood that the respondent fully understands the issues, that the researchers understand the responses, and that the response rate is increased. However, an important disadvantage is the expense of training and utilizing interviewers. Telephone interviews can be used as an adjunct to the mailed questionnaire methodology to increase the response rate and clarify ambiguous responses.

Mailed questionnaires. A survey instrument mailed to the sample population has the advantages of being cheaper and more objective, allowing respondent anonymity, and making possible computer analysis of data. Unfortunately, there are significant disadvantages to the method: the difficulty of designing an unambiguous but thorough instrument, the inability of some persons to interpret and respond to questions at an abstract level, and the typically low (as low as 35%) response rate. Despite its significant difficulties, this method is commonly employed. It necessarily becomes the modus operandi when researchers are dealing with a geographically widespread sample population.

Group processes. The primary purpose of group processes is to collect opinions or to focus expertise on a particular aspect of a problem. Methods that require group participation governed by rules and constraints in contrast to more unstructured, open discussions include brainstorming and the nominal group process.

Brainstorming involves soliciting group members' unrestricted, uncensored responses to a question. The objective is to get beyond the usual to the unusual perspectives—to describe the widest dimensions of the issue. Although a useful technique for getting planners out of stereotyped views of the problem, brainstorming seldom translates into action.

The nominal group process, on the other hand, offers planners a process through which problems are definitively described and then the described elements are prioritized through an individual and group weighting process.[2] This process helps the planner dissect the problem to avoid prematurely offering solutions. The process can increase the efficiency and effectiveness of planning committee meetings, consultant meetings, and similar situations in which a group is used to provide input to a problem.

Consultation

Whatever the process, planners with limited experience in research design should consult reference texts in educational research and survey methods and seek expert consultation before undertaking needs assessment studies.[1,10] This advice is not intended to discourage the neophyte, for most educators would agree that educational research competence is gained through experience.

Just like professional competence, research competence is best gained through guided clinical experience. The challenge for the educational planner is to translate the generalities presented here into a pragmatic approach to conducting needs assessments for the clinical component of the professional curriculum.

GUIDELINES FOR ASSESSING NEEDS IN CLINICAL EDUCATION

In assessing needs in clinical education, the educator may be attempting to answer such

questions as: What new programs should be instituted? What clinical experiences are prerequisite to professional proficiency? What are the strengths and weaknesses of the clinical component of the program? How does the program accommodate new professional responsibilities? Should it? To what extent can simulation replace actual clinical experience?

The process used to answer those questions will significantly affect the efficiency with which the answers are obtained and their validity. In planning a needs assessment study, the educator begins with the initial statement of the questions and then outlines the *where, who, what,* and *how*. The statement of the questions is critical. Asking the wrong questions sets in motion a time-consuming and expensive process that results in the wrong data being collected and the wrong program, if any, being developed.

The outline (see opposite page) is a delineation of the where, who, what, and how pertinent to the design of a needs assessment study.[8,13]

Location of the study (where)

In most instances, the study will be conducted in the area served by the program. Professional association studies, for example, are characteristically national in perspective, while single program studies are usually local, state, or regional in focus. One noteworthy exception, however, was a survey of a national sample of professionals to determine the real and ideal state of clinical competencies in order to determine the nature of a particular educational program.[11]

Again, the perspective of the planner determines the study population. If, for example, a comparison is sought between competencies gained in simulated and actual clinical experiences, the educator can focus on the indigenous clinical settings or look at other programs for a broader data base.

Time, expertise, and financial resources are obvious constraints. No doubt, most program directors will attempt to determine the clinical experience needs for a program with a defined service area (community) and will have limited time and money with which to

Guidelines for assessing clinical education needs

I. Where to conduct study
   A. Service areas of program
   B. State, regional, or national areas
II. Who plans and conducts study
   A. Study manager
      1. Program faculty
      2. Committee representing such groups as:
         a. Allied health profession educators
         b. Medical/dental profession—medical/dental societies, professional schools, practitioners in involved agencies
         c. Health facility/agency administrators and practitioners—graduates of program or sample profession, clinical supervisors
         d. Consumer/civic groups
         e. Government groups—licensure boards, public health departments, accreditation/certification boards
         f. Research consultants
   B. Manager activities
      1. Specify geographic area to be studied
      2. Define the study problem(s)
      3. Select study methods
      4. Establish study budget
      5. Maintain interagency communications
      6. Manage conduct of study through subcommittees
      7. Prepare report
III. What variables are studied
   A. State of the art of the profession
      1. Practice roles and activities of practitioner
      2. Content of clinical curriculum
      3. Clinical practice strengths and weaknesses
      4. Patterns of patient/client care
   B. Future of the art of the profession—the ideal
      1. Changing consumer attitudes
      2. Attitudes of influential health professionals, health service administrators, and educational personnel
      3. Projected plans for expansion/modification of health services
      4. Changing/expanding advocacy role by professional society or licensure boards
      5. Developing health care policy at regional, state, and national level
      6. Effect of emerging professions
      7. Effect of reassignment of health professional roles
   C. Efficacy of the educational experience
      1. Graduate satisfaction of the program
      2. Employer satisfaction with graduates
      3. Comparisons of graduate results on standard tests
      4. Comparison of educational program with the ideal
      5. Constraints on admission, progress, acceleration, and advancement
      6. Faculty specialty strengths and weaknesses
IV. How to use the data
   A. Determine the need for the existence of the clinical experience (program) in light of:
      1. The future role of the practitioner
      2. The effectiveness and availability of simulation experiences
   B. Define the needed clinical experience in light of:
      1. The efficacy of the present program
      2. Professional judgment
      3. The defined weaknesses of the existing program
      4. The defined professional role

conduct their study. Such educators are well advised to limit the geographical area of the study.

Research group conducting the study (who)

This important consideration often suffers from lack of serious consideration, even though it may ultimately decide the fate of an otherwise well designed study. A committee that represents the college and clinical faculty, agencies, and institutions that will be directly involved by the study or its results should plan and carry out the needs assessment. The breadth of that representative committee will parallel the degree of broadness of interpretation of the problem. For example, if the study is to assess the kinds of clinical experiences needed in a given area by physical therapy students, a narrow view of the practice area as only acute care health facilities will probably result in a narrow committee (that is, representatives of physical therapy departments in area acute care facilities, college faculty, and the medical profession). On the other hand, the graduate's practice area could be defined as the community at large, including private practices, extended and acute care facilities, neighborhood health clinics, rehabilitation centers, and the public school system. In this instance, the committee could include representatives from program graduates, special interest consumer groups, public school officials, and the comprehensive health planning agency, as well as the more obvious health professionals.

The object of a needs assessment study is, of course, to get the best data. Since data collection is time-consuming for everyone involved in the process, the quality of the data is reflected in the amount of time (commitment) given to the study. Individuals are more likely to exhibit commitment when they have been involved in designing the process. Planners should consider that the members must not only be knowledgeable in the educational and practice area in question but must also have the authority to expedite the study.

Planners should seriously consider the cumulative expertise of the research group in light of the sophistication of the research de-

sign. If an elaborate design is under consideration, does the expertise exist to actualize the plan? On the other hand, does the simplicity of the design reflect limited research skills? Some research groups might be well advised to consider using consultants to design and carry out their study. Faculty colleagues in systems analysis, computer science, psychology, sociology, etc., may also be of assistance to the group.

Object and design of the study (what)

As mentioned, the design of the study (the variables that are considered) are dictated by the perspective and knowledge of the planner. The interactive perspective will require examination of such data as: (1) changing social and cultural attitudes that may have an impact on the profession; (2) attitudes of influencial medical, health service, education, and consumer personnel; (3) present and projected plans for expanding pertinent health services; (4) patient care patterns and effects on those patterns; and (5) changes in other health careers that provide similar or equivalent services.

Regardless of the type of assessment project being considered, at the outset of the project a series of questions needs to be asked:

- What do we want/need to know?
- Why do we want to know it?
- How will the information be used once it is obtained?
- Where can we find the necessary data?
- How can we obtain these data?
- What useful data resources exist?
- How can we most effectively compile, analyze, and present the data?
- Should any other agencies, colleges, or departments be involved in the program?
- What will the project cost?
- How long will it take to complete?
- What is the source of financial and personnel resources?
- What consultant assistance is necessary?
- Where can it be found?
- What techniques and processes are available whereby findings can be translated

into programs designed to meet the needs?

Answering these questions systematically and completely will give the project focus and aid in its manageability. Resolution of these issues may result in a significant reduction in the need for original data collection. Pertinent data may be found to be already available. Educators too commonly undertake expensive, time-consuming studies in the face of existing pertinent data either because they lack knowledge of the data or because they doubt the validity of the data for their situation. Careful review of the literature and consultation with appropriate professional organizations and government agencies are, therefore, important first steps in defining and operationalizing a needs assessment study project.

The general focus of needs assessment studies in clinical education necessitates the collection of certain baseline data, such as the *current* state of the art of the profession and the nature and effectiveness of the current educational program, as well as the *anticipated* state of the art of the profession.

Collection of the data (how)

The data collection procedures selected for the study must be congruent with the type of data sought and the group expected to provide the data. Standard data collection methods are described in the previous section. Table 5 also lists methods of data collection that can be used at various stages of the study.

Interpretation and presentation of the data

After the problem is stated, the study designed, and the data collected, the ultimate task remains—interpretation of the data to answer the questions. The data sought in a needs assessment study are intended to aid educators in making decisions on whether a given clinical experience is necessary and precisely what that needed experience is.

Interpretation of data should be guided by knowledge of the biases, strengths, and limitations of the collection methodology used. Standard research handbooks should be consulted in the selection and implementation of the methodology, as well as in interpretation. The data may lend themselves to statistical analysis and requires that the researchers review current statistical methodology.

Table 5
Methodology and process for needs assessment studies

Process	Methodology	Respondents
I. Definition of the study	Brainstorming, nominal group process	Research committee and consultants
II. Data gathering		
A. Current state of practice	Interviews, questionnaires, task analyses	Professional experts
B. Effectiveness of current educational program	Interviews; questionnaires; proficiency, certification, and local exams; interviews, nominal group process	Graduates and employers, graduates and graduates of other programs, faculty
C. Future state of practice	Interviews, questionnaires, Delphi technique	Professional experts, consumer groups, community groups
	Review of literature and legislation	Research committee
III. Analysis of the data	Computer or hand tabulation, statistical analysis	Research committee
IV. Presentation of report		Research committee

Presentation of the data, together with recommendations, is the culmination of the study. Formal, written documentation, desirable even for the most limited study, provides a permanent record of the study. It also provides authorities an opportunity to offer interested parties a broader base of data from which to design their studies, programs, etc.

In brief, the final report should present:

- Purposes of the study—a brief outline of the major objectives of the study
- Background of the study—the results of the literature search and a rationale for the study
- Design of the study—a descriptive overview of how the research was designed and conducted
- Presentation of findings—an extended, descriptive, and, if possible, graphic presentation of the data
- Conclusions and recommendations—inferences of the findings and rank-ordered recommendations for action

SUMMARY

This chapter describes needs assessment, an integral part of systematic program planning, as a research and planning activity designed to provide data on the basis of which educators can: (1) identify the kinds of new clinical educational programs needed in a community and (2) evaluate systematically their existing educational programs in light of current professional practice. Inherently a research project, a needs assessment study includes the processes and methodology of social research. The efficacy of the implementation of the research project depends on the perspective and expertise of those designing and conducting it. This chapter outlines and describes those processes and methods essential to effective needs assessment.

REFERENCES

1. Babbie, E. R. *Survey Research Methods*. Belmont, Calif.: Wadsworth Publishing Co., 1973.

 A comprehensive handbook on methods for survey research. This handbook is a practical and realistic guide for the beginning researcher. Aspects treated include discussions on the scientific context of survey research, the design and analysis of survey research, and the social and scientific perspective of survey research.

2. Casbergue, J. P. The Nominal Group Process: An Effective Tool for the Instructional Developer. A paper presented at the Division of Instructional Development Concurrent Sessions at the Association for Educational Communications and Technology Annual Meeting, Dallas, Texas, April 14, 1975.

 Caspergue has refined the process originally described by Delbecq and Van de Ven, detailing a group process technique for identifying problems. The prioritized listing of problems resulting from the process provides groups with the framework for future problem-solving action.

3. Committee for Economic Development. *Building a National Health-Care System*. New York: The Committee, 1973.

 An often-quoted study of the health care system, which analyzes the causes of inadequacies and inequities in U.S. health services and proposes a program for improving their organization and financing. The committee proposes a national manpower program that has become the basis for current manpower legislation.

4. Grupenhoff, J. T., and Strickland, S. P. (Eds.). *Federal Laws: Health/Environment Manpower*. Washington, D.C.: Sciences and Health Communications Group, 1972.

 A comprehensive source book that deals with health manpower resources and the federal government's role in ensuring adequate numbers of health professionals. The editors discuss the history, intent, and authorizations of federal legislation related to the health professions, nursing, and allied health. The appendixes include nearly 200 pages of basic source documents: Presidential messages to Congress, reprints of legislation, and excerpts from Congressional committee reports.

5. Holloway, S. Trends in hospital-based health care and health manpower. In M. Boyles (Ed.), *Proceedings: Selected Papers from Health Manpower Education Conferences, 1974-1976*. Washington, D.C.: American Association of State Colleges and Universities, 1976.

 One of a series of articles addressed in the section "Clinical Resources and Community Relations." The author raises questions on health manpower in the light of current legislation and utilization trends. This brief article raises important questions that health manpower planners and educators should consider.

6. Joint Council for Continuing Education for Medical Laboratory Personnel. An Assessment of Continuing Laboratory Education Needs in Michigan. Committee on Needs Assessment. Lansing: Michigan Department of Public Health, 1977.

 A study of laboratory personnel serving small (100-bed) hospitals, private laboratories, and physicians' offices. The study, sponsored by a council representative of laboratory-related professional societies, public health departments, colleges and universities, and private laboratory directors, attempts to address the problem of assessing not only wants but needs in continuing education.

7. Lawler, R., and Hedl, J. J., Jr. Research design. In C. W. Ford and M. K. Morgan (Eds.), *Teaching in the Health Professions*. St. Louis: C. V. Mosby, 1976.

A discussion for beginning allied health researchers on the nature of the research process. The authors present general guidelines for that process. The text, of which the chapter is a part, should be considered prerequisite to the present one.

8. National League for Nursing. *Guidelines for Assessing the Nursing Education Needs of a Community*. New York: National League for Nusing, 1968. (Publication No. 11-1245)

A concise, useful outline of the process for assessing nursing education needs.

9. Regional Medical Programs Service: *Quality Assurance of Medical Care*. Washington, D.C.: Health Services and Mental Health Administration, 1973.

A document that reproduces papers originally presented at the Conference on Quality Assurance of Medical Care, which was sponsored by the Regional Medical Programs Service, January 23-24, 1973, in St. Louis, Missouri. The papers address a broad range of subject areas, including assessment, future needs of quality assurance, and the many aspects of criteria.

10. Travers, R. M. W. (Ed.). *Second Handbook of Research on Teaching*. Chicago: Rand McNally, 1973.

A standard bearer on teaching research. The editor critiques previous research efforts and advocates comprehensive approaches. Topics include "The Assessment of Teacher Competence," "The Teaching of Affective Responses," and "Research on Teaching in Higher Education."

11. University of North Carolina at Chapel Hill, Division of Physical Therapy. The Role of the Physical Therapist and the Training Needs of Those Working in Pediatric Programs. Report of Special Project No. 465, Division of Physical Therapy, School of Medicine, University of North Carolina at Chapel Hill, June 1969 to July 1970.

A report of a training needs assessment of physical therapists involved in pediatric service programs. The model includes determination of the present role of physical therapy in pediatric programs and of the future needs of physical therapists.

12. Vogt, M. Modeling techniques for allied health planning. In M. Boyles (Ed.), *Proceedings: Selected Papers from Health Manpower Education Conference, 1974-1976*. Washington, D.C.: American Association of State Colleges and Universities, 1976.

A refutation of past methods used to estimate health manpower requirements. The author suggests outcome-oriented health manpower planning, which is conducted by future-directed planners and which considers the changing profile of the community to be served. Described is a mathematics-based modeling technique for considering community variables, as well as manpower utilization patterns in manpower predictions.

13. Warheit, G. J.; Bell, R. A.; and Schwab, J. J. *Planning for Change: Needs Assessment Approaches*. Gainesville, Fla.: University of Florida, College of Medicine, Department of Psychiatry, Research Group, 1976.

A comprehensive handbook to needs assessment directed specifically to assessing mental health service needs and evaluating service programs. While not specifically directed to educational needs assessment, this document offers planners a practical model for needs assessment and a well documented, digested review of pertinent social research.

14. Weiss, A. T. The consumer model of assessing community mental health needs. In Needs Assessment Methods for the Community Mental Health Center. *Evaluation*, 2, 1975, 64-76.

A four-part article that describes four approaches to needs assessment specifically for mental health services: epidemiologic, social statistical, consumer, and the NIMH demographic profile system. The author's model may motivate educational planners to think of ways to get consumer input for future programming.

15. Yett, D. E.; Drabek, L.; Intriligator, M. D.; and Kimball, L. J. Health manpower planning: An econometric approach. *Health Services Research*, (Summer) 1972, 134-147.

The econometric model is described and critiqued.

16. Zacharewicz, F. A., and Coger, R. Educational needs assessment: A systematic approach. *Journal of Allied Health*, 6, (Winter) 1977, 54-60.

Presentation of a model for assessing educational needs and developing systems to meet those needs. This model, the first in allied health literature, provides a practical framework for educational planners and offers a base for further development of a comprehensive process.

2
LEGAL CONSIDERATIONS IN CLINICAL AFFILIATION AGREEMENTS

J. Kay Felt

In the past neither a health care institution nor a school was required to give much attention to formal contractual relationships for clinical experience. Few such institutions were responsible to third parties for the conduct of clinical education, and there were few cases holding supervisory employees or students responsible.

Most institutions were not susceptible to suit by virtue of two mechanisms: (1) the concept of *charitable immunity,* under which the resources of a nonprofit institution are to be spread among as many recipients as possible in order to do the most good rather than to be diverted from the principal charitable purpose by the payment of damages to an occasional injured recipient [1]; or (2) the concept of *governmental immunity,* under which a state agency is not susceptible to suit for actions taken in its governmental capacity unless it consents.*

Today, as applied to health care organizations, only a few states retain the charitable immunity concept in its purest form. In most states, the delivery of health care is viewed as a business, with the courts generally holding that nonprofit institutions engaged in a busi-

ness should be held to the same standard as their profit-making counterparts.[2] In a fairly large number of states, governmental immunity does not apply, under the theories that the rendering of health care is a proprietary (or business) function rather than a governmental function and that a state should be responsible for its conduct when it engages in a business.[3] The traditional immunities continue to apply to governmental[4] and nonprofit *educational* institutions in many jurisdictions, although the courts have begun to abrogate the concept of charitable immunity for nonprofit schools in more and more jurisdictions.[5]

The regulatory milieu in the past was such that little consideration was given to the requirements of (1) the state regulators of health care, for there were none in most jurisdictions; or (2) the educational authorities, for advanced educational programs were largely outside their jurisdiction. Instead, various educational accrediting organizations and, ultimately, hospital licensing and accrediting agencies have imposed the regulations that now exist.

This chapter is intended not as a complete review of all applicable legal considerations, but as a guide for hospitals and schools and their lawyers. The first portion surveys principles basic to the relationship of affiliating organizations, and the latter sections comment on typical contract provisions.

---

*Whether governmental agencies are generally susceptible to suit depends on the existence of a statute and the scope thereof. Even where there is immunity, it may be limited by court interpretation.

RESPONSIBILITY FOR THE QUALITY OF PATIENT CARE
Emerging institutional responsibility

Today most health care institutions are responsible for the quality of care rendered in them. In some states the courts have imposed the rule[6]; in others, the legislature has taken the lead.[7] Regardless of who imposed it, the rule provides that the *governing body of the hospital is responsible for the quality of care rendered within it and must adopt rules and regulations designed to facilitate the rendering of care in accordance with applicable standards of practice, whether that care is rendered by its employees* or by independent staff physicians, students, trainees, or other persons permitted to use the facility.*

One theory under which the hospital may be responsible for the conduct of persons other than its employees is that the patient or other injured third party is lead to believe that such persons are hospital employees. Since the hospital permits these persons to function in rendering patient care, it in effect represents or holds out to the public that such persons have been selected by the hospital and are capable of performing the functions assigned to them.

Under another theory, the hospital may be responsible for failure to use due care in the independent staff selection process. The same theory could be applied to the selection of students who are to participate in clinical affiliation programs.[8] This is not to say that the hospital is liable for every error of such a nonemployee, but it must use due care in selecting only qualified people to work in the institution and it must monitor their performance.

Even in those jurisdictions where neither the legislature nor the courts has spoken on this issue, a hospital is well advised as a matter of planning to preserve in its clinical affiliation contracts sufficient rights to meet the responsibilities to patients that may be thrust upon it by the courts.* At the same time, it should carefully word its contracts so that it does not, by virtue of a contract, assume responsibilities to patients that the courts have not imposed.†

Thus today in most jurisdictions *the hospital should be assumed to be responsible for seeing that the care rendered by anyone it permits to lay hands on patients, including students and their instructors, conforms to applicable standards of professional practice.* The hospital's responsibility is not automatic in every case of injury, but there should be rules, regulations, and policies by which its governing body can be assured that (1) only qualified persons will be permitted to practice and (2) persons demonstrating themselves to be unqualified will be removed from patient care situations. Otherwise, in the event of patient injury, the hospital itself, in addition to those persons individually responsible, may be liable to the patient for damages.

No contract can or should relieve a hospital of the basic responsibility to use due care to see that no harm comes to patients. Whether the school also is responsible for the quality of patient care, however, depends on the degree to which representatives of the school participate in rendering or supervising the rendering of care. The greater the extent of participation by the school's faculty in the clinical program, the greater the degree of the school's exposure to liability for the negligent rendering of patient care. To the extent that the clinical supervision of students is provided by hospital employees, the degree of the school's exposure is lessened. Liability might

---

*Every institution that is not immune from liability under the charitable or governmental immunity concepts is automatically responsible for the conduct of its employees acting within the scope of their employment under the concept called *respondeat superior*, meaning literally "let the master answer."

*Under the case law system derived from the English common law, the law is enunciated on a case-by-case basis with succeeding cases adding to the body of jurisprudence new rules that are based on the specific facts of each respective case. That a given type of case has not yet been brought to the high court of a particular jurisdiction does not mean that the institution would be absolved in future cases.

†It is assumed here for planning purposes that a hospital should assume that it is responsible as a matter of law for the conduct of students; however, this assumption should not be accepted as true without research of the laws of the individual state.

well be imposed, however, when school employees participate jointly with negligent hospital employees and the school employees fail to take action to prevent patient injury. Regardless of the degree of the school's exposure, however, the hospital is first and foremost responsible and cannot delegate to any other organization its basic responsibility.

Responsibility of trainees

In virtually all jurisdictions, responsibility is imposed on students for their own negligent conduct. A student is thus liable for any patient's injury proximately caused by deviation from or breach of applicable standards of practice. Not every injury that is sustained at the hands of a student entitles the patient to recover in damages, however. The student must be shown (1) to have owed the patient a duty to follow a certain standard of practice; (2) to have deviated from that standard in a way that (3) was a direct and foreseeable cause of the patient's injury; and (4) the patient must not have been guilty of contributory negligence or have assumed the risks of the injury that occurred. It must be emphasized that the student is not judged as a "learner" but is expected to perform in accordance with the standards applied to one who has already completed training and joined the profession or occupation.[9]

Responsibility of instructors and supervisors

An instructor (supervisor) is not automatically responsible for every negligent act of a student merely because of the instructor-student relationship unless the student is also an employee of the instructor.* Some independent act of negligence by the instructor must be shown in order for the instructor to be responsible: e.g., (1) the instructor's own failure to exercise proper supervision; or (2) the instructor's assigning the student to a task for which the student had not yet been trained or had been inadequately trained (assuming that the instructor was either responsible for the

inadequate training or knew or had reason to know of the inadequate training).[9] Generally speaking, an instructor (supervisor) is entitled to assume that a person who has successfully completed a particular course of training is competent to perform the tasks covered by the training program unless the instructor either knows or should know of some individual lack of competence on the part of the student. Of course, to the extent that the instructor also participates in rendering care to patients, the instructor must adhere to applicable standards of practice or be responsible to the patient in damages for any injury caused by deviation from the standards.

RESPONSIBILITY FOR THE EDUCATIONAL PROGRAM
Program quality

An educational institution that operates a hospital is responsible both as a health care organization and as a school. For educational institutions that do not operate their own health care facilities, the primary regulating forces are the accrediting organizations that approve the curriculum. Although in general no school can operate an educational program without recognition and approval by the state's education authorities, few states impose specific curriculum requirements on educational programs above the elementary and secondary school levels. Thus far, there has been no ground swell of judicial or legislative action to impose institutional responsibility (or individual responsibility, for that matter) for the quality of an educational program.

Some educational commentators, however, are beginning to fear such responsibility. There are reports of cases in the trial courts brought by students on the theory that their schools have an obligation to provide sufficient knowledge and experience to enable them to successfully complete licensing or certification requirements. These cases seem doomed unless the students can show that substantial numbers of their school's graduates fail to meet the requirements or unless they can show that school employees knew or should have known that a student was intel-

---

*If the student is an employee, the general principle of *respondeat superior* would apply.

lectually or otherwise incompetent and had a duty to warn the student. In any event, the best protection for the school seems to be *to provide clear warnings to students that completion of a course is no guarantee of successful licensure or certification and to emphasize the individual student's personal responsibility.*

Although not yet resulting in formal institutional accountability, demands are increasing from health care agencies that minimum standards of competence be imposed so that they can expect a minimum level of competence from the graduates they employ. Thus, just as students are beginning to demand some guarantees as to personal expectations from the course content and program completion, employers are beginning to demand similar guarantees as to performance levels of graduates. Whether the law will develop to accommodate these new concerns is unclear, but from the standpoint of planning, schools should (1) begin to pay close attention to their potential responsibility and liability for curriculum content and performance levels; (2) more clearly define course content and program goals; and (3) provide appropriate warnings to students and potential employers about the limitations of any educational program.

A school is far more susceptible to suits for injunctive relief compelling it to adhere to a specific, announced course curriculum or for the return of student fees and tuition than it is to suits for inadequate preparation of a student. Generally, although the institution can make minor deviations in curriculum and schedule, especially in the event of campus disturbances or other unforeseen disruptions such as natural disasters or strikes, the announced course curriculum cannot be terminated. In such instances, the courts require completion of the program or the return of student fees.[10]

Injury to third parties

Few cases deal with the responsibility of the school for the conduct of its students and for injuries its students inflict on third parties. Generally, a school is not automatically re-sponsible for student conduct in the way it is for its employees' conduct under the theory of *respondeat superior.* The reason: students are not agents or employees of the school. Nonetheless, the school could be responsible for other failures of school personnel with respect to student activities. For example, the assignment to a clinical program of a student known to be unqualified (by training or by some individual want of competence) could make the school liable to an injured patient. However, the school would probably not be liable for the negligent conduct of a student believed to be competent or unless the school had carelessly failed to ascertain whether the student was competent or unless school personnel failed to render appropriate levels of supervision.

The general rule is that an assignor of a task to a health care trainee is not responsible for the trainee's negligent conduct as long as the task assigned is one that such trainees have been taught to perform and the assignor has no knowledge of any individual lack of competence on the part of the assigned trainee.[9]

Injury to students

Care must be exercised by school personnel to see that no unreasonable risk of harm comes to trainees.[11] Certainly, a health occupations trainee can be deemed to have assumed the risks of contracting contagious diseases and of some degree of exposure to dangerous substances such as anesthetic gases in the operating room or nuclear materials in the radiology department. Nonetheless, a training program must be conducted in accordance with safety and other regulations. In the event of any deviation from applicable regulations that might cause an injury to a student, the program would probably be liable to the student. In this context, it should be noted that since students ordinarily are not employees of the school any injury sustained by them is not compensible under workmen's compensation laws. The school must, instead, provide monetary damages for injuries proximately caused by the school, which can be significantly higher than the workmen's compensation formulas would allow.

Privacy rights of students

Among the rights of students that may affect the responsibilities of both the health care institution and the school are rights conferred under a set of federal regulations designed for the twofold purpose of (1) permitting parents of students or students who have attained the age of 18 years to inspect, review, and amend the students' records and receive copies thereof and (2) requiring the school to maintain the privacy and confidentiality of those records.[12]

The regulations apply to all educational agencies or institutions to which federal funds are made available under any program for which the U.S. Commissioner of Education has administrative responsibility. They do not apply to a school solely because its students receive benefits under a federal program as long as the funds are not made available to the school itself. (Funds will be considered to have been made available if they are provided by grant, contract, subgrant, or subcontract or are provided to students attending the school when the funds may be paid to the school by the students for educational purposes such as under the Basic Educational Opportunity Grant Program and the Guaranteed Student Loan Program.) Thus these regulations apply to a broad spectrum of schools.

In addition, since the term "educational agency or institution" means any public or private school receiving funds under any federal program and since the term refers to the organization as a whole (including all of its components), the regulations apply even to educational programs that do not directly receive federal funds, but that are operated by an organization that does.

Although some exceptions exist, education records are generally defined as those directly related to a student and maintained by a school or by a party acting for it. The latter could presumably include a health care institution with which the school contracts.[12]

Each school covered by the regulations is required to formulate and adopt a policy of annually informing parents and students of their rights under the regulations and to for-mulate policies designed to comply with the regulations. Although a parent or student may waive any of the rights, a waiver will not be valid unless it is in writing and signed by the parent or student. A parent or student may not be required to waive any rights as a condition of entering a program.

An applicant for admission into a postsecondary school or a student at such an institution may waive individual rights to inspect and review confidential letters and statements of recommendation as long as the applicant or student is, upon request, notified of the names of all individuals providing letters or statements and as long as the documents are used only for their original purposes. Again, such a waiver may not be required by the school as a condition of admission to or receipt of any other service or benefit. Moreover, these waivers must be executed by the individual, regardless of age, rather than by the parent.[12]

Any agreement between a hospital and a school subject to the requirements of the federal regulations must specify clearly which party will be the custodian of all student records relating to the educational program. The agreement must also specify how evaluations of student performance will be maintained, and by which parties, so that the hospital does not inadvertently find that it is also subject to the federal regulations. Because of the nature of these regulations, the contract should require that the parties maintaining the records follow the provisions of the regulations.

Disciplinary rights of students

Additional concerns center around the emerging legal rights of students who are disciplined by or dismissed from educational programs. Public institutions are required to provide both substantive and procedural due process; i.e., to discipline or dismiss students only for reasons that are fair and reasonable and to follow rules of procedural fairness.

Generally, a student is not entitled to a hearing on issues relating merely to scholastic failure, but is entitled to a hearing where the dismissal is wholly or in part for behavioral reasons.[13] The standards of due process require at least that there be a notice of the charges against the student and an opportunity for the student to confront school officials who have knowledge of the facts.[14] The authorities are split on such other issues as whether there is a right to counsel at such proceedings.[15]

Generally, such a hearing should be before an impartial body that did not participate in the prior phases of disciplinary action. Total absence of prior knowledge of the matter is not necessarily required, however, since that may be impossible in an educational program. It is also desirable to permit an appeal to the governing body of the organization or a group designated by it if the hearing results are unfavorable to the student.

The hearing requirements applicable to private schools are less clear. Generally, a private school may not arbitrarily expel a student once it has contracted to accept the student, and there must be sound reasons for any expulsion. However, a hearing is not necessarily required as long as the student has a reasonable opportunity to offer his or her version of the matter.[16] A private school may, however, be required to provide a hearing if that right is contained in the school's contract of admission or rules and regulations. If the school is affected by so-called "state action," such as by having received substantial public aid or by being otherwise sufficiently imbued with a public interest, it may be required to provide a hearing. Although mere state regulation is not enough to convert a private school into a public agency, a private school may be subject to state action if it responds directly to the mandates of public officials.[17]

As a result, students may not be withdrawn or expelled from affiliation arrangements without some consideration of their rights to a hearing and procedural due process.

WHY A WRITTEN CONTRACT

The primary functions of a clinical affiliation agreement between a health care institution, such as a hospital, and a school should be to describe the relationship that actually exists between the parties, as well as their respective obligations and responsibilities. Lit-

tle is served by forcing the parties to sign contract forms designed for model programs, since each program has its own character, and the contract that does not reflect that character will be largely ignored or modified by custom and practice. Such a contract will be remembered by the parties only when their relationship has disintegrated or an unfortunate accident sends each to the printed form in an attempt to find the other fully responsible for the ensuing damages. Too often such a contract never did accurately reflect the parties' respective functions or, worse yet, has been modified by an oral agreement. The result is usually that the contract becomes an additional cause of, rather than a solution to, the parties' problems.

Because of individual variances among facilities, institutions, and programs, only general principles to guide the contracting process are enunciated in this chapter. Each contract should be tailored to the specific situation.

General principles of contract writing and suggested language are treated, first, in a section dealing with the concerns of health care institutions; second, in a section covering the concerns of schools; and third, in a section on the mutual concerns of both parties.

CONTRACT CONSIDERATIONS FOR HEALTH CARE INSTITUTIONS
Right to review the clinical program

Few health care institutions entering into an affiliation agreement want the obligation to be certain that the program satisfies all applicable certification and accreditation requirements. Nonetheless, because the hospital has responsibility for patient care and because it must plan for the allocation of its own personnel and resources, it should demand the right to review and develop the details of the clinical program. In particular, the hospital must be sure that it has the resources for an adequate clinical instructional program without compromising the quality of patient care.

One possible approach is for the hospital to require the school to notify it of the details of the clinical program and of the number of students to be presented for instruction well before the beginning of each instructional period. Alternatively, the hospital might set an upper limit on the number of students to be presented, so that its resources are not unduly taxed.

Insofar as other details of the educational program are concerned, the hospital must always retain the right to require the school to make modifications as necessary to accommodate the hospital's reasonable patient care requirements.

A typical contractual provision designed to provide the hospital with the type of information that it needs to plan for clinical rotation and to determine whether any modifications are required follows:

The college shall provide the hospital with at least _____ months advance notice of the details of the clinical affiliation program, including the objective of the program, the dates and times students will be presented for clinical affiliation, and the names of students and faculty participants, and shall modify the educational program as necessary to accommodate the reasonable requirements of the hospital.

Another typical way of handling the same issues is the following:

The hospital agrees to make facilities for inservice training available to the college, and the college agrees to present not more than a total of _____ students to the hospital during any instructional period. The college agrees to present new students for clinical training only at the beginning of an instructional period. As a condition precedent to the admission of any student, the college agrees to submit the names of the students it anticipates presenting to the hospital at least _____ weeks prior to the first day of the instructional period. The details of the clinical program and the instructional plan shall be mutually agreed upon not less than _____ weeks prior to the first day of the instructional period. In the event that the parties are unable to agree, this agreement shall terminate and neither party shall have any further obligation to the other.

Right to review the preclinical instructional program

Ordinarily it is not the function of the health care institution's personnel to establish the curriculum or to participate in the preclinical

instructional program; however, the hospital must be able to assure itself that the curriculum is adequate to prepare students to perform the tasks that will be assigned during the clinical affiliation.

Several approaches can be used. First, the hospital might demand participation in formulating the curriculum jointly with school personnel. Such an approach is ordinarily not desirable for either party. A more typical approach is to require the school to consult with the hospital about the curriculum and to give the hospital the power to require additions or changes. It is not unusual for the hospital's interest to be protected by service of hospital personnel on the school's advisory committees and planning bodies. A third approach is for the contract to require the school to "present only students who have had adequate preclinical instruction." This approach works well when the school is well-established in the offering of allied health education training. It has the effect of requiring the school to certify both the adequacy of the instuctional program and the adequacy of each student's individual preparation. A typical provision under this approach is the following:

The college agrees to provide adequate preclinical instruction to each student, in accordance with standards mutually agreeable to the college and the hospital, and to present for clinical experience at the hospital only those students who have satisfactorily completed the preclinical instructional program.

As a practical matter, the hospital may not want extensive participation in specifying curriculum content unless the school lacks experience in establishing programs. Whatever arrangement is used, the hospital's role should be specified in the agreement.

Right to refuse to accept certain students

Occasionally, a health care institution may find that a school will present for clinical affiliation former hospital employees who are now enrolled in its training program. Usually, the hospital welcomes such former employees as students. Occasionally, however, the school may present a student who was formerly terminated for cause, reassigned under questionable circumstances, or given the opportunity to resign. The agreement should preserve the right of the hospital to refuse to accept any such students. The hospital will be well advised to exercise that right only in circumstances where the reason for the adverse action is reasonably related to the student's ability to perform in a hospital. Only in cases in which the student's conduct while an employee was such as to jeopardize the quality of patient care or to cast doubt on the student's integrity should the student be denied the opportunity to demonstrate the ability to satisfactorily complete the program. Nonetheless, the hospital will be well advised to require inclusion of a statement such as the following:

No provision of this agreement shall prevent the hospital from refusing to accept any student for the clinical program who has previously been discharged as an employee of the hospital or who has been removed from or relieved of responsibilities for cause by the hospital or who has been refused employment by the hospital.

Right to provide or approve faculty

Regardless of whether its own or the school's personnel are supervising students in providing patient care, the health care institution should assume that it may be responsible for any failure to provide adequate supervision. Thus the hospital should either require that it provide the supervisory personnel itself or demand the right to approve any faculty provided by the school. A typical contract provision that puts the burden on the hospital to supply the personnel is the following:

The hospital shall plan and administer all aspects of the patient care program and shall provide qualified supervision of all patient care activities.

An alternative course of action puts the burden on the school, but preserves substantial rights for the hospital:

The school shall provide adequate numbers of qualified supervisory personnel to supervise the students in rendering patient care. The hospital shall have the right to review the qualifications of and approve or reject all supervisory personnel provided, to require the replacement of any personnel deemed unsatisfactory, and to require the

school to provide additional qualified supervisors if the numbers provided are inadequate in the judgment of the hospital.

As a general matter, to the extent that the hospital can provide its own employees as supervisors, problems in contract administration will be minimized. Of course, the school also has an interest in the quality of supervision, and the contract should reflect that interest.

Right to require compliance with rules and regulations of the health care institution

Generally, a health care institution does not wish to assume the responsibilities of the school in exercising disciplinary control over students. Today, hospitals have sufficient problems in administering the various disciplinary actions that are brought against their own employees and staff members without assuming primary responsibility for complying with the various laws, rules, and regulations that apply to disciplinary actions brought against students, particularly at public schools. Thus the hospital will want to avoid responsibility for the disciplinary process to the greatest extent possible.

Informing students and faculty of the hospital's rules and regulations and requiring compliance with them are basic principles that the school should follow. The following contract language would be appropriate:

The school shall inform all students and faculty of the rules, regulations, policies, and procedures of the hospital and shall require such students and faculty to comply with them. Specifically, without limitation on the generality of the foregoing, the school shall inform the students of the scope of the responsibility and authority of the hospital's staff for patient care, hospital administration, and confidentiality of hospital records and shall inform the students of the scope of the rights of patients to require privacy and confidentiality of patient records and information.

In order to fulfill its responsibility for patient care, however, the hospital must retain the ability summarily to remove a student or faculty member from any patient care setting at any time, particularly when the hospital's supervisory personnel determine that the presence of the student or faculty member constitutes a threat to the quality of patient care. Language such as the following should be satisfactory:

Any other provision to the contrary notwithstanding, the hospital personnel may at any time summarily relieve a student or faculty member of any specific assignment, or request such a person to leave any patient care area for any reason such personnel deem to be related to the quality of patient care.

In addition, the hospital should generally retain the right to request that a student who fails to perform satisfactorily be withdrawn from the clinical affiliation program. Such a right should not be exercised frivolously, but for reasons related to the rendering of patient care. Because of the substantial responsibility that the hospital has for the quality of patient care, it should retain the final authority to determine who shall remain in the program. Of course, the school may fear that the hospital could pursue wrongful dismissal of a person from the program; as a result, it is not unreasonable in an appropriate circumstance, for the hospital to assume responsibility for an unlawful termination. A provision such as the following is appropriate:

The school shall promptly consider any complaints made by the hospital against any student, in accordance with the school's standards and procedures for disciplinary actions that are applicable to complaints involving the school's students. In addition, the hospital may submit a written request to the school for the withdrawal of any student from the clinical affiliation program, and the school shall promptly so withdraw the student. Any such student may be reinstated to the program only upon terms and conditions satisfactory to the hospital.

Alternatively, the language can be modified to provide for a limited hearing procedure before a determination is made about whether or not a requested withdrawal shall become final. The modified language might read as follows:

The hospital may submit a written request to the school for the withdrawal of any student from the hospital. The school shall immediately withdraw the student until there can be an investigation of the matter and a final determination can be made as to the student's future status. Upon completion of the investigation, the school shall inform the hospital of its findings in the matter, and the hospital may thereafter make a final decision on whether it will require the permanent withdrawal of the student from the hospital or whether it will authorize the reinstatement of the student and whether terms and conditions will be attached to the reinstatement.

Whether or not a hearing is available to the student will depend on the reason for dismissal (is it academic failure or an alleged behavioral problem?). In a case involving pure academic failure, hearings are not required. The status of the school as a public or a private agency is also relevant. For these reasons, it is difficult to propose with any degree of certainty contract language that will suit all possible circumstances. If the school does afford hearings to its students, the contract should refer to the hearing process and to the status of students pending the outcome. Whether a student should remain in the program until completion of the hearings depends on the extent to which the allegations against the student relate to the student's ability to render quality patient care.

One additional matter that should be considered is whether or not the hospital should be responsible for any damages that the school may incur in the event of a wrongful withdrawal caused by the hospital. Contract language such as the following could be considered:

In any case in which the hospital requests that a student be permanently withdrawn from a program or that the student be disciplined and the school does not agree with the request, the school shall inform the hospital of the basis for the disagreement. Thereafter, if the hospital continues to request the withdrawal of the student, the school shall act in accordance with the request, provided, however, that the hospital will defend, indemnify, and hold the school harmless for any claim arising from such withdrawal of a student in any case in which the hospital is determined by any court or administrative agency of competent jurisdiction to have acted in an unlawful manner in requesting the withdrawal. The school shall advise the hospital promptly if any such claim is brought and shall provide the hospital with an opportunity to defend the claim. No settlement of any such claim shall be effected without the consent of the hospital.

Right to enforce patients' rights

Increasingly, hospitalized patients can expect information about them to be held in confidence. In certain circumstances, a patient who is diagnosed, treated, or referred for alcohol or drug abuse can expect that even the most minimal identifying information, such as the patient's name, address, and fact of treatment, will be confidential.[18] In many states, an obligation of confidentiality is imposed by statute, but even where there are no statutes, courts have held that patients are entitled to expect that no information from their records will be made available to third parties. Contract language to require schools to inform students and faculty members of the rights of patients and to enforce compliance with the policies, procedures, rules, and regulations of the health care institution is suggested in the preceding section.

In addition, it must be remembered that a patient even has the right to require that only those persons whose presence is necessary for the carrying out of a medical treatment be present. Specifically, in the absence of an agreement to be a teaching patient in a teaching hospital, the patient can demand that persons not required for the treatment be excluded.

Whether a patient is an appropriate candidate by reason of psychological or emotional conditions to be a teaching patient is a medical question. The attending physician must retain the authority to designate patients as being inappropriate for a teaching program. It is, therefore, almost mandatory that a provision such as the following be included in any agreement:

> Any provision of this agreement to the contrary notwithstanding, no patient shall be prevented from requesting that the patient not be a teaching patient, and no member of the medical staff shall be prevented from designating any patient as a nonteaching patient.

CONTRACT CONSIDERATIONS FOR SCHOOLS
Quality of the educational program

Explicit language to the effect that the school "shall plan and administer the educational program" for its students, including the portion of the program that relates to the clinical experience of the student at the health care institution, is necessary in any contract. Although the school may collaborate with the hospital concerning the details of the educational program and may modify the program as necessary to accommodate the hospital's reasonable requirements, responsibility for the quality of the program should be retained by the school. Even in circumstances in which the clinical supervision is provided by hospital employees, the school should retain the right to have its faculty present at the hospital at all times when students are present. Language such as the following is appropriate:

> The school shall provide one or more faculty members in attendance at the hospital at all times when students are present. The faculty members shall be responsible for the students' educational experience and training.

In situations in which the clinical supervision is provided by the hospital, the following language is appropriate:

> Subject to the provisions of this agreement relating to the rights and responsibilities of the hospital for the quality of patient care, the hospital's supervisory personnel shall cooperate with faculty members to the end that the students' clinical experience shall be appropriate in light of the objectives of the educational program.

When such matters are a problem, it may be wise to have the contract clarify that school faculty cannot use affiliation time for their own private pursuits and that they must be present, in fact, for supervisory purposes. Similarly, hospital personnel cannot abdicate their regular patient care responsibilities simply because faculty and students are present.

Because of the school's potential responsibility to students and employers for the quality of preparation of the student, either the agreement itself or the literature provided to students and prospective employers should specifically state that successful completion of the program and the clinical affiliation component does not constitute any guarantee that a student will be able to pass licensing or certifying examinations or perform successfully in practice. In the past, few contracts have explicitly dealt with this issue.

Privacy rights of students

Many schools are subject to the requirements of the federal regulations[12] entitled "Privacy Rights of Parents and Students." Since the primary burden for enforcement of those rights is placed on schools, safeguards should be provided in the agreement to assure that all educational records relating to the individual student be maintained in a central place and that the custodian of the documents be required to comply with all laws relating to the maintenance of, confidentiality of, and access to such records. Certainly, the federal regulations are of overriding interest to most organizations. However, careful consideration should be given to whether or not in any given state other requirements apply. Language should be inserted in the contract containing at least the following provisions:

The school shall maintain all educational records and reports relating to the clinical affiliation program and shall comply with all statutes, rules, and regulations relating thereto. The hospital shall forward to the school copies of all confidential letters and statements of recommendation relating to any student for maintenance in the school's files, and each party shall comply with all applicable requirements relating to the maintenance and release of such confidential letters and statements.

In order to minimize the potential effect of the regulations on hospitals not otherwise required to comply with them, it is certainly appropriate to place the sole burden for compliance on the school. If the following language is used, however, the personnel of the hospital must understand that all requests for information about a student must be redirected to the school, and the hospital's personnel should supply no information whatsoever:

The school agrees to maintain all records and reports relating to the clinical affiliation program. The sole responsibility of the hospital in such respect shall be to provide evaluations of each student on evaluation forms provided by the school at the end of each instructional program. Such evaluation forms shall be retained permanently in the files of the school, and the hospital shall have no responsibilities in such respect. The school agrees to maintain such records in accordance with all applicable statutes, rules, and regulations relating

thereto and to comply with all applicable statutes, rules, and regulations relating to the release thereof.

Disciplinary rights of students

Of particular importance are the ability of the school to carry out its own disciplinary proceedings and the necessity for it to require that disciplinary action be taken only for reasons related to the competency of the student to perform in the clinical setting. Although behavioral problems may require disciplinary action, such action should be taken *only* when the nature of the behavior compromises patient care or violates explicit rules and regulations. Whatever contract provisions are agreed on, their primary thrust must be to protect the health care institution from liability to a patient and the school from liability to a student for wrongful withdrawal caused by the hospital. Suggested contract language appears elsewhere.

Access of students to the facilities of health care institutions

Many contracts deal with such issues as the terms and conditions for student use of cafeteria, recreational, lounge, restroom, locker, and other facilities of the health care institution. Ordinarily, it is not essential that such matters be treated in the documents, particularly if the hospital and school have had a long relationship and no problems have arisen in the use of such facilities. Such facilities are often accessible to students on the same basis as they are to hospital employees. Only where gross distinctions are to be made between students and employees is it important to cover these issues in the contract.

Of far more importance is the matter of access by the student to emergency and other health care facilities of the hospital. Ordinarily, a student will be required to submit to the same sort of periodic physical examination and immunization requirements as hospital employees, and the agreement should so provide. The agreement should also deal with the conditions under which a student who becomes ill or who is injured on the job will be treated in the emergency room. Some contracts provide that the students will receive emergency treatment at no cost. Others require the student to pay the hospital's reasonable charges. Whatever arrangement is chosen, the contract should deal with the issue.

In addition, because students are not employees and, as a result, are not ordinarily entitled to the benefits of workmen's compensation laws, the contract should require that students have health insurance protection. Otherwise, in the event of a severe injury or illness, the hospital may be confronted with the legal or moral obligation to provide free care since most students would be rendered indigent by a large medical and hospital bill.

MUTUAL CONCERNS
Civil rights

In almost all jurisdictions, both educational and health care institutions are prohibited from discriminating because of religion, race, color, creed, national origin, and sex in the selection of students or the operation of a program. Various states prohibit discrimination on the basis of such additional factors as age, height, weight, and marital status.[19]

Moreover, although the traditional rule has been that a person could be excluded from an educational or training program for having a handicap that would impair the person's ability to obtain employment,[20] recently promulgated federal regulations potentially prohibit such exclusion.[21] Generally, they prohibit discrimination against a qualified handicapped student in recruitment, admission, and retention by a training program on the basis of the person's handicap. Some states have also promulgated similar statutes and regulations.[22]

Although it is not appropriate for a school or a hospital to provide factual information about licensing and certification requirements that may present obstacles to handicapped persons, it is mandatory that a person not be counseled for more restrictive career opportunities than a nonhandicapped student with similar interests and abilities.[23]

Admission tests may not be used if they have a disproportionate effect on handicapped persons unless the tests have been validated to show that they acccurately predict academic success. Also, they must be given in places accessible to handicapped persons. In the administration of admissions and other examinations, the school must provide methods for evaluating the achievements of students who have a handicap that impairs sensory, manual, or speaking skills.

Preadmission inquiries may not be made as to whether a person has a handicap unless the inquiry is for the purpose of taking voluntary action to overcome the limited participaton of a handicapped person and for making necessary accommodations.

Moreover, a school that is affected by the regulations is required to modify the academic program as necessary to ensure that academic requirements do not discriminate or have the effect of discriminating on the basis of handicap against a qualified applicant or student. *A school need not, however, modify essential academic requirements.* The regulations specifically provide that modifications may include changes in the length of time permitted for completion of the course, substitution of specific course requirements, and adaptation of the manner in which courses are conducted. The school must also provide auxiliary aids so that no student is denied the benefit of participation. These can include taped texts, interpreters, readers, and other similar equipment. The school is not required, however, to provide individually prescribed devices and readers for personal use or study or other devices or services of a personal nature.

A school must also take special care not to discriminate in the provision of nonacademic services such as physical education.[24]

These regulations will be of particular concern for allied health education programs because of the inability of a hospital to subject its patients to the risk of injury resulting from the students' physical or mental limitations. Close questions must always be decided in favor of safeguarding the patient at the expense of the students' clinical experience. Because of the newness of the regulations, it is difficult to predict how far schools will be permitted to go in foreclosing handicapped persons from clinical experiences. If hospitals are pressured to accept students presenting substantial risks, however, they will refuse to enter into affiliation agreements at all.

Under some circumstances, alcohol and drug abusers are also handicapped persons, which presents special problems for the hospital setting.

As these regulations are interpreted by the courts and their effect becomes clearer, careful planning will be required by the parties to screen from clinical programs persons presenting serious risks, and the advice of legal counsel will be essential.

For any contract document to deal specifically with all of the various statutes, rules, and regulations prohibiting discrimination is obviously impossible. However, the contract should impose upon each party the obligation to comply with whatever state or federal statutes and regulations exist. Thus language such as the following is appropriate:

Each party shall be separately responsible for compliance with all laws, including antidiscrimination laws, which may be applicable to their respective activities under this program.

Employment responsibilities

Responsibilities inherent in the employer/employee relationship include the obligations of the employer to compensate its employees and to provide fringe benefits under its employment policies and applicable labor contracts. In addition, employers are required to comply with workmen's compensation, unemployment compensation, minimum wage, and other laws that may be applicable. The last include state and federal laws relating to taxation and withholding of certain taxes from an employee's compensation. Because of the nature of these responsibilities, only one employer should be responsible for any individual employee, so that there is no duplication of the various requirements. Although the respective agencies will look to the realities of each situation to determine whether each party has complied with applicable requirements, the contract should specify which party employs each category of personnel.

The clinical affiliation agreement should specifically indicate whether students are deemed to be employees and which party is their employer. It may reflect that the students are not employees of either the school or the hospital. If that is the case, the materials provided to students should also reflect that the students will not be entitled to any benefits under the respective workmen's compensation, unemployment compensation, or other acts regulating the employer/employee relationship. Contract language such as the following is appropriate in such cases:

Students and faculty of the school shall not be deemed to be employees of the hospital nor shall employees of the hospital be deemed to be employees of the school for purposes of compensation or fringe benefits or within the terms of any federal or state statutes or regulations relating to fair labor practices, workmen's compensation, unemployment compensation, or the withholding of income and social security taxes. This provision shall not be deemed to prohibit the employment of any student or faculty member of the school by the hospital under a separate employment agreement or to prohibit the employment by the school of any employee of the hospital under a separate employment agreement.

Reimbursement between contracting parties

Typically, clinical affiliation agreements provide that no monetary consideration be paid by either party to the other. Such an arrangement is deemed to be mutually beneficial to both institutions. Third-party reimbursing agencies will ordinarily not inquire into the scope of educational costs, as long as there appears to have been a fair allocation between the two institutions of their respective responsibilities, and as long as the costs of education are borne primarily by the school. However, if it appears that the costs of education are being shifted to the health care system, reimbursement authorities will generally object.

The expenses of hospitals that participate in consortia with hospitals and schools that are designed to provide shared educational services have been denied by the reimbursing agencies in many situations. Thus a hospital should not enter into a clinical affiliation agreement without understanding that certain of its costs may be disallowed by reimbursing agencies.

To date, it has not been typical for such agreements to require that a school reimburse a hospital in the event that the hospital is determined by applicable reimbursing agencies to have inappropriately expended its resources for educational purposes. Unless the cases pending are resolved in favor of third party reimbursement of such costs, hospitals will be forced to look to the schools for reimbursement in the future.[25] To the extent that each individual contract can specify the responsibilities of each institution, placing upon the hospital responsibility *only* for supervising and monitoring the quality of patient care activities, the risk of denial of reimbursement is minimized.

It may also be somewhat helpful for the contract to specify that the clinical affiliation program is for the mutual benefit of each institution.

Indemnification and insurance

To attempt to set forth general rules concerning insurance and indemnification to be applicable to all programs is unrealistic. Each contract must be tailored to the realities of the individual situation.

The affiliation agreement should specify whether one or both of the parties are responsible for obtaining liability insurance coverage for students. It is frequently appropriate for either the school or the health care institution to carry insurance and for the party that procures insurance coverage to indemnify the other. Assuming that insurance coverage is available, the contract should be negotiated so that the party able to procure insurance coverage at the least cost is responsible for procuring it. In such a circumstance, if the hospital procures the insurance, the school should reimburse the hospital for a proportionate part of the cost in order to avoid any attack on the reimbursibility of the hospital's costs. The matter is much more difficult when insurance coverage is either unavailable or is available only at substantial premiums.

Whether the party that provides insurance coverage may indemnify the other party is a question of local law, as are the issues raised in situations where limited or no insurance coverage is available. Specific situations must be dealt with on a case-by-case basis. As a general rule, however, to the extent that a hospital assumes responsibility for the acts of persons that are not its employees, it can expect to be reimbursed by the third-party payers for the cost of insurance only if some form of compensation is provided by the school for its proportionate part. An institution should not agree to indemnify another unless the agreement is reviewed by general counsel.

Compliance with federal and state laws

Since it is impossible to recite in any contract all of the laws that may govern the conduct of the respective parties, it is sufficient for a contract to provide simply that each party shall be required to comply with all statutes, rules, and regulations that relate to its performance under the contract.

Third-party rights

Under existing contract law in most jurisdictions, a person who is not a party to an agreement, but for whose benefit an agreement is created, may be entitled to enforce the provisions of the contract under a "third-party beneficiary" theory. In effect, the third party is entitled to demonstrate to a court that the contract was created for the third party's benefit.

Examples of contracts in which the rights of such a party have been vindicated are legion. Since such cases proceed on the theory that the parties to the contract intended to benefit the third party, third-party-rights should be excluded by the language of the contract. Accordingly, language such as the following is appropriate:

This contract is intended solely for the mutual benefit of the parties hereto, and there is no intention express or otherwise to create any rights or interests for any party other than the hospital and the school. Without limiting the generality of the foregoing, no rights are intended to be created for any patient, student, employer, or prospective employer of any student.

Contract modifications

If the parties decide that it is important to have a written contract, it is equally important that any modifications of the document be in writing. Unless the contract specifically provides to the contrary, even a written document can be amended by a verbal agreement. Accordingly, language such as the following is suggested:

This contract constitutes the entire agreement between the parties, and all prior discussions, agreements, and understandings entered into verbally between the parties are hereby merged in the contract. No amendment or modification to this agreement, including an amendment or modification of this paragraph, shall be effective unless the same is in a written document signed by the party to be charged.

Independent contractor status

Under some circumstances, parties that participate in a joint program are deemed to be joint venturers, each becoming the agent of the other under certain circumstances and thus assuming liability and responsibility for the actions of the other. In order to minimize this possibility, it is advisable to insert a provision in the contract such as the following:

In the performance of their respective duties and obligations under this contract, the school and the hospital are each independent contracting parties, and neither is the agent, employee, or servant of the other. Each is liable only for its own conduct and responsibilities.

Contract term and termination

The ideal length of the term of an agreement is a matter on which the parties are not likely to agree. The health care institution will want to establish a term that is short enough for it to make other arrangements for the use of its facilities and resources unless it derives special prestige or benefit from the existence of the agreement. Thus the hospital will ordinarily want a short term.

The school will not want to be bound for periods exceeding the time frame within which it usually plans, such as one or two years. Once the school identifies an appropriate clinical affiliation site, however, it will want to bind that site to participation in the arrangement for as long as possible. Even when short termination provisions are allowed, the school will want to be certain that its students who are participating in a clinical rotation at the time of termination are permitted to complete the rotation.

One trap for the unwary in such contract provisions is the automatic renewal clause. As a general principle, parties should avoid contracts that renew themselves automatically unless one party or the other gives written notice of its intention not to renew within a specified period of time prior to the expiration of the current agreement. For example, parties *should generally avoid* language such as the following:

This agreement shall be for a period of one year from the _____ day of _____, and shall be renewed automatically from year to year thereafter unless either party shall give the other party written notice of its intention not to renew not less than _____ days prior to the first day of _____ of any year.

Although no one effective way in which to handle termination provisions exists, language such as the following is appropriate:

This agreement shall be effective for a period of one year from the _____ day of _____, _____ (the "basic term"), and shall continue from month to month thereafter. Either party may terminate the agreement during the basic term or thereafter upon written notice to the other party which is mailed not less than _____ days prior to the effective date of such termination; provided, however, that the students then receiving instruction in any program shall be given an opportunity to complete the current instructional period. This agreement may also be terminated by mutual consent of the parties at any time.

Power to negotiate and sign a contract

Both parties will want to be certain that the person negotiating for the other side and signing the contract has the authority to do so; otherwise, the contract will not be binding. The most effective way to obtain such assurance is by receipt of a certified copy of a resolution of the governing body of the agency conferring such authority on a specified individual or category of individuals.

SUMMARY

Although the general guidelines provided in this chapter can be useful in negotiating clinical affiliation agreements, they are no substitute for specific advice provided by attorneys for both parties. On any questions of local law, the advice of a local attorney is essential.

REFERENCES

1. *McDonald* v. *Massachusetts General Hospital*, 120 Mass 432 (1876).

2. *Parker* v. *Port Huron Hospital*, 361 Mich 1, 105 NW2d 1 (1960); *Bing* v. *Thunig*, 2 NY2d 656, 143 NE2d 3, 163 NYS2d 3 (1957).

3. See generally 57 Am Jur2d 1.

4. *Davie* v. *Board of Regents*, 66 Cal App 693, 227 P 243 (1924); *Wolf* v. *Ohio State Univ. Hospital*, 170 Ohio St 49, 9 Ohio Ops2d 416, 162 NE2d 475 1959; 33 ALR3d 703, 722.

5. *Georgetown College* v. *Hughes*, 76 App DC 123, 130 F2d 810 (1942); *Univ. of Louisville* v. *Hammock*, 127 Ky 564, 104 SW 219 (1907); *Roberts* v. *Kirksville College of Osteopathy & Surgery*, 16 SW2d 625 (Mo App 1929); 15 Am Jur2d CHARITIES §189; ALR3d 480.

6. *Darling* v. *Charleston Community Memorial Hospital*, 33 Ill2d 326, 211 NE2d 253, 14 ALR3d 860, *cert den*, 383 US 946, 16 L Ed2d 209, 86 SCt 1204.

7. Michigan Hospital Licensing Law; MCL 331. 422; MSA 14.1179(12).

8. *Joiner* v. *Mitchell County Hospital*, 125 Ga App 1, 186 SE2d 307, 51 ALR3d 976 (1971); *Ferguson* v. *Gonyaw*, 64 Mich App 685, 236 NW2d 543 (1975).

9. See generally, *Nursing and the Law*, The Health Law Center, Aspen Systems, pp. 10-11 (2d Ed 1975). The rules applied to students are in conformity with the general rule that an unlicensed person who performs the functions of a licensed person will be held to the standard of practice of the licensed person. *Thompson* v. *Brent*, 245 So2d 751 (La App 1971).

10. *Zumbrun* v. *University of Southern California*, 25 Cal App3d 1, 101 Cal Rptr 499, 51 ALR3d 991 (1972); *Paynter* v. *New York University*, 66 Misc Ed2d 92, 319 NYS2d 893 (1971); *DeVito* v. *McMurray*, 64 Misc2d 23, 311 NYS2d 617 (1970); *Harte* v. *Adelphi University*, 63 Misc2d 228, 311 NYS2d 66 (1970).

11. See generally, 38 ALR3d 830, 841, and 38 ALR3d 908, 923.

12. "Privacy Rights of Parents and Students," 45 C.F.R., Part 99, which were promulgated under Section 438 of the General Education Provisions Act, Title IV of Public Law 90-247, as amended, 88 Stat. 571-574 (20 U.S.C. 1232g).

13. *Mustell* v. *Rose*, 282 Ala 358, 211 So2d 489 (1968), *cert den* 393 US 936 (no hearing or dismissal of medical student for academic reasons); *Militania* v. *Univ. of Miami*, 236 So2d 162 (Fla App 1970); *Brookins* v. *Bonnell*, 362 F Supp 379 (DC Pa 1973) (hearing required for dismissal of nursing student for failure to submit transcript and reports and for poor attendance). *Bd of Curators, Univ. of Mo.* v. *Horowitz*, US Sup Ct No 76-695, decided March 1, 1978.

14. *Graham* v. *Knutzen*, 362 F Supp 881 (DC Neb 1973) *Soglin* v. *Kauffman*, 295 F Supp 978 (DC Wis 1968); *Dixon* v. *Alabama State Board of Education*, 294 F2d 150 (5th Cir 961).

15. See generally 33 ALR3d 229.

16. *Mitchell* v. *Long Island Univ.*, 62 Misc2d 733, 309 NYS2d 538 (1970).

17. *Coleman* v. *Wagner College*, 429 F2d 1120 (2d Cir 1970).

18. 42 C.F.R., Part 2.

19. MCLA §37.2205; MSA §3.548 (205).

20. *Davis* v. *Southeastern Community College* (424 F Supp 1341 (ED NC 1976).

21. §504 of the Rehabilitation Act of 1973, 29 U.S.C. 794, and the rules and regulations promulgated thereunder (45 C.F.R. §84.1 *et seq.*).

22. See MCLA §337.1101 *et seq.*; MSA §3.550(101) *et seq.*

23. 45 C.F.R. §84.44.

24. 45 C.F.R. §84.47.

25. *The Oklahoma Group* v. *Blue Cross and Blue Shield of Oklahoma*, PRRB Hearing Dec. No. 76-D22 (June 4, 1976), reversed by the Commissioner of Social Security (August 3, 1976), now the subject of judicial review; *Provider Reimbursement Manual* HIM-15 §404.2; Blue Cross Association, *Administrative Bulletin* nos. 834 and 834-A.

3

CLINICAL CONTRACTS AND AGREEMENTS

Alan L. Hull
Leonard E. Heller

Recently, tremendous growth has occurred in the variety and number of allied health programs. As reported in *The Study of Accreditation of Selected Health Educational Programs*,[3] the total number of accredited programs had increased from 2,855 in 1965 to 3,666 in 1970 and was projected to be 4,974 by 1975—a growth of 74% in a ten-year period. These programs are, in turn, offered by a wide variety of institutions, including junior colleges, four-year colleges and universities, vocational/technical schools, and hospitals. Furthermore, clinical facilities, which are an integral part of allied health programs, are as varied as the institutions offering the programs. They include community hospitals, tertiary care hospitals, medical laboratories, and private professional offices.

NEED FOR FORMAL AGREEMENTS

The usual problems of education are compounded by the involvement of two different organizational entities in the clinical affiliation. Each entity has its own values and goal priorities. The primary goal of the educational institution is education and research; the primary goal of the clinical facility is patient care. Since the ultimate responsibility for the education of the student lies with the educational institution, the educational program director has the responsibility to develop a sound formal agreement with the clinical facilities to ensure the quality of learning experiences.

Such an agreement or contract between the institutions is a method of specifying and controlling the relationship between the participating institutions.

Many accrediting agencies have begun to require formalized agreements between educational institutions and their clinical affiliates. These agencies require that clinical learning experiences provide "an adequate range and variety of clinical material, both normal and abnormal" (p. 215).[2] The accrediting agencies often look for formal agreements in order to ascertain whether the minimum requirements concerning number of patients, procedures, bed size, and location are met.

The American Hospital Association revised its 1967 *Statement on Role and Responsibilities of the Hospital in Providing Clinical Facilities for a Collaborative Educational Program in the Health Field* in 1976 to "emphasize the shared responsibility of hospitals and educational institutions regarding curriculums, clinical facilities, and costs."(p. 1).[1] The primary mission of the hospital is to provide quality patient care which, in turn, depends largely on competent health professionals practicing in the hospital. Therefore, it is in the best interest of a hospital to participate in allied health education programs. The guidelines point out that the hospital has a responsiblity to understand the philosophy, objectives, and goals of the educational program as well as the resources and capabilities of the educational institution to conduct the program. The guidelines also state that a written contract should be arranged between the hospital and educational institution.

The federal government, through the Division of Associated Health Professions within the Bureau of Health Resources Administration, has also been instrumental in fostering the use of formal, written affiliation agreements between educational and clinical institutions. Educational institutions requesting federal support for allied health special projects and postprofessional training must supply copies of their clinical affiliation agreements. These agreements stipulate:

1. The responsibilities of each institution
2. The procedure used to coordinate the institution and the students' clinical experience
3. The resources used
4. The approval of a teaching plan for the clinical component by the faculty from both institutions

In this manner, the best interests of the students and patients are protected.

According to Moore and coworkers[5] the written affiliation serves several functions: it facilitates joint efforts and actions, establishes common objectives, and leads to understanding of each institution's goals. Thus the written contract provides a base for the development and operation of a program involving two institutions.

Some educational institutions require all their departments to use the institution's standard affiliation agreement, based on the assumption that such an agreement is adequate for all situations. General purpose contracts produce problems in the health professions in such areas as determining who pays for malpractice insurance. Also, some local, state, and federal agencies (such as Veterans Administration hospitals) require the use of contracts developed for the particular agency. Although the practice is diminishing, some health facilities pay stipends to students during their clinical training, which may also necessitate special contract clauses. If the educational institution follows the practice of using a standard contract, problems may arise when ei-

ther the educational institution or the clinical facility wishes to make revisions. Since intrainstitutional approvals must be sought, considerable time and effort will be spent by the program's director. The use of a standard affiliation agreement with specific program riders is a way to overcome this problem (see Appendix A, pp. 54 to 57).

Any contract containing specific information can cause problems, since the contract must be renegotiated each time the contract lapses or a characteristic of the agreement (such as the number of students) changes. The best solution for the program director seems to be to develop one contract that contains the continuing policies and practices for the specific affiliation and to develop an addendum incorporating the specific characteristics that change frequently. Examples of continuing policies and practices are the benefits of the affiliation to each party; the general responsibilities of each party; the principles to be followed concerning such things as student conduct, grading, and nondiscrimination; and an indication of how frequently the specific affiliation characteristics will be revised. The specific characteristics are such things as numbers and educational levels of students; stipends, travel payments, and supplies to be made available to students; and how often the educational coordinators from both institutions will meet. These issues are detailed in a clinical education publication, as described by Ford in Chapter 13.

The long-term agreement can then be negotiated once and be effective until some distant point in the future (either a specified date or a period of time after one party notifies the other that it no longer wishes to continue the agreement). The agreement of the specific characteristics can be renegotiated each year and made an addendum to the primary agreement. See Appendix B, p. 58, for an example of a program affiliation agreement.

AFFILIATION AGREEMENTS AS LEGAL CONTRACTS

The law requires that only three activities need occur to develop a contractual liability[8]:

1. An offer
2. An acceptance
3. Some kind of monetary or nonmonetary consideration, such as a promise to render a service, granting of special privileges or honors

The occurrence of these three activities implies that the parties have negotiated and understood the terms of the agreement.

Furthermore, the persons who eventually act as agents for their respective institutions must have the authority to do so. In most states, an entire institution will be considered to be an individual entity, with rights and privileges similar to those of an individual in that state.[5] Thus a department chairperson or program director signs a contract not only for that department or program, but also for the whole institution. For that reason, the body that holds the ultimate responsibility for the institution, usually the board of directors, must first grant an individual the authority to sign.

Affiliation agreements vary in the degree of formality, the amount of detail specified, and the form that they take. As long as both parties have agreed to an affiliation agreement, it is legally binding, whether it is an oral or written contract and whether it is formulated with or without the help of legal staff. There are four basic types of affiliation agreements[5]:

1. Gentlemen's agreement
2. Business letter
3. Memorandum of agreement
4. Contract

The gentlemen's agreement is usually an oral agreement, and the affiliation usually develops over a period of time between two institutions. Although this method will avoid the immediate difficulties of agreeing on most aspects of the affiliation at one time, all the issues will eventually have to be decided. The time saved initially may not be worth the possible problems and misunderstandings in the future. Further, the pressures of the accrediting agencies and the federal government to develop written contracts will remove this option for the health professional educational administrator.

The business letter was the first step in the evolution of the formal affiliation contract; it formed the basis for many medical school/hospital affiliations in the late 1800s and 1900s. Moore's study[5] of physical therapy affiliation agreements shows that this method is still heavily relied on by program directors, but that the letters usually leave many issues undecided which must be decided in a gentlemen's agreement format. The study points out that the law states, "whatever is left out of a written agreement is considered legally ineffective if it is inconsistent" with existing agreements or policy (p. 38).[5]

The two most complex forms of written agreement are the memorandum of agreement and the contract. They differ primarily in the amount of input by each institution's attorneys. The memorandum will usually be developed by an administrator and then checked for legality, consistency, and completeness by the institution's attorney. The contract is the most explicit and comprehensive agreement and is almost always developed with the help of the institution's attorney.

If a dispute does have to be settled in a courtroom, however, any one of the four agreement types will be considered binding by the court.

The legal implications of the affiliation agreement are of concern to the allied health program director. Problems that may lead to legal confrontations can arise from two general areas: (1) problems between the two institutions, and (2) problems involving student and/or faculty interaction with patients. The former should result in very few problems having to be resolved in the courtroom. The process of developing an agreement should provide a forum for the discussion of most problem areas, and the contract should include mechanisms for resolving conflicts once the program is in operation. If the problem does have to be resolved in a courtroom, the affiliation contract is a potent tool for the resolution of the problem. An arbitrator or court may be required to interpret clauses in the contract that are unclear. In cases in which an item is simply not understood by one institution, however, the institution must comply with the contract.[8] Therefore, program directors should fully understand the language and implications of each affiliation contract.

Numerous problems can arise in student/faculty/patient interactions. Unless otherwise stated in the affiliation agreement in a "hold harmless" clause, both institutions would most likely be liable if a student were involved in an action that caused injury to a patient if the student were acting within the scope of his or her clinical responsibilities. For example, if excess radiation were given to a patient in the performance of the student's job, the institution would be liable. However, if a student strikes a patient, the student would probably by liable, since the student would not be following prescribed patient care practices.

Unlike the professional standards that have been set for most health professionals, there are no set standards for professional care for students. As a result, this area is legally uncertain. If the student tells the patient, "I am a physician," the student will be held to the same standards as a physician.

If a lawsuit develops from related activities involving a patient and a student, faculty member, or program director, the institutions with which the person is associated (i.e., either the hospital or educational institution or both, depending on the affiliation agreements) will be liable. These institutions may, in turn, sue the person if the institution feels it is justified.

CONTENTS OF AFFILIATION AGREEMENTS

The growth in the number of allied health roles and programs, coupled with the pressure for each program to maintain written agreements with its affiliated clinical facilities, requires allied health program administrators to be knowledgeable in the legal and educational issues surrounding affiliation agreements. The relationship between two institutions involved in an allied health program is complex. Researchers have been studying this relationship with the hope of finding common components among all the affiliations. One such study of medical school/hospital affiliation during the early 1960s suggests that a minimum of nine key issues should be explored and settled in an affiliation between a medical school and a teaching hospital.[4] Although the study involved only medical schools and hospitals, the nine issues are of concern to all allied health program directors developing an affiliation agreement.

1. Shared goals. Shared goals should be understood by both parties. This implies that the institutions must clearly identify their individual goals and priorities. Clear understanding of each party's goals and priorities is necessary in order to ensure that the institutions can work together for the benefit of the students, the profession, and the community. These goals include patient care, education, research, and community service.

2. Faculty and hospital staff. Faculty and hospital staff appointment policies should be well documented. The central issue is the amount of independence or input each party will have in the selection and appointment of the staff members who will be directly responsible for the education of students at the clinical site. The positions of educational coordinator at the clinical facility and the clinical coordinator at the educational institution are probably most important in this respect since these persons will function as the liaisons between the two institutions.

The educational institution must also take into account the requirements of professional accrediting bodies. Accreditation for a given program may require that the educational or clinical coordinator have a minimal level of experience and training. It may even require that the clinical instructors have an academic appointment with the educational institution. Such appointments must be arranged through the chairperson of the academic department and meet the standards of the educational institution.

In addition, the agreement should provide for recruitment and selection of the clinical personnel involved in the education program through a process that allows the faculty and the clinical staff to have input. Seaton discusses in Chapter 12 five role models for individuals involved in providing clinical education.

3. Other clinical staff. Clinical staff such as

nurses and residents have a direct responsibility to the hospital or clinical facility in which they work, yet they will have no formal responsibility to a program for the training of students. This point may be more of a problem for the medical school/hospital relationship than for the allied health programs, but the clinical facility's selection criteria for these personnel should include the applicant's ability to work with and train students.

4. Students managing patients. The level of involvement by the students in the management of patients is an issue that should be understood by both parties. The preclinical phase in a health professions curriculum usually consists of observations of a patient being treated by the clinical staff. During the clinical phase, the student is involved in direct patient care under the supervision of the clinical staff. During this phase, the student will encounter a broad range of problems, and consequently, the proper amount of supervision by the clinical staff is critical. Since the student is at the clinical facility primarily to learn and secondarily to provide patient care, provision must be made to ensure that the student is not used to perform routine duties because of a personnel shortage. Performing routine duties prevents students from experiencing the full range of patient problems that they will encounter in practice, and the patient will be receiving care from students not closely supervised by a professional. Scanlan in Chapter 9 and Pierce and Eichenwald in Chapter 10 relate these issues in more detail as they discuss integrating clinical experience with didactic education.

5. Patients. The type of patients who will be involved in the clinical education program should be identified. The questions that must be answered include:

1. How many patients will be available to students during their clinical experience?
2. What patient problems will students see?
3. When in their clinical sequence will students see each type of patient problem?

The suggestion made for the medical school/hospital affiliation was that any patient admitted by the clinical facility would participate in the teaching activities, so that students could see the interaction between health professionals and their private patients. The patients, however, should be advised that they are participating in the teaching of students and should be made aware of the important function they are serving.

6. Patient care versus teaching. Differentiation between patient care and teaching components of the clinical facility should be discouraged. The clinical facility should not establish for students clinics or experiences that are geographically separate from the clinics or activities normally performed by the facility. The objective is to enable the student to use the discipline's theory in the practical treatment of all types of patients in a closely supervised, natural setting. The students should also be able to experience or at least understand all the popular theories appropriate to their allied health field that are used in treating patients. The two institutions involved should also realize that their staff and students can help disseminate new theories and policies in health care, a process that can be inhibited if the learning and patient care components are separated.

7. Research. The allied health professionals interested in conducting clinical research should have a mechanism for initiating such projects. The issues such as informed consent, subject description, drugs, and potential risks should be discussed between the two institutions. A committee composed of faculty and staff members from both institutions should review research proposals and their impact on patients. The benefits to the faculty, students, and institutions should encourage faculty research on the theoretical and practical aspects of the discipline as well as on the delivery of patient care by the individual professions.

8. Ancillary educational space and facilities. A student's clinical experience usually requires some independent study and consultation with faculty members. The facilities and space that will be made available by the clinical institution for individual studying, reading, and group discussions should be noted. In addition, the clinical sites in which students will be learning within the facility should also be identified.

9. Affiliation agreement. The issue of the type of affiliation agreement must be discussed. The question of whether to have a written agreement seems to be an academic one, since sources external to the educational and clinical facilities (such as the accrediting agencies and the federal bureaucracy) are strongly encouraging some kind of written agreement. The requirements of the individual institutions should be well understood and the specificity of the contract agreed to by both parties.

The specificity and duration of the contract that are agreed to will result in differing solutions, depending on the institutions, program directors, allied health profession, and allied health professionals involved.

The topics identified in the 1962 study of medical school/hospital agreements[4] are here elaborated and expanded to include the issues that must be considered in all allied health program affiliation agreements. These issues should be considered by both institutions *before* contract negotiations begin, for they must eventually be considered by both parties.

CONTENT OF AGREEMENTS

The point that has been emphasized by most authors concerning affiliation agreements is that there is no standard contract or practice to follow. Each affiliation is a unique relationship requiring separate negotiations, understandings, and administrative practices. Providing several different types of clinical facilities in order to ensure a wide variety of professional activities is to the advantage of the educational institution. Clinical facilities also benefit from affiliating with more than one type of allied health education program. For example, a clinical facility may affiliate with a community college offering the occupational therapist assistant program and with a four-year institution offering the occupational therapist program. The interactions of students and staff allow for discussion of the various levels of responsibilities and profes-

sional roles, as well as discussion of how the profession provides total patient care.

Moyer[6] suggests that several content areas should be included in affiliation agreements between medical schools and hospitals. These content areas encompass the issues already discussed and can serve as a guide for the development of affiliation agreements between allied health educational programs and their affiliated clinical facilities. The following sections and accompanying suggestions, some of which are discussed by Moyer, should be included in the affiliation agreement.

Introduction. A statement should be included that names the two institutions and departments or sections involved.

Objectives. The institutions should state the goal priorities of each institution and the objectives of their joint ventures in a concise manner. This is the point at which the differences in goals and objective priorities should be identified and a consensus reached to ensure a successful program.

Corporate interrelations. The way in which the two institutions will interact should be identified. Most likely the two institutions will be independent of each other except for the affiliated program, but in some cases the clinical facility may be a separate part of the same educational institution (for example, a student health service or university hospital).

Financial relationship. A statement describing the financial responsibilities that are shared by the institutions is often required. The affiliation agreement can include any of three types of financial arrangements: direct payments to the clinical facility; indirect payments, such as payments for staff positions at the clinical facility; and payments to students. Other financial arrangements that should be considered are payments for student uniforms, meals, travel, and housing (depending on the distance between the clinical facility and the educational institution). The agreement that these payments will or will not be made should be included in the general contract. Specific dollar amounts should be included in the addendum, which should be updated each year.

In some cases, the institutions will not be involved in a direct cash transfer. For example, an educational institution may finance the position of educational coordinator at the clinical facility. This person may be paid from funds provided by the educational institution, but be responsible for coordination of the students' experiences at the clinical facility. Such arrangements should be clearly specified in the contract, especially since there may be confusion on the part of the educational coordinator concerning institutional priorities.

The number of clinical facilities that require reimbursement from educational institutions for the clinical education of students will probably increase. Hospitals now look to third-party payments for much of the cost of patient care; some hospitals look to Blue Cross/Blue Shield, Medicare, and Medicaid for payment of 65% to 70% of their patient charges.

The policies set by Medicare for the payment of patient charges are used as the basis for payments made by several other programs. Medicare does not provide for any reimbursement for educating medical students, although it does provide for some reimbursement for educational costs related to house officer education and some approved allied health programs. This is important to the hospitals since the Medicare program specifies which costs it will consider in calculating payments to the hospital. These costs include direct costs (such as some equipment purchases) and overhead charges (such as maintenance and administrative costs). The Medicare program will then pay the hospital the lower of either the acceptable costs or patient charges for patients covered by the program. In some states there are limits to the increased amount that will be reimbursed by the Medicare program to an individual hospital each year.

The implications of these forces on hospital- and other clinic-operated educational programs are substantial. Clinical administrators must cut back some health care programs to maintain others or to develop new programs. Identifying the financial and educational commitments the educational and clinical facilities make to each other in an affiliation agree-ment is one method for protecting the quality and stability of the educational program.

Professional requirements. The method that will be used to recruit staff, as well as a description of the professional qualifications the primary personnel involved in the educational program should have, must often be spelled out. If the staff at the clinical facility desire adjunct academic appointments in the educational institution or the faculty in the educational institution want to be able to perform their professional activities in the clinical facility, written provisions must be made. Another important consideration in this area is the requirements that may be placed on the program personnel, specifically on the educational coordinators, by accrediting bodies. The agreement should reflect not only the needs and requirements of the two institutions, but also the needs and requirements necessary to maintain the educational quality of the interinstitutional program.

Communication between institutions. The mechanisms for setting policies and administering the program should be carefully negotiated and clearly stated in the affiliation agreement. An open communication process between the two institutions is critical to the success of the program. Even though all of the problems that will arise from an affiliation between two institutions cannot be discussed before the agreement is signed and the program begins, the ability to resolve potential problems is an important function of the communication and personnel involved, and a communication mechanism to solve these problems should be established so that the problems can be dealt with quickly. Frequent meetings between the institutions should be mandated by the contract. In instances where more than one affiliation agreement exists between the educational institution and the clinical facility, a committee that includes the dean of the educational institution and the director of the clinical facility should be established. This affiliation committee would meet at least four times a year and be responsible for the long-term planning for all affiliated programs, as well as mediate problems that may arise between educational and clinical departments.

A subcommittee of the affiliation committee for each program may also be productive. The subcommittee would be composed of departmental faculty members and chairperson(s) from the educational institution, faculty and staff from the department or section in the clinical facility, and students. This subcommittee would meet regularly to resolve specific problems and to suggest modifications in the program and affiliation. These representatives could also serve as a steering committee to deal with such specific problems as curriculum development, clinical educational development, staff recruitment, and intradepartmental evaluation.

In a study of interdepartmental conflict, researchers found that status incongruities and the incompatibility of some coordinators' personalities were important factors in influencing interdepartmental conflict.[10] In order to reduce the possibility of interorganizational conflict, the staff members who work with staff members in another department or institution should be at the same status level within their respective organizations. For example, department heads who may serve on the affiliation committee should not send a subordinate to the meetings if the other institution is represented by its department head. The incongruity of status also leads to problems if the clinical department head is in the position of having to regularly communicate with faculty members at the educational institution instead of with the department chairperson. In short, individuals in two institutions who have the same status within their organization should communicate with one another.

A mechanism for the resolution of problems should be included in the affiliation agreement. Most problems should be resolved in meetings between the departments, although some will require the attention of the affiliation committee. If that committee cannot resolve a specific problem, some prespecified arbitration method should be followed. In order to preserve a good relationship between the two institutions, the arbitration should be speedy, fair, and thorough. The method may differ from institution to institution. The institutions may choose an organization such as the American Arbitration Association to resolve the problem. If it is an agreement between public institutions, a public official or committee may be specified. An example of a problem that may require outside arbitration occurred when a student who had completed the necessary course work and was ready to begin the clinical rotation was arrested for a violation of drug laws. The clinical facility did not want to place the student in a situation where patients could be endangered. In this case, the student and the educational institution maintained that the student had entered into a contract with the educational institution and therefore was entitled to the clinical education. The arbitration agency to which the case was submitted decided that since the student had not been convicted of the drug charges, the clinical facility had acted prematurely. The arbitrator ordered the student reinstated in the clinical facility on a day shift so the student could be carefully supervised.

This example points up the problems of different priorities in organizational goals and objectives. The educational institution was primarily interested in the education of the student, while the clinical facility wanted to assure the good care of its patients. In some cases, these conflicting priorities require an impartial ouside agency to resolve the problem; this agency or organization should be specified in the contract.

Exclusivity of the clinical facility. Moyers[6] points out that when more than one institution affiliates with a clinical facility, problems are likely to arise. These problems are most likely to occur in the areas of student conduct, faculty appointments, and financial commitments. However, as mentioned earlier, there is an advantage to students and faculty members if they have an opportunity to experience the interaction of the various kinds of responsibilities in the allied health professions. Therefore, if possible, clinical facilities should affiliate with several educational institutions for several different allied health programs, but not with more than one institution for each type of program.

Duration of the agreement. Depending on what works best for both institutions, the contract can specify either a termination date or process agreed to by both parties (for example, one academic year after either party notifies the other that its administrators wish to terminate the agreement). The addendum that contains the specific details of the agreement should be renegotiated at regular time intervals, perhaps each academic year.

The program directors who are responsible for developing a new affiliation agreement should appreciate the importance of having a detailed process for terminating the contract. If the accrediting bodies suddenly require additional facilities or educational activities that would necessitate sending students to clinical facilities with advanced equipment or larger patient populations, a new affiliation may need to be negotiated. In some cases, the old affiliation could be salvaged by changing it to meet the needs of a program that trains professionals at another level of responsibility within the allied health profession. If the accrediting agency requires that all programs training professionals at a particular level of responsibility be offered by a particular type of institution (for example, a four-year college or university instead of a two-year community college), a new affiliation may need to be negotiated.

Institutional and program accountability. All segments of our society are calling for increased accountability for institutions supported by public funds. Educational institutions, especially those that are public, are increasingly being made to justify their programs. Institutions, in turn, should be requiring their departments to evaluate, justify, and defend their individual programs. Since any decision becomes an important component of an affiliation agreement, the criteria that will be used to evaluate the objectives of the affiliation should be agreed on and included in the contract before the affiliation begins. Since the criteria to be measured and the levels of attainment may change from year to year, a statement agreeing only that the evaluation process will occur and who will be responsible for conducting it should be included in the

master agreement. The specific objectives and criteria used should be renegotiated each year and included in the addendum to the affiliation agreement.

SUMMARY

No single contract will work in all cases for all programs. The process and people involved in developing the affiliation agreement are the most important factors in establishing and maintaining a good process. Sheps[9] and Pascasio[7] have suggested processes for the development of an affiliation agreement. Pascasio specifically cautions that a sequence should be used as a guide to developing an affiliation or program at a specific institution, since each institution will have its idiosyncratic program and administrative needs (see Appendix B, p. 58). Briefly, the process for developing an agreement is as follows:

1. Draft a general agreement that concentrates on the purposes, objectives, and obligations of the affiliation, but which mentions all nine topic areas. This draft will be examined and refined by the affiliation committee, composed of all the major subunits (e.g., fiscal affairs, academic affairs, student affairs, etc.). The temptation to borrow language from other agreements should be avoided in order to make the affiliation agreement meet the specific needs of the affiliation.

2. This initial statement should then be reviewed by the chief executives of both institutions and their controlling boards for their agreement in principle to the affiliation.

3. An attorney should then be sought to help draft the final agreement, including the addendum. If it appears that an existing contract will suffice, then it should be used. The final contract should be in agreement with the principles approved by both boards.

4. Once the general contract has been approved by the appropriate people in both institutions, items included in the addendum must be agreed upon by the two institutions. Then all people af-

fected by the affiliation should receive copies of the contract.

REFERENCES

1. American Hospital Association: Guidelines: *Mutual Responsibilities in Educating Health Manpower.* Chicago, Ill.: American Hospital Association, 1976.

   This statement updates a 1967 AHA statement on the Role and Responsibilities of the Hospital in Providing Clinical Facilities for a Collaborative Educational Program in the Health Field. *The purpose of the statement is to assist hospitals and other health care agencies in developing cooperative programs with educational institutions to train and educate health care personnel.*

2. Council on Medical Education, American Medical Association: *Allied Health Education Directory/ 1974.* Chicago: American Medical Association, 1974.

   A directory that describes how 30 organizations cooperate for medical education; presents enrollment and program data by state; describes the 24 programs accredited by the organizations, the approval process, and essentials; and lists the individual programs. A 1976 edition is now available.

3. Council on Medical Education, American Medical Association: *Study of Accreditation of Selected Health Educational Programs, Part One.* Washington D.C.: National Commission on Accrediting, 1971.

   A series of working papers prepared by the staff of SASHEP to assist the members of the study committee as they consider the issues of structure, financing, research, and expansion in relation to the accreditation of health educational programs.

4. Graduate School of Public Health, University of Pittsburgh: *Study of Affiliations between Medical Schools and Teaching Hospitals.* Evanston, Ill.: Association of American Medical Colleges, 1962.

   A description of the types of hospitals with which all the medical schools existing in 1962 were affiliated, the relationships between the hospitals and medical schools, and key issues found to be common to all medical school/hospital affiliations.

5. Moore, M. L.; Parker, M. M.; and Nourse, E. S. *Form and Function of Written Agreements in the Clinical Education of Health Professional.* Thorofare, N.J.: Charles B. Slack, 1972.

   The results of a workshop session and survey analysis of affiliation agreements for clinical education in physical therapy. The authors present tentative guidelines (in the form of a checklist) for developing interinstitutional agreements.

6. Moyer, J.H. Affiliation agreements: Medical school-community hospital. *Pennsylvania Medicine, 76* (October) 1973, 45-46.

   The author describes the individual objectives, roles, characteristics of, and the interrelationships between community hospitals and medical schools involved in a clinical education affiliation. A guide is provided for drawing up an affiliation agreement.

7. Pascasio, A. Clinical Facilities, in Ford, C. W. and Morgan, M. K. (Eds). *Teaching in the Health Professions.* St. Louis: C. V. Mosby, 1976.

   This chapter focuses on four major concepts in establishing clinical facilities: (1) Determining sites; (2) Selecting sites; (3) Contracting for sites; and (4) Evaluating results.

8. Schaber, G. D., and Rohwer, C. D. *Contracts in a Nutshell.* St. Paul, Minn.: West Publishing Company, 1975.

   A text that attempts to provide "a good overview and an accurate general analysis of the more frequently encountered problems of contract law." It is written for use by lawyers and law students.

9. Sheps, C. G.; Clark, D. A.; Gerdes, J. W.; Halpern, E.; and Hershey, N. Medical schools and hospitals: Interdependence for education and service. *Journal of Medical Education, 40* (September) 1965, Part 2, 144.

   A report based on data collected for the study completed by the University of Pittsburgh Graduate School of Public Health (see Reference 4). The report presents an in-depth discussion of the key issues identified in the first study of medical school-hospital affiliations: shared goals, faculty and hospital staff appointments, patients and teaching, medical students and patients, interns and residents, patient care, research, and affiliation agreements.

10. Thomas, K. W., Walton, R. E., and Dutton, J. M. Determinants of Interdepartmental Conflict, in Tuite, Mathew, Chuholm, Roger, and Radner, (Eds). *Interorganizational Decision Making.* Chicago: Aldine, 1972, 66-67.

    Examines reasons for department conflict in volume representing an interdisciplinary approach to the study of interorganizational decision making. Examples include interaction between business groups, governmental groups, and business-government activities.

APPENDIX A

Affiliation agreement*

Institution	Date
Program Director(s)	
Dept. Head, Hospital & Health Related Programs	
Institutional Administrator	Dean, School of Allied Health

Agreement

This agreement is concerned with the clinical experience of Ferris State College students in the following programs in the School of Allied Health, Department of Hospital and Health Related Programs.

Student capacity

☐ Respiratory Therapy   Special rider page __ ____
☐ Radiologic Technology   Special rider page __ ____
☐ Health Services Management   Special rider page __ ____
☐ Medical Lab Technology   Special rider page __ ____
☐ Medical Technology   Special rider page __ ____
☐ Nuclear Medicine Technology   Special rider page __ ____
☐ Medical Record Technician   Special rider page __ ____
☐ Medical Record Administration   Special rider page __ ____

A. This agreement shall continue in effect per enclosed riders. Either party may terminate this agreement if notice (in writing to the appropriate signature above) is given at least twelve (12) months prior to the date on which the termination becomes effective. In the event of such a termination, the students currently assigned to the affiliating agency shall be granted the right to complete the program under the conditions set forth in the agreement.

B. This agreement shall be reviewed on request and subject to change by the mutual consent of the parties; any such changes shall become part of this agreement.

C. All students shall conform to standards of dress and conduct as established within the affiliating agencies.

D. Student vacations and holidays—see individual riders, Item 2.

E. According to accreditation policies and eligibility for degrees, the student must be enrolled at Ferris State College during the entire educational program, unless otherwise specified in rider.

F. The college and the affiliating agency shall not exclude persons on the grounds of sex, race, creed, color, or national origin from the programs endorsed by this agreement and agree to comply with the provision of Title IV of the Civil Rights Act of 1964.

Ferris State College agrees to:

A. Assume final responsibility for the educational programs.

B. Assume administrative responsibilities (recruitment, records, placement, program change, fees, etc.). (See riders for any additional details of supervision.)

*This form is used by some programs offered by the Department of Hospital and Health Related Programs, School of Allied Health, Ferris State College, Big Rapids, Michigan.

C. Furnish the affiliating institution with required student records.

D. Arrange for meetings of college and affiliating institutional staff.

E. Have on file the proof of state registration, current licensure, and/or certification of all faculty engaged in clinical supervision.

F. Terminate any service provided by the student to the patient when in the judgment of affiliating institution personnel the activities of the student and/or faculty are detrimental to the patient.

G. Provide Ferris faculty and student liability insurance during the clinical experience.

H. Provide medical care for students in accordance with the current college bulletin. (Off-campus students must carry their own hospitalization insurance.)

The affiliating agency agrees to:

A. Furnish clinical facilities required for student experience.

B. Make available a classroom facility to conduct formal instruction.

C. Provide facilities and services (e.g., dressing room space) that are available to other institution personnel.

D. Advise the College of anticipated changes in institutional policies and procedures that affect the student's program, within a reasonable time prior to such time the changes take effect.

E. Make available institutional staff as resource persons in accordance with a planned schedule approved by the institution.

F. Refrain from imposing upon the student fees other than for room and/or board and/or laundry service and hospital medical service.

Respiratory therapy rider

Respiratory Therapy Program Department of Hospital and Health Related Programs School of Allied Health

1. Both institutions shall comply with accreditation policies as established by the Council on Medical Education of the American Medical Association and as outlined in the Essentials of an Accredited Educational Program in Respiratory Therapy.

2. The clinical education program shall be nine (9) months (1,200 hours). The exact amount of holidays and vacations shall conform to the Ferris State College academic calendar. All sick days shall be made up as determined by the adjunct clinical instructor and the clinical coordinator. The clinical experience shall consist of 1,200 clock hours with 960 clock hours being in clinical instruction and 240 clock hours being classroom instruction.

3. Students will be rotated through each hospital on a predetermined schedule to enable them to obtain as much educational clinical experience as possible.

4. Ferris State College shall grant an Associate Degree to each student who successfully completes the required academic and clinical credits.

Medical record technology rider

Medical Record Technology Program Department of Hospital and Health Related Programs School of Allied Health

1. Both institutions shall comply with the accreditation policies established by the Council of Medical Education of the American Medical Association and the American Medical Record Association as outlined in the Essentials of an Accredited Program in Medical Record Technology.
2. The students must complete 360 hours of clinical affiliation; any absence including sick leave must be made up.
3. Students will have a 40-hour week arranged by the hospital.
4. The affiliating institution may accept students from other college programs.
5. The Ferris State College medical record coordinator shall visit the students at the affiliating institution at least once each quarter.
6. Both Ferris and the affiliating institution reserve the right to dismiss a student promptly for infraction of student regulation or for reason of unsatisfactory academic work. Such action will be preceded by consultation between authorities of the two institutions.
7. Ferris State College shall grant an Associate Degree to each student who successfully completes the required academic and clinic credits in medical record technology, not depending upon passage of certification examinations.

Medical record administration rider

Medical Record Administration Program Department of Hospital and Health Related Programs School of Allied Health

1. Both institutions shall comply with the accreditation policies established by the Council of Medical Education of the American Medical Association and the American Medical Record Association as outlined in the Essentials of an Accredited Program in Medical Record Administration.
2. The student must complete during the fourth year 320 hours of clinical affiliation; any absences including sick leave must be made up.
3. Students will have a 40-hour week arranged by the hospital.
4. The affiliating institution may accept students from other college programs.
5. The Ferris State College medical record coordinator shall visit the students at the affiliating institution at least once each quarter.
6. Both Ferris State College and the affiliating institution reserve the right to dismiss a student promptly for infraction of student regulations or for reason of unsatisfactory academic work. Such action will be preceded by consultation between authorities of the two institutions.
7. Ferris State College shall grant a Bachelor's Degree to each student who successfully completes the required academic and clinic credits in medical record administration, not depending upon passage of certification examinations.

Nuclear medicine technology rider

Nuclear Medicine Technology Program Department of Hospital and Health Related Programs School of Allied Health

1. Both institutions shall comply with accreditation policies as established by the Council on Medical Education of the American Medical Association and as outlined in the Essentials of Accredited Educational Programs for the Nuclear Medicine Technologist and the Nuclear Medicine Technician.
2. Sick leave and holiday policy shall comply with established hospital policy, except that any prolonged sick leave shall be made up before completion of program.

3. The affiliating hospital or institution shall provide a minimum of 1,500 hours of clinical experience, which shall:
   - Be under direct supervision the first 50 percent of the clinical experience
   - Be a planned part of the educational program
   - Have the work of the student evaluated, and the results used in the overall evaluation of the student.
4. The affiliating hospital shall provide a minimum of academic instruction and procedures critique as listed below:
   - 9 hours of Basic Pathology
   - 2 hours of Orientation
   - 9 hours of Therapeutic Radionuclides
   - 10 hours of Basic Laboratory Techniques, including 4 hours of Instrumentation
   - 3 hours of Radiation Protection, including 1 hour of Radiopharmaceuticals
   - 38 hours of Radionuclides, Clinical Application
5. The students will have four quarters of academic instruction and three quarters of clinical education. The final three quarters of the program, the student will pay tuition and be enrolled at Ferris State College. An Associate Degree in Nuclear Medicine Technology will be awarded by Ferris State College to students successfully completing the total program.

Medical technology rider

Medical Technology Program Department of Hospital and Health Related Programs School of Allied Health

1. Both institutions shall comply with the accreditation policies established by the Council on Medical Education of the American Medical Association as outlined in the Essentials of an Accredited Educational Program in Medical Technology.
2. Vacations, holidays, and sick leave will conform to institution and board of school's policy.
3. Ferris State College shall grant a baccalaureate degree to each student who successfully completes the required academic and clinical credits. The baccalaureate degree will be granted regardless of how well the student does on the Board of Registry Certification examinations.
4. Credit for the clinical subjects shall be given for each segment of the program.
5. The affiliating institution may accept students from other college programs.
6. The Ferris State College medical technology coordinator shall visit the students at the affiliating institution at least once each quarter or semester.
7. Both Ferris and the affiliating institution reserve the right to dismiss a student promptly for infraction of student regulations or for reason of unsatisfactory academic work. Such action will be preceded by consultation between authorities of the two institutions.
8. The institution shall administer examinations covering the lecture material in each of the subjects and forward the grades received on these examinations, along with the grades earned in the practical laboratory work, to the college.
9. The affiliating institution shall forward a copy of the results of the student's Board of Registry Certification examination to the college for the student's permanent record file.

APPENDIX B

University of Pittsburgh
School of Health Related Professions
Contract processing request

Hospital/Agency _____ Hospital/Agency Administrator _____

Address _____ Name of Contact Person _____

City, State, Zip Code _____ Position of Contact Person _____

Area Code _____ Telephone _____ Date of Contact _____

1. Was verbal _____ or written _____ contact made with Hospital/Agency?
   (check one)
   If written contact was made, please attach a copy of correspondence.
2. Is the Administrator aware of contractual agreement? _____
3. Are you requesting any special consideration? _____
   If so are you requesting:
   Use of Cafeteria at the expense of students _____ Hospital/Agency _____
   Housing at the expense of students _____ Hospital/Agency _____
   Stipends (please specify) _____
   _____

   Other _____

NOTE: Please do not send sample
      contracts. Upon receipt of   _____
      this form, this office will   Submitted by
      follow through.
          _____
          Department

          _____
          Date

4
INTERDISCIPLINARY CLINICAL EDUCATION

Jo Ivey Boufford

The clinical segment of all health professions education is designed to prepare students to be sensitive and skillful practitioners of their respective disciplines.

Many methods are used to implement the clinical education experience. The requisite knowledge, skills, and attitudes are more or less clearly defined by faculty members and presented to students through various teaching exercises: rounds, conferences, seminars, patient interviews, tutorials, self-instructional methods. Readings are assigned. Role models in the student's discipline are provided, so that students learn their roles by observing experienced professionals delivering care to patients. Service obligations are carefully defined for students to provide them with the opportunity to learn by doing—by actually delivering services to patients—under the appropriate supervision of members of their own discipline. Evaluations of the student's level of accomplishment are obtained by observations, chart reviews, oral or written examinations on clinical subject matter, and/or a definitive certifying examination for entry into the profession.

A missing element in much of this educational experience for the majority of health professions students is learning about the roles of other health professionals in the care of the patients to be served. The delivery of medical care—diagnosis, treatment, and long-term management—has become an increasingly complex process for the acutely ill. As expectations for health maintenance services, preventive services, and rehabilitative services have expanded the range of responsibilities of the health care delivery system, coordination of the resources of multiple health professionals has become increasingly necessary. Truly skillful and sensitive practitioners of one discipline may not be providing the best care to patients in the broadest sense unless they (1) are aware of the resources that other health professionals can provide to a patient and (2) coordinate *their* care of the patient with that of other involved professionals. For these reasons, interest in and pressure for interdisciplinary educational experiences for health professionals are increasing.

To date, these interdisciplinary educational experiences have taken a variety of forms, many reflecting the need to work within the limitations of the "separationist" structure that exists in most health science centers. Under this structure, "interdisciplinary" education occurs largely by chance in clinical settings where the needs of the patient or the situation compel traditionally oriented professionals to work together. Increasingly, however, educators in the various health professions are attempting to develop explicit, predesigned learning experiences for interdisciplinary groups of students.

PREPROFESSIONAL SCHOOL LEVEL

The Health Sciences Program at the University of Nevada, Reno, currently features a common core curriculum that extends from

59

college entrance to graduation for all students planning to enter a health profession. A lower division, horizontal core consists of basic courses in the biomedical sciences common to all health fields and required for entry into several of the existing clinical programs. A vertical core of interdisciplinary team teach ing and classroom and community-based experiences extends throughout the program's preprofessional and professional education.[1]

Lehman College of the City University of New York jointly sponsors with Montefiore Hospital and Medical Center the Health Professions Institute at Lehman.[2] In this program, B.A. level social workers, R.N. nursing candidates, and B.S. candidates in medical services administration learn together in special sections of basic science courses. They also share a core group of courses in community health and a classroom laboratory experience in their third year. Interdisciplinary teams of these students joined by fourth-year medical students from the Albert Einstein College of Medicine spend their fourth year in a clinical primary care experience in a field setting. The field settings are currently operating as team-oriented delivery systems within the Montefiore Hospital and Medical Center complex.

Although the Reno model has been highly successful in classroom and community-based interdisciplinary teaching for several years, neither of these preprofessional programs has yet operationalized a *clinical* component within their interdisciplinary educational experience. They do, however, reflect two of the more comprehensive models for interdisciplinary education at the preprofessional level.

PROFESSIONAL SCHOOL LEVEL
The classroom course

At the professional school level, many institutions have developed classroom courses for interdisciplinary groups of students. These are programmatically the easiest to organize and can be run as electives. The goal of these courses is usually twofold: (1) to provide students with some information about one anoth-

er's professional training and skills and (2) to provide a forum for interdisciplinary discussion of general issues in health care important to all health professions, for example, practitioner/patient relationships, medical ethics, and organization of the health care delivery system. In this type of course, no actual task requires collaboration by the students. The interdisciplinary exposure is primarily intended to increase the future professionals' ability and willingness to collaborate with one another in the care of patients.

The project-based course

The project-based educational experience, another model developed for interdisciplinary training, is an attempt to provide a task focus for the training of interdisciplinary groups of students. Widely used by the American Medical Student Association in its Appalachia summer program, it has been extended to a year-round community-based program for students from all health professions.[3] This model has also been used in the successful Kentucky January program run by the University of Kentucky College of Allied Health Professions.[4] Both programs involve students from different health professions in the design and implementation of a project in conjunction with individuals or groups from the host community.

Project-based courses are wide ranging. They can focus on projects such as health fairs, screening programs, development of patient education materials, and continuing education for area health professionals. The projects should have one critical characteristic: the successful completion of the project should *require* collaboration of the various health professions students in the course. This one characteristic increases the likelihood of the students' enjoying a truly interdisciplinary experience in which they explore one another's abilities and cooperate to attain their defined goals. A field faculty member from any one discipline who has some basic skills in group dynamics and knowledge of the team development process can serve as faculty facilitator for the student team as its members develop, implement, and evaluate the project.

The clinical team practicum

The most challenging interdisciplinary educational experience is the clinical practicum. In it, interdisciplinary education truly becomes a *team* educational experience in the real world setting of the health care delivery system. Before educators can clearly identify the characteristics of and implement an interdisciplinary clinical practicum, they must understand some of the basic characteristics of team delivery of health care.

The definition of a team must come first. Whenever two or more persons *must* work together to get a job done, that job requires a team. If one person can do the job alone, a team is unnecessary. Trying to develop a team structure around a task that does not require it results in wasted human resources, unnecessary fragmentation, and conflict. Thus in the clinical setting the first responsibility of the educator is to identify the clinical task(s) (for example, the service to be provided) and to determine whether a team approach is required.

If a team approach fits, the educator must next determine who is on the team. The membership of a clinical team is established by defining the needs of the patient population to be served. Once these needs are defined, the resources required can be identified. From that step, the professionals best able to provide the appropriate resources can be selected to form the team. For example, a learning disabilities team might include a pediatrician, clinical psychologist, speech therapist, and social worker. A geriatric home care team would more likely include an internist or adult nurse practitioner, physical therapist, occupational therapist, and social worker.

For a student to have a meaningful experience as a member of a clinical team, there must be a clear role for the student's discipline on that team. If there is not, the student will not be needed to perform the clinical task and thus will not have the experience of functioning interdependently with other professionals—the critical requirement for a truly interdisciplinary team educational experience.

If the clinical task clearly requires a team and the student's discipline is appropriately represented on the team, the next requirement for an interdisciplinary team clinical experience is the presence of students from other appropriately selected disciplines on that clinical service.

Scheduling is often the major obstacle to most interdisciplinary clinical experiences. Health professions schools run on several different academic calendars: medicine in eight to twelve-week rotational blocks, social work in semesters, nursing and allied health in terms. Coping with this problem means being prepared to work with limited time resources. Ideally, students' schedules should be coordinated to the maximum extent possible, assuring *at least* one block of time in common during each week of the experience.

A clinical model suited to a situation in which there is limited time for student interaction is that of the *mixed clinical preceptorship project*. In such a design, the student is precepted in the clinical encounter by a faculty member in the student's own discipline during the times in which other students may be either out of the clinical site or in the site in clinical precepting sessions with a faculty member from their own discipline. During some of these individual sessions, the student can observe preceptors in other disciplines to learn what they do in the clinical setting. During the sessions in which all students are present, the interdisciplinary experience can be focused on a discrete project related to that clinical setting. For example, if a team consisting of a medical student, nursing student, health educator student, and physical therapy student is working in an arthritis clinic, a common project might be developing a patient education booklet for clinic patients. The resources of each discipline would be required, and the project would relate to the clinical setting in which the students were placed. The teaching of team skills by one or more faculty members could then occur around the project activity, while individual clinical teaching could occur independently as students learn from their own faculty preceptors or observe preceptors from other disciplines.

If schedules can be worked out to permit

students greater shared time in the clinical setting, a more ambitious educational experience, the *clinical team practicum,* can be attempted. In this model, the students form a team and actually assume responsibility for the care of a defined number of patients or families on an ongoing basis. Although the optimal time commitment for such an experience is not set, one full day or two half days per week (the same day or days each week) is probably the minimal feasible time. Less than an eight-week experience does not seem to allow for any meaningful patient follow-up.

In addition to time availability, the clinical team practicum has another important requisite for success: the availability of a faculty team who can serve as role models for the student team in the clinical task. Because quality clinical training is so dependent on the presence of role models who can represent in action the kind of professional behavior desired in students, the presence of faculty members who actually function interdependently in the care of patients rather than just *talk* about the team approach is a critical variable in this model for teaching in the clinical setting. In the Institute for Health Team Development[3] project in five universities around the country, just such courses have been attempted in primary care settings.

The actual training of the faculty as a practice and/or teaching team is a critical first step in the effort.[2] If the faculty members do not actually experience the process of developing as a team and practicing or teaching as a team, they cannot model the behaviors so critical to the teaching of students in this setting. These critical behaviors appear to be (1) demonstration of knowledge of and respect for the differentiated roles of other team members and (2) the ability to openly manage conflict between team members and to use the differences identified to obtain richer solutions to problems. These behaviors can be direct outgrowths of the team development activities conducted with faculty members as they experience working together as teachers and deliverers of health care.

Although some teams that have been working together over an extended period may develop a level of role differentiation and trust, many need to focus on the *explicit development* of these aspects of team functioning. This requires a commitment of time and energy by faculty or service personnel. The teaching faculty, who in many health professions institutions have no role in direct patient care, may decide to take on at least a part-time (one day per week) service commitment as a team with faculty members from other disciplines to model a team delivery approach. Or they may decide to arrange release time for the delivery personnel who normally work at a clinical site so that those personnel can work to improve their own team's functioning and, in turn, serve as models for the student team. Ideally, these delivery personnel can have faculty appointments and be both teachers and service providers. If they are not able to serve as faculty members, however, a relationship between the delivery team and field faculty in the student's discipline must be developed that is complementary. The delivery team can provide the appropriate range of clinical precepting and team development training around the clinical task while the field faculty members can supplement the student's training in their own discipline and/or in specifically identified interdisciplinary content areas.

If faculty or service personnel are willing to commit themselves to development as a team, how can their development be facilitated? The process is usually called team development. In simple terms, this means that team members *explicitly* define the ways in which they will work together to perform their jobs (in this case, the clinical delivery of care and/or the teaching of students) most effectively and efficiently.

The techniques for accomplishing this process have largely been borrowed from the fields of social psychology and organizational development, where work or task group analysis and team development have been used with success in the business world for many years.[7,8] Methods vary from self-instructional modules that permit a team to conduct its own development without a consultant[5] to methods involving a team development consultant that are as varied as the consultants themselves.[6] All approaches include some common elements: the process of goal setting (what does the team see as its conceptual mission and its operational objectives?); the process of role negotiation (who will do what on the team to accomplish the goals?); the team maintenance (how will the team get its work done, set the agenda, run meetings, follow up on assigned tasks, make decisions, manage conflict, etc.?); and interpersonal process (how should individuals interact with one another as they do their work?). The team must set aside some time for initial development in these general areas and decide on a regular time (e.g., weekly team meetings) for ongoing team maintenance so that the team can continuously pay attention to how it functions and what it is accomplishing.

As the faculty or service delivery team defines its own functioning, it in a sense develops the interdisciplinary curriculum for the student team in the clinical setting. If the student team is to take care of patients as a team, it must go through the same process of goal setting, role negotiation, and team maintenance. Because the faculty members or service personnel have experienced this, they can serve as facilitators for the student team. This facilitation should occur as the student team develops—cares for its assigned patients; performs the necessary diagnostic work-ups; develops a treatment plan; and, with the approval of the faculty team and the cooperation of the patient, implements a management plan and evaluates its results. Team development thus occurs around the actual patient care task instead of as a separate project.

Certain elements of an interdisciplinary core curriculum should be defined by faculty and taught to students of all disciplines represented in the primary care setting. This teaching can occur in seminar or didactic sessions that ideally build on problems uncovered in patient care sessions or as part of separate laboratory sessions taught by individual faculty members or by the faculty team as a whole. As an example, in the primary care setting, a common interdisciplinary core curriculum

might be: knowledge of the other disciplines on the team; the skills of team development; the health worker/patient relationship (interviewing skills, etc.); family dynamics; and primary care delivery systems (problem-oriented medical records, epidemiology of primary care, economics of primary care, etc.). Core areas of common interest to all involved disciplines can be likewise identified for a given secondary or tertiary care clinical experience.

The extent of the clinical training to be accomplished in the individual student's own discipline during the team experiences must be defined and time must be allotted for this activity, which may largely occur with an individual faculty preceptor in the student's discipline. If the team experience is also to serve as the major field experience in the clinical training of the student, sufficient student time and faculty support must be provided to assure a high quality experience in both the team and clinical specialty areas.

STRATEGIES FOR PROGRAM DEVELOPMENT

As is apparent, a great deal of time and energy is required to develop a true interdisciplinary team experience for students in the clinical setting, especially one in which faculty members are functioning as an interdisciplinary team. Since most clinical settings are still rather traditional, what are strategies for implementing the best possible interdisciplinary experience within the existing limitations?

Clinical settings need to be selected where sufficient physical space is available and where the patient care task lends itself to the team approach. Most practitioners in these settings will, at least, consider themselves a loosely defined team in their work and the presence of interdisciplinary groups of students will seem sensible.

The identification of and contact with faculty members from other appropriate disciplines within the institution who are interested in interdisciplinary education are equally important. These faculty members must be willing to work out the coordination of the clinical placement of students.

It is important to negotiate the clinical precepting time for students with the staff of a potential site. The student experience will most likely have to be structured to complement the existing schedules of site staff. Scheduling, as much as possible, should conform to the needs of the on-site clinical staff. These individuals may, then, be more open to departures from this schedule for team education time.

Negotiation should concentrate on sites that provide the opportunity for at least a half day per week in a full-time rotation or some proportionate block of time in a less than full-time experience in which *all* students can be released together. In a mixed clinical preceptorship project, such block time can be used for a collaborative project by the students that the faculty members can use as a vehicle for the teaching of skills. If service delivery personnel can be involved in the identification of appropriate projects for the students that will be of benefit to the site, they may be more open to permitting and facilitating joint release time. If they are involved as consultants in implementation of the projects (e.g., a health fair or screening program), they will be exposed to the student team in action and perhaps become interested in the team development activities the students are experiencing. This may, at some future time, lead them to greater involvement in their own internal team development.

Development of the delivery staff of a clinical site as a team or development of a team of teaching faculty who will practice part-time to provide a clinical experience for students are both *major* undertakings. Clinical site staff should not be pushed to go through team development. The commitment of energy and time required must be clear and the on-site delivery staff, *with* the administrative support of their facility, must be allowed to buy in on their own. Otherwise, commitments to team development will dissolve under the pressure of service or other demands. Faculty teams that can implement this model must likewise be committed to a service role and be granted the necessary release time to undergo team training, to practice part-time, and to do the necessary curriculum development work. Administrative support for these efforts is also critical.

Although not all health teams require physician involvement, to the extent that a clinical team experience depends on the cooperation of a physician or involves medical students, the medical school faculty member or delivery physician is the key person to influence. Because physicians are often the most resistant to the team approach and, rightly or wrongly, by tradition may be considered the team leader, their willingness to initiate team development of delivery staff or a faculty team or to permit medical student involvement can often be the deciding factor. Leadership from physicians can often facilitate successful entry into a site and the successful development of a team educational experience in the clinical setting.

SUMMARY

To develop significant numbers of clinical sites that are truly team oriented in their care of patients is time consuming. To train significant numbers of health professionals who have a truly interdisciplinary orientation also takes a considerable amount of time. Questions often asked are: Once trained in the team approach, where will students find jobs? Since few team-oriented clinical sites exist, is it really worth all the trouble to develop these educational experiences and risk student disappointment?

The answer is emphatically, *yes*. The basic goals of interdisciplinary education and team development can be summarized as: increasing the individual professional's knowledge of other disciplines, their training, and their roles in patient care; developing in each professional a positive attitude toward the idea of collaborating with other professionals in caring for patients; inculcating in each professional the skills necessary to facilitate this collaboration (clear communication, goal setting, role negotiation, problem solving, decision making, leadership, and conflict management skills). No matter what the clinical setting or nature of practice, any professional with this additional knowledge and these attitudes and skills is better prepared to function as a skilled and empathic practitioner in the coordinated care of patients. In addition, an individual who has learned to communicate with and collaborate openly with other health professionals is better prepared to communicate and collaborate with patients in a similar way.

Students who experience these new educational models and find that they lead to greater personal and professional satisfaction can use the skills they have gained to act as change agents: to move the institutions that educate health professionals and the health care delivery system in new directions to improve the care of patients.

REFERENCES

1. Baldwin, D. C., Jr. Interdisciplinary education in the health sciences: A program for learning how health teams function. *Health Team News,* 1 (October 1), 1974.

    A description of the structure and operation of the interdisciplinary teaching program in the health sciences at the University of Nevada, Reno. Curriculum, organization, and teaching methods are briefly outlined.

2. See Boufford, J. I., and Eichhorn, S. F. *Interdisciplinary Health Teams: Their Education, Training and Practice.* Bronx, N. Y.: Institute for Health Team Development, 1978.

    Summary of the activities of the Institute for Health Team Development at Montefiore Hospital and Medical Center over the years of funding by the Robert Wood Johnson Foundation.

3. Eichhorn, S. F. *Becoming: The Actualization of Individual Differences in Five Student Health Teams.* Bronx, N.Y.: Institute for Health Team Development, 1973.

    A record of Dr. Eichhorn's experience as team development consultant with five student health teams placed by the American Medical Student Association in various communities in Appalachia during a summer field-work program. The development, problems, and accomplishments of each team are traced, and general conclusions on the process of team development are formulated.

4. *Kentucky January Program Description and Evaluation Summary, 1972-1976.* Lexington, Ky.: University of Kentucky, College of Allied Health Professions, Office of Special Programs, 1976.

    A booklet that describes four years of experience in the Kentucky January program run by the University of Kentucky. Program philosophy, organization, curriculum and evaluation design are presented.

5. Rubin, I., Plovnick, M., and Fry, R.: *Improving the Coordination of Care,* Cambridge, Mass.: Ballinger Publishing Company, 1975.

    A self-instructional team development manual based on the work done by Dr. Rubin and his colleagues at the Martin Luther King Health Center. This book can serve as a guide to delivery teams in their own team development process.

6. Shaevitz, M. The care and feeding of a consultant. In J. Royer and J. Boufford (Eds.), *The Conference as a Tool for Change.* Carnegie Foundation, 1973.

    An overview of the potential and pitfalls of hiring a consultant. This chapter outlines the various types of consultants available and the process for picking the one for your needs.

7. Tichy, M. K. (Ed.). *Behavioral Science Techniques: An Annotated Bibliography for Health Professionals.* New York: Praeger Publishers, 1975.

    An annotated bibliography organized around the major issues facing a health team in its development, from goal setting to conflict management. Relevant references from the applied behavioral sciences literature are provided for the health professional.

8. Wise, H., Beckhard, R., Rubin, I., and Kyte, A.: *Making Health Teams Work.* Cambridge, Mass.: Ballinger Publishing Company, 1974.

    A book built on the foundation of the team development efforts at the Martin Luther King, Jr., Health Center. It presents discussions of health team development from the viewpoints of various authors.

part two **DESIGNING LEARNING AND ORGANIZATIONAL STRATEGIES**

5

EARLY EXPOSURE AND FIRST-LEVEL EXPERIENCE

Clair Agriesti-Johnson

CHANGING OF CLINICAL EDUCATIONAL PATTERNS

The responsibility for educating allied health professionals has customarily been shared by two institutions: colleges or universities have had major responsibility for didactic learning; health care facilities have provided for clinical experiences that give students the chance to work with allied health practitioners. The responsibility for indoctrinating students into a system of values continues to be shared by both institutions. Today, there is a movement toward even closer coordination and integration of didactic and clinical learning in the allied health fields.

Professional and lay publications currently reflect concern for the development of individuals capable of providing better health care for more citizens at lower cost to the consumer.

The era of preventive medicine has also ushered in changes in clinical education. Health maintenance demands that consumers of health care services assume major responsibility for their own care. This is a departure from the practitioner-managed health care delivered in crisis care settings. Allied health professionals, with the prime function of helping people formulate and achieve specific health goals, have a definite role in this preventive approach. If health maintenance is to become a reality, allied health professionals will need to add the dimension of counseling to their existing therapeutic and technical roles.

CONFLICTS WITHIN CLINICAL EDUCATION PATTERNS

In the last decade, the belief has been promulgated that acquainting students with realistic situations strengthens their learning. However, that belief has been broadened to include the concepts of instructional coordination and educational accountability, so that today allied health educators more and more tend to coordinate didactic and clinical learning earlier and earlier into the professional curriculum, rather than at the completion of professional course work.

Although these influences have accelerated needed changes in clinical education, they have produced certain problems as well. Earlier clinical experiences mean students are in a position to deliver health care before they have mastered the scientific learning sufficient to ensure patient safety. This, in turn, implies closer supervision of younger students at the same time service and educational institutions are forced to introduce economies. The tutorial relationship between students and preceptor has traditionally been costly; however, the introduction of such a relationship even earlier in the curriculum further increases the cost of allied health education.

Resolution of this dilemma is clearly a societal responsibility. Yet, it is just as clear that the system of allied health education must grapple with this problem well before the dilemma is resolved. This chapter offers a systematic way to help plan and handle early clinical training without sacrificing patient safety or inflating patient care costs.

PLANNING EARLY EXPERIENCES

In the planning of early clinical experiences for allied health students, certain steps are critical[3]:

1. Developing a conceptual frame of reference based on professional practice
2. Developing objectives that consistently focus on professional practice
3. Organizing clinical experiences to facilitate the concurrent acquisition of knowledge, attitudes, and skills critical to professional practice
4. Selecting clinical teaching methods compatible with the limitations on resources
5. Developing criteria by which the student will be evaluated

These steps represent a process, not a solution. Their use can result in a number of solutions. Some examples are provided for the purpose of clarification and for generating ideas, but the unique needs, problems, and resources of each educational program will generate other possibilities.

Developing a conceptual frame of reference

A critical first step in the planning process is assessment of the professional practice for which students are being prepared. Changing needs may dictate changing practices. In diagnosing curriculum needs in order to ensure ideal rather than actual clinical practice, it is important to review the literature, compare opinions from a variety of sources, and subject these data to critical analysis on a continuing basis[3] (see pp. 5 and 6).

Before developing a competency-based education project, six divisions within the Ohio State University's School of Allied Medical Professions took this first critical step. Their early experience suggests that:

- Allied health professionals practice within four contexts: *preventive, crisis, rehabilitative,* and *long-term health care.*
- One of three specialty roles is specific to each allied health discipline: *clinician, technologist,* or *therapist.*
- At least three process domains are common to all allied health specialties: *management, education,* and *research.*
- Four competencies are inherent in each process domain: *assessment, planning, implementation,* and *evaluation.*
- Content common to all allied health specialties in management, education, and research is usually provided in the preprofessional curriculum.
- Content specific to each discipline is usually provided in the professional curriculum.
- Process domains provide a conceptual frame of reference particularly suitable for planning early clinical experiences, and these must interface with specialty content in order to ensure patient safety.

Developing objectives

The unique role specific to allied health disciplines involved in delivering direct patient care is the role of *clinician.* This specialty role is evident, for example, in medical dietitians, occupational therapists, and physical therapists. The clinician role should serve as a central focus for developing objectives.

The major goal of clinical experiences is to foster an environment that enables students to become competent providers of quality health care and to make the transition from student to practitioner. Historically, the gap between academia and the real world of practice has been wide. Coordinated education and competency-based education have served to narrow this gap. Both models are essentially competency-based and include objectives. Although the terms *competencies* and *objectives* seem synonymous, a competency is usually broad in scope and may encompass several objectives in various learning domains, whereas objectives tend to reflect smaller learning units. Competencies are professional entry-level behaviors that the learner should, upon completion of a professional program, be able to perform independently. Objectives are more appropriate to early clinical experiences than competencies and should serve three major functions: (1) to provide a consistent focus on competencies, (2) to guide content selection, and (3) to guide evaluation.

Table 6 demonstrates the articulation of competencies and objectives within the *clinician* role according to the Stufflebeam model.[10] Inspection reveals that, though competencies are presented in functional order, they tend to proceed from most basic to most complex. Therefore, when planning early clinical experiences, presenting them to the student in this order results in (1) a logical frame of reference for the student, and (2) an experience that tends to be the least threatening for the student. For example, a first clinical experience that involves a medical record would be less threatening than one that involves a patient or an allied health professional.

Table 6

Articulation of competencies for clinician role

Competencies	Objectives
Assess patient status	Collect, analyze, and interpret patient based data to identify need.
	Prioritize needs according to urgency and opportunities to respond to needs.
	Identify client goal(s).
Plan patient care programs consistent with the needs and potentials of individuals and groups	Identify medical goal.
	Develop evaluation criteria.
	Develop plan of action.
	Select most cost-effective strategy to implement plan.
	Acquire human and material resources necessary to implement.
Implement health care plan	Delegate functions and responsibilities.
	Allocate resources.
	Establish method and channel of communication.
	Provide leadership in delivery of health care (decision making).
	Coordinate or assist in coordination of team activities.
	Monitor activities of program.
	Organize and record or present relevant data to justify activities.
Evaluate activities in light of alternatives available or potentially available	Assess context data and make decisions on: Physiological and psychosocial needs Environmental factors Goals
	Assess input data and make decisions on: Plan of action Resources Morale Efficiency Side effects
	Assess product data and make decisions on: Intended outcomes Unintended outcomes

Organizing experiences

Taba[11] suggests that learning experiences or skills should: (1) be required, (2) be needed, (3) be learnable, (4) promote active learning, (5) serve multiple objectives, and (6) promote learning of main ideas. Clinical time is wasted if the skills are not required or if the student already possesses the skill. It is also wasted if the student is not ready to master the skill; in other words, experiences should be organized from simple to complex and from known to unknown to prepare the student. The clinical skill should be interfaced with specific content the student is currently acquiring so that it promotes active learning. The clinical instructor should help the student to coordinate several process skills with specific content and thus to simultaneously acquire several important clinical skills. The instructor should also promote the learning of main ideas by helping the student reason from a specific problem to a class of problems.

Organizing clinical experiences, then, calls for an academic faculty skilled in educational management. Because of the shortage of such faculty members, allied health programs have been forced to recruit from the practitioner population. But allied health practitioners have not customarily been prepared for this role, either. So academic faculty need to acquire the educational theory necessary for the task, as well as the attitudes and skills needed to plan inservice education programs for participating clinical faculty.

Both academic and clinical faculty should operate from a similar conceptual frame of reference. On the surface, this may seem an impossible demand. Yet, there should be a one-to-one relationship between standards of practice and the competencies taught. The mechanism that assures this is the inclusion of academicians in development of the standards of practice for professional organizations. The same mechanism can be used to ensure that the standards of education reflect the needs of changing allied health practices. In addition, at the institutional level, it is critical that practitioners, students, and other special interest groups be involved in planning clinical experiences that meet those standards mutually set.

Selecting clinical teaching methods

Clinical teaching is often viewed as a *method* of teaching. Yet, there are many methods that can be used in the clinical setting, and most are a variation of the on-site problem-solving method. This method is similar to the laboratory method in that it offers students supervised, individualized, direct experiences in the hospital, but is broadened to include health care settings as diverse as the home, community agencies, schools, children's camps, and health spas, as well as rehabilitative and extended care facilities.

To design early clinical experiences in a variety of such settings is particularly important. Yet, each setting has its unique administrative and social structure, climate, and philosophy. While crisis care settings tend to foster the development of therapeutic skills, preventative, rehabilitative, and long-term settings provide climates that tend to foster interpersonal, education, and counseling skills.

Resourceful teachers also arrange experiences to utilize resources outside these conventional institutional settings. Other possibilities include:

Retail outlets: Here, students can research such areas as cost and availability of health foods, over-the-counter drugs, exercise equipment, toys, and crafts.

Special interest group meetings: Students from a variety of allied health disciplines can team teach topics of interest to parents, teachers, hospital employees, and members of other special interest groups such as local diabetes, kidney, and cerebral palsy associations.

Rap sessions: Bringing the patient to students can be as effective as and more efficient than bringing the students to the patient. A group of students can interview a member of a free-living population to ascertain the needs, problems, and resources most critical to patient-managed health care in that most primary of all health care settings—the home.

For teachers limited to the resources within a medical center, the site becomes less critical than the patient chosen. Preventive care can be delivered in a crisis setting, and crisis care in a preventive setting.

Schweer[9] states that until research evidence clearly substantiates the belief that certain teaching methods produce better results than others, teachers must rely on currently available information and their own resourcefulness in the selection of teaching/learning methods. Clinical teaching methods depend for total effectiveness on availability of necessary resources at a given place and time. Resourceful teachers utilize and manipulate those resources to meet the objectives of the clinical program, not vice versa.

Developing evaluation criteria

Evaluation of clinical performance is an integral part of any baccaluareate program that prepares functional allied health practitioners. The teacher's ongoing descriptive evaluations of student achievement can be a far more important contribution than a final grade. In such programs student-teacher conferences can be held to provide students with a framework for evaluating their progress toward the goals specified.

Since professional clinical performance is characterized by flexibility and independence, measurement of such performance involves the observation of an almost infinite number of behaviors by a variety of raters making inferential and intuitive judgments.[4] The judgments are also being made in a particular environment with the added dimension of an interpersonal encounter. The dynamics of clinical evaluation, therefore, include students operating in and with a changing environment that consists of patients, clinicians, and faculty as well as abstract ideas and concrete things.

Because inference depends heavily on analysis into elements and association by classes, while intuition, by contrast, is global and complete, the evaluation of clinical performance based on operationally defined objectives is more of an analytical process than an intuitive one. Yet, intuitive judgments should not be ignored.

Precise statements of what the instructor expects may make things easier on the student as well as the instructor, but further teaching opportunities may be lost. A student who refrains from discussing patients in public places may only be complying with the instructor's wishes. The instructor who focuses only on the narrow objective is not likely to be able to guide the student toward higher level ethical concepts such as integrity.

One attempt to find a reasonable compromise between vagueness and overprecision in objectives is domain-referenced testing (DRT).[1] It deals with both content and form and provides a way to integrate testing and instruction so that evaluation data can diagnose the student's learning deficit.[8] The DRT approach is currently being developed as a means of evaluating competencies in a variety of allied health professions.[7] Although it produces only test items, not on-site evaluation strategies, the DRT movement and the theory it is based on have particular relevance for evaluating first-level clinical experiences.

In the DRT approach a domain consists of a subset of knowledge, attitudes, and skills for which essential attributes of content, behavior, and context are carefully described. Domain-referenced evaluation integrates five domains: (1) *objectives,* or what we do; (2) *knowledge,* or what we know; (3) *products,* or what we can possibly do, demonstrate, or produce with the means available; (4) *instruction,* or what we actually do with the means available; and (5) *test items,* or what we measure with. There needs to be a correspondence between at least two pairs of these domains before strong inferences can be drawn. For example, there should be as close a correspondence between what we want to do in terms of objectives and what we actually do as there is between what we actually do and what we measure with.[5]

A detailed discussion on DRT is not within the scope of this chapter, but practical suggestions from the DRT movement are incorporated in the planning process outlined. In that process, curriculum development does not proceed in a linear fashion. Often, two or more components of the plan are developed simultaneously. This is particularly true of the development of objectives and the development of evaluation criteria; objectives are only statements of intent unless evaluation criteria are also stated.

A statement of what students are expected to do and in what *context* they will be evaluated provides a description of the behavior and experience as well as implying content the student needs to master. If the mission of allied health education is "to assure effective and efficient health care to populations served," then a goal that is generalizable to all allied health education programs is "to prepare practitioners who provide or assist in the provision of health care." When this goal is examined in detail four competencies or abilities emerge: the abilities to assess, plan, implement, and evaluate. A functional ranking of these competencies reflects a hierarchy of behaviors. For example, a student might logically need to assess client-based data before selecting a treatment method.

But further effort is necessary in order to determine first-level objectives and their component behaviors. If students are to assess data, they must first demonstrate the ability to gather it. In order to do this, they need to be able to determine which data are relevant to a particular client's care and which are not. This implies that the student has mastered quite a number of complex skills with a subset of clinical behaviors that can be organized into a learning hierarchy. But clearly, the first-level student does not have this frame of reference; therefore, the clinical instructor must provide it. At this stage, the behavioral approach to clinical evaluation is very relevant.

By delineating the steps that lead to the complex behavior, the instructor provides the frame of reference the student needs. For example, the following cluster of clinical behaviors—gathering, recording, and assessing client-based data—reflects a learning hierarchy. It is also generally consistent with educational objectives in the cognitive domain and implies affective development as well.[4]

Level 1: "Using only resources that are suggested, gathers and records standard information with little variance from prescribed method. Makes little effort to interpret data."

At this level the instructor initiates the ideas, and the students follow through. The students demonstrate that they know exactly which information is needed to deliver health care, but not why the particular information is needed. The emphasis is on recognition or recall of terminology, specific facts, criteria, principles, and generalizations—the *knowledge* stage of cognitive development.[2]

Another element emerges, that of affect or values. The emphasis is on sensitivity to the importance of certain patient and practitioner behaviors to the delivery of health care. This is demonstrated when the students are aware of what is expected of them, are willing to receive guidance, and give controlled or selected attention to the tasks at hand—the *receiving-attending* stage of affective development.[6]

Level 2: "Seeks and records pertinent information from records and persons on own initiative. Requires guidance to interpret data."

At this level the students begin to supplement standard information with suggestions. The emphasis is on translation, interpretation, and extrapolation of data—the *comprehension* stage of cognitive development. The verb *seeks* implies that the students are beginning to value the importance of the activity to the delivery of health care. The emphasis is on active attention demonstrated by a willingness to respond—the *responding* stage of affective development.

Level 3: "Seeks and records the most pertinent information. Initiates own interpretation of data, but seeks guidance in relating information to total client problem."

At this level the students are beginning to judge the relative importance of data. This suggests that they can use knowledge in unfamiliar situations—the *application* stage of cognitive development. In seeking guidance, the students demonstrate a developing value system that reflects a willingness to learn to be better. The emphasis is on the acceptance of a value—the first level of the *valuing* stage of affective development.

Level 4: "Seeks, records, and interprets data.

Relates information to total problem. Validates information with instructor or other specialists, as necessary."

At this level the students demonstrate the ability to synthesize information by analyzing a situation into its component parts, sifting relevant from irrelevant data, judging the relative importance of data, and relating this information to the total problem. The emphasis is on relationships—the *analysis* stage of cognitive development. When the students validate conclusions with a specialist, they are beginning to show preference for a value—the second level of the *valuing* stage of affective development.

Level 5: "Using own experience base, seeks, records, interprets, and validates information to formulate an accurate assessment of the problem. Seeks assistance only when faced with unusual problems."

At this level the students demonstrate the ability to evaluate judgments. In so doing, they use human and facilitating resources. Chief among these are the client or the community, the team, records, texts, and current research. The emphasis is on preliminary planning and judgment—the *synthesis* and *evaluation* stages of cognitive development. In seeking assistance when faced with problems out of their own therapeutic range, the students also demonstrate a commitment to values related to self, clients, and profession—the third level of the *valuing* stage of affective development.

Some may question the specificity of the evaluation provided at each level. For those committed to the objectives approach to clinical evaluation, this criticism is legitimate. For those who have been grappling with the dichotomy inherent in teaching both technical and professional skills simultaneously, it is not.

The criteria presented look incomplete until the term *prescribed method* is clarified. Fig. 5 is one portion of a prescribed method of data gathering, an interview form. Although it communicates to a student the precise information to gather, it does not specify *how* to gather the data. Yet the evaluator must be able to judge both the quality of the history and the quality of the interview. The history the student submits may meet all the criteria of a complete history, but the manner in which the data were elicited may have annoyed the client. The prescribed method must delineate two sets of criteria.

Criteria related to the process of interviewing should parallel the purpose for the interview. If the interview is conducted to *elicit* information, then the student will likely do most of the listening. If the interview is conducted to *give* information, then the student will likely be doing most of the talking. And what of the content of the student's verbalizations? Is the student's information valid? Are questions open or closed, cognitive or affective? The focus depends on the purpose for the interview. Some points to judge during the history-taking process are: (1) Who did the talking and who did the listening? (2) Did the student respond to or ignore client verbalizations? (3) Were the student's verbalizations affective or cognitive, exploratory or nonexploratory? When evaluating a process, the evaluator must assess the value of prescribed behavior in the context in which it is demonstrated. To illustrate, a student who elicits a complete history from a client who is critically ill is not demonstrating competence any more than the student who continues to ask open-ended questions of a client who is begging for information.

The instructor has the responsibility to give first-level students something they do not have—precise evaluation criteria interpreted in light of purpose and context. First-level students need such criteria; professional entry-level students should not. An analogy comes to mind. Musicians must *first* practice their scales and subsequently refine their technique over a lifetime. The first step is critical if the musician is ever to be able to improvise, interpret, or compose. Professional musicians are rarely evaluated on their ability to play scales, but beginners are. So too, first-level allied health students should be evaluated on their ability to demonstrate prescribed behaviors, but the professional entry-level students should not. It is the re-

Dietary data needed	Yes	No	Implied
1. Name			
2. Home address			
3. Diagnosis			
4. Diet prescription			
5. Height/weight			
6. Ideal weight			
7. Preferred weight			
8. Daily dietary intake:			
a. Kind			
b. Amount (metric)			
c. Time (daily)			
d. Time (weekly)			
e. Supplements			
9. Weekend dietary intake			
10. Marital status			
11. Number in family			
12. Education level			
13. Occupation			
14. Activity/work schedule			
15. Food preparation			
16. Storage/shopping			
17. Meaning of food			
18. Previous modification			
19. Evaluation of dietary intake and potential for change			

Fig. 5

Interview form for gathering data needed to evaluate a dietary history.

peatability of the *results*, not the repeatability of the *process*, that assures the instructor that the student knows the theory undergirding the technique as well as the theory underlying professional practice.

If a student "involves clients in planning their own health goals at least 80% of the time," then the instructor can say that the student meets that criterion. But, is the student competent to provide health care? To answer that question, students must be viewed more globally, yet no less precisely, as they proceed through the curriculum. As students near graduation, evaluation efforts should focus increasingly on results in patients. As the Professional Standards Review process becomes a reality, the allied health professional will be evaluated via both process and product criteria. One dimension of a competent health care practitioner is the ability to demonstrate results as measured by client self-sufficiency, including such variables as increased mobility, weight loss, or occupational rehabilitation. Such criteria apply to the evaluation of both students and their instructors, to both experiences and clinical facilities.

SUMMARY

Individual allied health programs can use the planning process to develop early clinical experiences. These experiences should proceed from a common frame of reference reflecting the standards of practice of the allied health specialty for which students are being prepared. Since practice requires both technical and professional skills, process should be coordinated with content, and the functional ordering of process skills should reflect a learning hierarchy. Some practical suggestions are implied: (1) the inclusion in the planning process of those persons who will be most involved in the evaluation process—at a minimum these are academic and clinical faculty as well as students; (2) the organization of objectives from most basic to most complex or from specific to general; (3) the broadening of the concept of *clinical* to include any experience that provides a practical focus (students might be required to practice on one another, in simulated clinical settings, or on simulated clients, with objectives matched to resources and students to objectives); (4) the movement from general technical skills to specific therapeutic skills through professional practice skills; and (5) the initial evaluation of process and products separately, progressing to a more global and integrated evaluation of both.

REFERENCES

1. Baker, E. L. Beyond objectives: Domain-referenced tests for evaluation and instructional improvement, *Educational Technology*, 15 (July), 1974, 10-16.

   First of several articles in a special issue on domain-referenced testing (DRT). It attempts to explain the technical contract between DRT construction and the commonly accepted rules of thumb used to develop objective-based tests.

2. Bloom, B. S. (Ed.). *Taxonomy of Educational Objectives: The Classification of Educational Goals.* Handbook I: *Cognitive Domain.* New York: David McKay Company, 1956.

   A basic handbook, which proposes a hierarchial arrangement of behaviors as a basis for writing educational objectives and developing test items at various cognitive levels.

3. Johnson, C. A. The development of a research method for the improvement of health science curricula. *Journal of Allied Health*, 2, (Fall), 1973, 168-172.

   A description of a practical method for determining the clinical performance activities inherent in allied health practice. The method described was tested within a specific allied health specialty, and the assumption is made that it is generalizable to other health professions.

4. Johnson, C. A., and Hurley, R. S. Design and use of an instrument to evaluate students' clinical performance. *Journal of the American Dietetic Association*, 68 (May), 1976, 450-453.

   A description of the development and testing of a clinical evaluation instrument. Problems inherent in clinical evaluation and limitations of the instrument are discussed.

5. Johnson, T. J. Program and product evaluation from a domain-referenced view-point. *Educational Technology*, 15 (July), 1974, 43-48.

   An article that discusses how DRT can be utilized as a framework for the evaluation of products and programs. The focus of attention is the evaluation of hard products (machines, devices) and the products (textbooks, curriculum materials) that form the program of instruction.

6. Krathwohl, D. R., Bloom, B. S., and Masia, B. B. *Taxonomy of Educational Objectives: The Classification of Educational Goals.* Handbook II: *Affective Domain.* New York: David McKay Company, 1964.

A handbook of educational objectives in the affective domain which builds on the first handbook by Bloom et al.

7. LaDuca, A., Madigan, M. J., Grobman, H., and others: *Toward a Definition of Competence in Dietetics: An Interim Report.* Chicago: University of Illinois, Center for Educational Development, 1975.

   A monograph that presents a conceptual framework for developing domain-referenced tests.

8. Nitko, A. J., and Hsu, T. C. Using domain-referenced tests for student placement, diagnoses, and attainment in a system of adoptive, individualized instruction, *Educational Technology, 15* (July), 1974, 48-54.

   An article that describes the role of DRT in helping students wend their way through a complex hierarchy of predefined skills. Though examples are from the author's association with elementary school arithmetic curricula, the process described has implications for other curricula as well.

9. Schweer, J. E. *Creative Teaching in Nursing.* St. Louis: C. V. Mosby, 1968.

A classic book primarily designed to assist the teacher in exploring the concept of creativity as it applies to the functions of clinical teaching. Though nursing is the focus, the principles can be easily applied to clinical situations specific to allied health. This book is a must for the new clinical instructor.

10. Stufflebeam, D. L. (Ed.). *Educational Evaluation and Decision Making.* Itasca, Ill.: Peacock, 1971.

    A description of a model for descision making that assumes four areas of evaluation: context, input, process, and product.

11. Taba, H. *Curriculum Development: Theory and Practice.* New York: Harcourt, Brace and World, 1962.

    A discussion of the role of objectives in curriculum development in light of the needs of society and accepted learning theory. This classic book is particularly suited to the needs of allied health practioners involved in curriculum development.

6
ACCOMMODATING PREVIOUS LEARNING

Phyllis Drennan

The principal objective of this chapter is to examine the accommodation of previous learning experiences. With some difficulty, a model that accommodates previous learning experiences can be constructed, specifically as the term relates to clinical practice evaluation. That sort of activity (model building) fits nicely with the contemporary predilection for constructing models. What is more difficult is trying to bring to light assumptions about the nature of those phenomena before building models of them.

A FUNDAMENTAL DILEMMA

Ascribing competency is an abstract concept and investigating competence for the purpose of equivalency evaluation of clinical performance is a process that assumes competencies are known. This creates a dilemma. Instead of existing as an isolated process, equivalency evaluation is also embedded in the context of existing academic procedures, policies, and people. Further compounding the dilemma is recognition of the impossibility of equating competence in theory with competence in clinical practice.[12] Menges[9] relates that the distinction between knowing subject matter and knowing how to apply subject matter is a subtle one. The distinction is somewhat artificial since both typically use paper-and-pencil instruments and the results of both are usually combined and reported in one score. The major difference may be that knowledge of subject matter items requires only the lower level cognitive skills of recall and recognition, whereas assessment of the ability to apply subject matter requires the more complex skills of analysis and synthesis of previously learned material.

Sagen[11] suggests that retention and understanding of material previously acquired are major variables in performance. Several major features of the health professions compound the dilemma of investigating clinical performance for equivalency evaluation. Sagen[11] describes four characteristics of health professions education that have relevance for accommodation of previous learning experiences:

1. *Task complexity.* Evaluation is complicated by the multidimensional professional tasks that involve psychomotor and affective competencies as well as cognitive skills and knowledge.
2. *Long-term retention of detailed material.* Evaluation of performance in a clinical situation usually requires significant amounts of detailed factual and theoretical knowledge.
3. *Linear nature of subject matter.* If the clinical situation being evaluated requires knowledge of the biological and physical sciences (whose logical structure is essentially linear), the testing situation may be limited by the students' science background.
4. *Standards of performance.* Ability to solve problems in a brief period of time

is usually a part of the accepted definitions of performance now embodied in health science certification standards.

A CONTEXTUAL FRAMEWORK

A place to begin is the meaning of the key words and concepts. According to one dictionary, to accommodate means to make fit, bring into agreement, or give consideration. Thus the underlying problem is to identify a mechanism by which to quantitatively relate random work experiences to structured educational activities. The question becomes, "Is it possible to have equivalency evaluation for clinical practice?" The simplicity of the question obscures the complexities involved in the evaluation of those competencies an individual may have gained through previous education and experience. The complexities of equivalency evaluation are multifaceted; only the more salient ones are discussed.

Assessment of the clinical competence of students entering an education program is difficult because each student is unique. However, criteria used for assessing the clinical competence of individual students are usually the course or program objectives that have been designed for groups of generic students. Some authorities suggest that the domain from which clinical tasks for evaluation should be chosen is the intersection of the expected accomplishment in professional practice and the content of the particular instructional unit being used for placement.

The expected competencies in clinical practice are multidimensional (psychomotor, affective, and cognitive) and are evaluated in relatively open systems. For some areas of instruction and evaluation, the Mager model works well for procedures. However, the knowledge utilization model is more applicable to clinical learning and evaluation. The assumption is made when relatively simple, direct instruction and assessment are replaced by more open, intricate systems, problems of evaluation go up exponentially.

Another complexity involved in equivalency evaluation for clinical practice is the commitment of faculty time. Faculty members involved in the equivalency evaluation process usually carry full teaching loads. Providing time to spend with individuals for the evaluation of clinical practice competencies is usually done on an overload basis throughout the contract year. Providing time in the agency for the evaluator to sufficiently sample the performance behavior(s) required is difficult. Usually clinical practice is evaluated on the basis of a few hours in an unfamiliar hospital or agency setting.

Wilson[16] suggests that site selection is a critical variable in equivalency evaluation for the clinical component. She suggests that sites other than the ones used for the regular program should be utilized. Unless the other site environment is known to the evaluator, an incongruency exists; the environment should be known by both the evaluator and person being evaluated. Of course, these assumptions are predicated on the evaluation of clinical practice being implemented in a direct care situation.

Evaluation skills of the evaluators, who are usually faculty members, are another critical variable adding to the complexity of the clinical equivalency evaluation process. The judgment of the evaluator is usually relied on for evaluation of the student's clinical performance. Reliability and objectivity of judgments are questionable. Scriven[13] suggests that two of the fundamental issues in educational evaluation arise from attempts to justify value judgments and the problems of obtaining unbiased information—in this case, the value judgment and unbiased information about an individual's competence in the clinical setting for placement in a specific educational program.

Evaluators need a clear understanding of practitioner roles and the clinical objectives. The clinical objectives may show variation in their actual implementation and subsequent evaluation. The variation often results from the demand of patient/client care rather than the evaluation needs of the student.

Assumptions about the phenomena are as critical as understanding of the complexities. For example, the assumption that faculty members have the knowledge and ability to accommodate previous learning experience is basic. Dewey asserted that one can learn by doing; faculty members must *learn* to accommodate the previous learning experiences of students by doing just that.

Another critical assumption undergirding the whole concept of equivalency evaluation is that the faculty member's beliefs and values are congruent with the concept. Wilson[17] makes the case that *equivalency* means equality in value, degree, effect, and significance. The assumption follows that *equivalency evaluation* connotes the verification of competencies and attributes of like value and significance to those acquired through a formal education program. Faculty members must agree on the value and purpose for accommodating previous learning experiences.

THE IDEA EXAMINED

If the hallmark of a good idea is the number of thoughts and actions it generates, then the notion of equivalency evaluation is a promising one indeed. However, a legitimate task of education is an attempt to correct popular beliefs by subjecting them to rigorous examination in the light of factual evidence. Bruner states that "we should have the courage to recognize what we do not understand and to permit ourselves a new and innocent look" (p. 171).[3]

Ideas have a momentum of their own; they are integral factors in an interdependent system of relationships. The search for how educators are evaluating clinical practice to accommodate previous learning experiences yields many and varied means. However, the literature reveals limited evaluations of the methodologies. People are writing primarily about what and how they are trying to cope with equivalency evaluation problems.

In a 1976 statement about the open curriculum in nursing education, the National League for Nursing Board of Directors indicated: "In any type of nursing program, opportunity should be provided to students to validate previous learning and facilitate advanced placement."[10] Ozimek admonishes nursing educators that "exit behaviors are considered the most important educational goals and serve as the basis for education."[10]

Wilson[16] suggests that equivalency evaluation should be viewed not so much as an activity that reveals what a student does not need to take, but rather as a way of identifying what educational experience the student still needs in order to become an able practitioner.

Conceptualization of the process of clinical equivalency evaluation, whether stated as accommodating previous learning experience or viewed as what the student still needs in relation to exit behavior, requires measurement, assessment of prior learning, and experience. Developing useful ways of assessing knowledge, attitude, skills, and other behaviors can be very tricky business. Instructional objectives, whether normative or criterion-referenced, dominate the literature on evaluation as modes for quantified measurement.

Bruner states, "we need a theory of instruction, because techniques of evaluation derive from it; evaluation has to do with measurement in the classic psychometric sense and the relation of such measurement to theory" (p. 171).[3] The idea of equivalency evaluation in its current form is best examined as a policy principle rather than a philosophy and as an ideology rather than a theory. The current stage is one of comment, reporting, and limited analysis. However, going beyond the weakness, vulnerabilities, untested assumptions, and the less than perfect procedures, many educators are attempting to define the process of equivalency evaluation for clinical practice.

SYSTEM RELATIONSHIPS

In system terms, outputs are usually examined; in the case of equivalency evaluation, input characteristics—the capabilities of the learner for advanced placement—are examined. The present use of system strategies exhibits a marked inadequacy in the assessment of the input competence. A statement of expected input competence is an assessment of the capabilities of the learner in relationship to the inventory of clinical performance expectations.[1]

In systems theory the purpose and performance expectations of the system must be identified before the parts that make up the whole can be developed; yet clinical performance relies on the totality of its parts. How clinical performance expectations interact and interface with the system for the purposes of achieving the goal of the system is what is important. A great deal has already been written about how these performance expectations must be stated specifically enough (in criterion-referenced measures) to reveal when they have been met.

THE PROCESS EXAMINED

In essence, the performance to be evaluated is situationally dependent, since equivalency evaluation for clinical practice is usually a performance examination in an actual patient care setting. Both the performance to be measured and the criteria for adequate performance must be specified.

Although evaluation of the student's performance is both a formative and a summative tool, as Wilson[17] suggests, application of knowledge is integrative. The student in the clinical performance examination confronts a new situation that must be dealt with by analysis or synthesis or evaluation of previous learning experiences. There is a high probability that the conditions in the clinical setting are not identical to any met before in a previous learning situation. In order for the equivalency evaluation to provide formative or diagnostic or summative data choices must be made about numerous data possibilities. The evaluator must determine which data have the greatest relevance, and which of the infinite behavior measurements are most germane to the pertinent evaluation questions. Once these choices have been made, the criteria for student performance, the clinical situation, and the particular means of measuring can be explicitly agreed on.

Most authorities agree that clinical evaluation should be criterion referenced rather than normative referenced. However, some argue that the equivalency evaluation process must have a normative reference against which to measure; that a student's performance should be compared with some Platonic, ideal performance. The essence of the process rests with assessment of competency-based performance vis á vis clear goal expectations. One way of defining evaluation is $E \equiv (P \cong O)$, with P defined as performance and O defined as the objectives. An advantage of this congruency definition is a high degree of integration within the instructional process; however, a disadvantage is that evaluation focuses narrowly on objectives, and the evaluation of behavior becomes the ultimate criterion of every educational action.

In evaluation of clinical performance and estimation of a student's skills, data should be gathered, but their interpretation and use inevitably depend on the value judgments of qualified persons. An inherent obstacle to the acceptance of professional educators' value judgments is that the educators are not disinterested parties and their credibility can at times be questioned.

In the many approaches to equivalency evaluation for clinical practice, course objectives, program goals, and expectations of the practicing health providers form the basis for the process. In nursing, instruments to measure clinical performance focus on abilities to plan, implement, and evaluate nursing care in a variety of situations. Clinical performance evaluation in nursing uses a variety of approaches: (1) a faculty member directly evaluates the student's nursing practice in a clinical setting; (2) a faculty member directly evaluates the student's performance in a simulated learning laboratory; (3) the student is required to take teacher-made examinations; and (4) a faculty member combines all of the preceding.[4]

Undoubtedly, the New York Regents external degree program for nursing has been the most rigorously planned and designed effort in nursing. Bevil's[2] article published in *Nursing Forum* and *Nursing Digest* describes the philosophy and the planning process underlying the technical external degree. Bevil also raises many critical questions about the program and its graduates.

In an article about the external degree program, Lenburg[8] relates that it took three years and $105,000 to create a test to measure clinical nursing competence. Lenburg makes particularly valuable suggestions for developing competency evaluations for large numbers of students seeking advanced placement. The one-on-one (student and evaluator) clinical performance examination she describes extends over two and one-half work days (twenty hours) and covers five patient situations. Two nurse examiners observe the student's clinical performance and document their findings in writing. The student must perform at the 100% level of competency each of the critical elements identified by the faculty.

The nursing faculty of California State College, Sonoma, uses the National League for Nursing achievement tests as one means of determining each student's knowledge base.[14] To assess competence in the clinical areas of nursing, faculty members observe the student in practice and assign a letter grade based on standards derived from faculty expectations and leveled behavioral objectives.

Computerized examinations for clinical decision making and their potential for use as challenge examinations are discussed by Sumida.[15] Two groups of students at the University of Hawaii, associate degree and baccalaureate degree students, were used to evaluate a computerized branching progression test design for clinical situations. The advantage of a branching progression test design for clinical performance is that the student's response made to the initial situation determines subsequent action. The purpose of Sumida's study was to evaluate nursing students' clinical competence upon graduation; however, she recommended the examination be developed into a challenge examination to measure knowledge of essential content and concepts in required courses.

A master grid for dietetic scenarios is described by LaDuca.[6] These scenarios are analyzed to produce specific statements of knowledge and skills called for by each student. Approximately 3,000 specific statements were reduced to approximately 100 general statements. He utilizes the same format, the professional performance situation model (PPSM) in describing a clinical evaluation model used by occupational therapists. LaDuca suggests that the consequences of pres-

ence or absence of critical behavior in performance can be observed; however, he cautions that performance constitutes only one side of the coin. Performance in the clinical setting is situationally dependent; in essence, the situation must first be defined, then the performance specified.[7]

Menges[9] emphasizes readiness for practicing certain helping professions, in which the practitioner interacts directly with the client/consumer: medicine, nursing, dentistry, clinical psychology, teaching, social work, and the ministry. While Menges' focus is on assessing individual readiness for professional practice, many of the data presented are applicable to understanding the accommodation of previous learning. The author reviews how to assess readiness in relation to the definition of effective professional practice, discusses instruments developed based on the definitions, and describes how the instruments should be assessed through predictive validity studies.

Of special interest to health provider educators is Menges' discussion of an oral examination to measure subject matter knowledge. He states that such an examination has not been shown to reliably assess complex clinical skills. The bedside examination used for medical boards was discarded in 1963, after a three-year study during which 10,000 examinations showed agreement between the two judges to be only at the level of chance (correlation of 0.25).[9] Menges suggests that oral and written examinations are often used to evaluate or to assess ability to apply subject matter. He also cautions that the student's responses on such examinations do not assess what the student would do in such a situation; all that is known is what the student says would be done.[9]

Branching simulation exercises and a computer-based examining technique are described in detail by Menges. Considering the cost involved ($105,000) in generating the assessment methods of the New York external associate degree program, a question could be raised about the heavy use of human resources and nonuse of computer technology. Advantages of the computer-based examination are that it can simulate patient situations in a clinical setting in greater detail than paper-and-pencil examinations; it can generate data about the examinee and it does not necessarily compare candidates. Evaluation of performance in the clinical setting by a faculty member, on the other hand, lacks adequate reliability and validity.

Clinical algorithms may be an assessment technique for clinical evaluation that needs further investigation, specifically, where carefully circumscribed critical performance situations can be identified. Clinical algorithms were developed for instruction of medical problems in a physician's assistant program. The computer is used to assess the assistant's accuracy in completing a medical record form according to the algorithm.[9]

From a review of how educators are trying to accommodate previous learning experiences, similarities emerge: they are using direct observation and evaluation of the candidate in the clinical setting, simulated laboratory experiences, and written and/or oral examinations. They are placing emphasis on discrete behaviors and characteristics rather than global behaviors. The literature does not reveal that checks for a representative sampling of performance, reliability, and validity of assessment are occurring.

THE INDIVIDUAL AND THE PROCESS

The relationship between the individual and the institution is not easily defined morally. Allowing for individual experiences in a structured setting has been a concern of educators for years as evidenced by the volume of literature discussing individual differences and instructional strategies. Sagen[11] specifically discusses individual differences and instructional strategies as they relate to the health professions. He concludes:

Until more is known about individual differences as they relate to instruction, and until the quality of student assessment is improved, most individualization should provide for broad options at the course level of instruction and for assignment to instruction based on differences in prior learning, differences in basic aptitudes and abilities, and most importantly, differences in individual preference.[11]

Sagen cautions that individualization in health professions education must continue to maintain reasonable performance standards to protect both the public and the profession.

Irby and Dorner[5] suggest that the purpose of evaluation is for decision making, and the quality of decisions is assumed to be improved by having valid and reliable information on student progress. Similar concepts could be stated for equivalency evaluation for clinical practice; however, from the literature review, the need for validity and reliability checks on the methods of assessment is evident.

THE NEED

Equivalency evaluation for clinical practice must be understood at a fundamental level; for now, only the process is being explored. Equivalency evaluation must become a balance of common sense and academic commitment, an ideology. Research and evaluation studies are needed to more fully explain the phenomenon. The methodology should become as value-free as possible and the variables more precisely defined, because they influence the results. The following hypothesis needs to be examined: The ambiguous goals and value characteristics of the clinical practice system are antithetical to the proclaimed pattern of subsystem organization and evaluation.

SUMMARY

In summary, the accommodation of previous learning experience by equivalency clinical evaluation is plagued by a fundamental dilemma: juxtaposition of an abstract concept and a process. The equivalency evaluation idea is embedded in traditional educational processes making it very difficult to evaluate. The instruments and methodologies employed to accommodate previous education and work experiences primarily use course objectives and professional judgment(s). These two methods may meet the criteria for face and construct validity, but not for reliability and validity of measurement. The course objectives or criteria for equivalency evaluation may satisfy the immediate objectives for placement, but where is the interface with expected ultimate professional practice? Anything beyond relatively simple and direct instruction in an open system results in problems of evaluation that increase exponentially.

The process in its present form uses both formative and summative evaluation concepts. The New York Regents have shown that designing equivalency evaluation methods takes time and is costly.

Branching simulation exercises and computer-based examining techniques may hold promise for evaluating (1) the candidate as an individual, (2) the course objectives, and (3) the performance expectations.

We have the courage to recognize what we do not understand and we also recognize the challenge as ours.

REFERENCES

1. Banathy, B. H. *Instructional Systems.* Palo Alto, Cal.: Fearon Publishers, 1968.
   An excellent book for an educator who wants to use a systems approach in designing a curriculum.
2. Bevil, B. *The New York Regents external degree in Nursing. Nursing Digest,* Summer, 1976, 16-19.
   A description of the philosophy underlying the external degree in technical nursing as well as the planning process. Discussion of the practical performance evaluations for clinical nursing may be helpful to allied health educators. The complete article appeared in Nursing Forum *13, November 3, 1974, 216-239.*
3. Bruner, J. *Toward a Theory of Instruction.* Cambridge, Mass.: Belknap Press, 1966.
   If we have a sense of what is worth measuring, we shall measure better.
4. Donnelly, G., and Heffernan, E. *Report of a Survey Regarding Policies and Methods for Evaluating the Competencies of Registered Nurse Students.* Villanova, Pa.: Villanova University, 1976, mimeo.
   A survey resulting from a faculty debate about the effectiveness of methods for testing for credit-specific nursing courses with a concurrent clinical practice course.
5. Irby, D. M., and Dohner, C. W., Student clinical performance, in Ford, C. and Morgan, M. K. (Eds.), *Teaching in the Health Professions.* St. Louis: C. V. Mosby, 1976.
   An overview of the structure and critical variables in health provider education.
6. LaDuca, A.: *Toward a Definition of Competence in Dietetics.* Chicago: University of Illinois, Center for Education Development, 1975.
   A description of a master grid for didactic scenarios and procedure for developing professional performance situation models. The scenarios are analyzed to produce specific statements of knowledge.
7. LaDuca, A. *Professional Performance Situation Model for health professions Education: Occupational Therapy.* Chicago: University of Illinois, Center for Educational Development, 1975.
   An excellent resource that describes how some evaluation and curriculum specialists attempted a design for proficiency/equivalency test system. The paper describes a conceptual model labeled "professional performance situation system (PPSM)."
8. Lenburg, C. The external degree in nursing: the promise fulfilled. *Nursing Outlook,* 24, July, 1976, 422-428.
   A discussion of how the clinical performance examination was developed and their final formats. Educators will be interested in the cost of developing the exams. State board results and follow-up studies of the first 42 graduates are also discussed.
9. Menges, R. Assessing readiness for professional practice. *Review of Educational Research,* 45, Spring, 1976, 173-207.
   An excellent resource for health educators. The author discusses techniques that define effective practice by what professionals do and the duties the author perceives to be important. Surveys, observations, and correlational research are reviewed and illustrations presented. Validity of tests of subject matter and tests of ability to apply subject matter are discussed at length.
10. Ozimek, D. *Relating the Open Curriculum to Accountability in Baccalaureate Nursing Education.* New York: National League for Nursing, 1976.
    A brochure that states the philosophy of the National League for Nursing regarding an open curriculum. The discussion of the issues is provocative.
11. Sagen, H. B. Individual differences and instructional strategies, in Jacobs, R. M. (Ed.), *A Flexible Design for Health Professions Education.* New York: John Wiley & Sons, 1976.
    A book based on papers presented at a conference in Iowa City in 1975. The authors discuss the critical issues associated with flexibility of medical, dental, pharmacy, nursing, and allied health education and provide data about practical approaches from planning through evaluation.
12. Schweer, J. E., and Gebbie, L. M. *Creative Teaching in Clinical Nursing,* 3rd ed., St. Louis: C. V. Mosby, 1976.
    Although the authors focus primarily on clinical teaching in nursing, other health related faculties should find Unit III on aspects of design helpful in evaluating teaching/learning experiences.
13. Scriven, M. Evaluation bias and its control, in Glass, G., Ed., *Evaluation Studies,* I, Beverly Hills: Sage Publications, 1976.
    A comprehensive review of exemplary works in evaluation research.
14. Searight, M. *The Second Step, Baccalaureate Education for Registered Nurses.* Philadelphia: F. A. Davis Company, 1976.

While the book is about baccalaureate curricula for registered nurses (diploma and associate degree), it will prove valuable for other health professionals faced with or involved in the process of devising an open curriculum model for the certified/registered practitioners seeking a baccalaureate degree.

15. Sumida, S. A computerized test for clinical decision making. *Nursing Outlook,* 20, July, 1972, 458-461.

A discussion of the development of a computerized test for clinical decision making which utilizes a branching progression. Two clinical situations are reported: one with associate degree students' responses and the other with bachelor of science students' responses. The potential as a challenge exam was discussed.

16. Wilson, M. Equivalency testing development of health practitioners. *Journal of Allied Health,* Spring, 1974, 103-129.

A survey of 150 institutions to determine the state of equivalency testing in higher education. The comment sections raise critical issues and provide cautions for health care educators.

17. Wilson, M. *Equivalency Evaluation in Development of Health Practitioners.* Thorofare, New Jersey: C. B. Slack, 1976.

An excellent resource for all health educators. This book explores evaluation and the expectations of faculty members. The student is central throughout the book.

7
GRADUATE LEVEL EXPERIENCES

Richard D. Kingston

Graduate degrees in allied health should not be considered merely the equivalents of advanced degrees in traditional academic areas. A majority of them also represent a higher level of training in an allied health profession. Thus, the graduate clinical experience is not an incidental requirement for the completion of an advanced degree; it is an integral part of the preparation necessary to achieve increased professional competency and career advancement as an allied health practitioner.

Several types of graduate degrees are available in the allied health professions. To determine the kind of clinical experience they represent, each must be examined. This chapter describes basic methods that can be used to systematically structure and manage clinical education in all major types of allied health graduate programs. Many of the methods outlined here are no doubt already in common use. This discussion is intended to bring together those methods and to present them in a unified approach that can provide the type of clinical experiences that will most benefit the graduate student, the degree-granting institution, the allied health profession, and the general public.

THE GRADUATE LEVEL IN ALLIED HEALTH: A DEFINITION

Few areas of higher education offer such a large variety of degrees or include as many levels of training as the allied health professions. The requirements for certification range from associate or two-year degrees in some professions to four-and five-year bacca-

laureate degrees in others. Such variation in the amount of training required to obtain a basic professional degree makes it necessary to establish a definition of the term "graduate level" as it relates to allied health.

Two basic interpretations of the concept of a graduate degree may be applied. The first is the traditional definition: a graduate degree is any degree that can be obtained beyond the baccalaureate level. A second definition has emerged to explain a degree situation found almost exclusively in the allied health professions: a graduate degree is any degree that can be obtained beyond the basic preparation required for practice in a profession. In professions that require only an associate degree for certification, a baccalaureate degree is a postprofessional degree and is therefore sometimes considered a graduate degree.

The interpretation of the term "graduate level" used in the present discussion is the traditional one. This chapter is concerned with the methods for providing meaningful clinical experiences in any degree programs beyond the baccalaureate level. The approach to clinical education described should, however, also be pertinent to most allied health programs offering postprofessional baccalaureate degrees, since significant parallels exist between the methods for handling allied health clinical education at the graduate and postprofessional levels.

GRADUATE DEGREES IN THE ALLIED HEALTH PROFESSIONS

Rosenfeld[4] describes the recent growth of the allied health education system as being

Topsy-like. His description would certainly apply to the development over the past ten years of most new graduate degree programs in allied health. New graduate degrees have been offered through whatever department or college could arrange them and in whatever curriculum design was available. While this spurt of growth has been necessary, given the pressure for more qualified personnel in many areas of the health care delivery system, the lack of comprehensive planning has produced a variety of new advanced degree programs whose location and content must be described as irregular at best. (The quality of these programs is an additional issue.)

An obvious result of the random growth of many of the new graduate programs is the lack of uniformity among them. To refer to a degree offered at one school with the assurance that allied health educators and students at other institutions will be able to recognize the type of program it involves is not always possible. The basic reason for the dissimilarity in the programs lies in a lack of influence by many national accrediting bodies over their content.

In spite of this often confusing situation, four basic types of graduate degrees are commonly held by members of the allied health professions. They are: (1) the basic science degree, (2) the advanced skills degree, (3) the general education or administration degree, and (4) the education or administration degree designed specifically for allied health needs. Further examination of these basic degree offerings is necessary to establish the role of clinical education in each type of program. For the sake of brevity, only graduate programs at the master's level will be discussed although the points covered generally apply to similar programs at the doctoral level. Doctorates in the allied health professions are available in a number of institutions, but they are not pursued frequently enough to warrant separate consideration. In addition to the graduate level, the 2 + 2 baccalaureate will be briefly considered.

Basic science degree

One option for those seeking an advanced degree in allied health is the type of program that offers study in an area of science directly related to the technical basis of a particular profession. Such a program leads to a basic science degree at either the master's or doctoral level. Examples are a master's program in microbiology for medical technologists, graduate study in head and neck anatomy for dental hygienists, and a master's program in physiology for physical therapists. With this type of degree, allied health practitioners can increase their professional qualifications by acquiring background in the sciences basic to the health care skills of their disciplines. In most cases, a basic science graduate degree is sought as preparation for a teaching career in a particular profession. For this reason, some institutions allow allied health graduate students in basic science programs to take minor areas in education.

The typical allied health basic science program does not include clinical experience. The curricula for most such degree programs consist almost entirely of academic courses in the health-related sciences. Although this approach usually provides little time or justification for requiring a component that involves advanced training in allied health clinical skills, some institutions do consider clinical education an essential part of the preparation in master's level, basic science programs. A clinical experience is most often required when the basic science degree is offered through a college or department of allied health rather than under the auspices of a school or college of medicine, as is generally the case. The institutions that require a clinical experience usually recognize that a majority of their graduates with basic science degrees will be asked to teach in their profession at some time during their careers.

If a clinical education component is included in the curriculum for a basic science degree, the results are a refining or expanding of the professional skills of allied health practitioners. An an example, a dental hygienist working on a basic science degree in pharmacology or histology might be expected to acquire clinical skills beyond those required to enter professional practice. Also, a medical technologist might be required to refine the laboratory skills related to a basic science degree in microbiology or clinical chemistry. However, clinical education is generally considered secondary to the purpose of a basic science graduate program.

Advanced skills degree

A second option might be considered the basic allied health graduate degree since it is the type of program designed to prepare allied health professionals to enter specialty practice areas of their professions. Numerous examples exist. Typical programs would be the master's degrees in orthopedics and pediatrics available to physical therapists, graduate degrees in the clinical skills related to children's dentistry or periodontics offered to dental hygienists, and advanced skills degrees in blood banking and hematology for medical technologists. Allied health practitioners who obtain these degrees commonly find careers in the areas of clinical specialization, research, and teaching.

Clinical education must be considered an essential component in any advanced skills graduate program. A basic requirement for the completion of such a degree is generally that students demonstrate not only a high level of proficiency in the advanced skills of their specialty but also the ability to practice those skills with professional competency. The clinical component of an advanced skills program is usually designed to provide students with several opportunities to show they can function as competent practitioners in actual clinical settings. The typical mechanism for providing this clinical experience is to assign graduate students to internships after they have completed mandatory instructional courses.

General education or administration degrees

Before the recent development of graduate programs specifically designed to prepare allied health educators and administrators, a traditional education or business administration degree was one of the few options available to allied health practitioners seeking the credentials for career advancement. These programs do not, however, deal directly with specific professional skills for teaching or ad-

ministering in the allied health field. They offer, instead, advanced preparation in general principles of education or business administration.

This does not mean that such degrees are of limited value to allied health professionals who wish to teach or serve as administrators. In fact, a few colleges of education and business administration have developed medical educator and public health administrator degrees that offer training for meeting the general problems of the health care system. But even in these programs, allied health graduate students find they have to translate their knowledge into the specific needs of their professions. In addition, no components in programs of this type provide allied health graduate students with clinical experiences to expand or refine their skills as practitioners.

The education and administration degrees that can be obtained entirely outside the discretion of a college of allied health or medicine do not relate directly to the present discussion of clinical education and thus require no further consideration here.

Education and administration degrees for allied health

One of the most positive developments during the past ten years has been the growth of a number of graduate programs designed specifically to train educators and administrators for the allied health professions. Spurred by reports such as that made by the Allied Health Professions Education Subcommittee of the National Advisory Health Council in the U.S. Department of Health, Education and Welfare,[1] many institutions have moved to provide more allied health personnel and programs by creating degrees to prepare educators and administrators for the allied health education system. The W. K. Kellogg Foundation has been a leader in this effort, primarily through its funding of Allied Health Instructional Personnel Centers across the country. As a result of the growth in the number of institutions offering this type of degree, programs in graduate level educator and administrator preparation are available regionally to a majority of the allied health professionals in this country.

The typical degree is a joint offering by a college of medicine or allied health and a cooperating college of education or business administration. In most cases, the curricula for these degree programs consist of a major area of study in either education or administration and a minor area of advanced training in an allied health discipline. The education or administration is usually taught in the cooperating college. Ideally, it includes courses designed especially for the allied health graduate student. The participating college of medicine or allied health is naturally responsible for determining and providing the curriculum for the advanced professional skills minor. The degree itself is normally conferred through the cooperating college of education.

The allied health professional minor in most education or administration graduate programs consists of some level of advanced skills training. The clinical component is usually much the same as that required for completion of advanced skills graduate degrees. The student is expected to develop advanced or specialized skills in a profession and demonstrate the ability to apply them competently in the clinical setting. While few programs of this type require a full clinical internship, most involve a clinical practicum in which the student is evaluated on skills proficiency and professional competency.

Many allied health educators have noted with interest the use of experimental clinical programs as alternatives to the regular advanced skills components in some educator and administrator preparation programs. One of several examples would be those programs that offer expanded functions training for dental hygiene graduate students. The main controversy over the use of expanded functions training concerns whether or not it should be offered since the practice of expanded functions has not been fully authorized in many states. The rationale commonly given for providing expanded functions training as an advanced skills option is that program graduates will most likely teach in their professions and thus need a level of knowledge and skills competency above that expected of their students.

The possibility also exists that the practice of expanded functions will be liberalized in the near future and thus necessitate trained personnel.

2 + 2 programs

Closely paralleling the education and administration graduate programs are the recently initiated 2 + 2 programs. These offer education or administration preparation to allied health practitioners who have only the two-year or associate degree required for certification in some professions. The curriculum of the 2 + 2 programs also consists of an education or administration major combined with a professional minor in advanced skills. Because of the numerous similarities between 2 + 2 programs and education and administration graduate programs, the discussion of methods for structuring and managing clinical experiences that follows should apply in most instances to the clinical components of 2 + 2 programs. These programs have proved extremely valuable in preparing educators for associate degree professions. Therefore, graduates of 2 + 2 programs should also have the benefit of meaningful clinical experiences as part of their advanced professional training.

CLINICAL EDUCATION IN ALLIED HEALTH GRADUATE PROGRAMS

The basic methods for managing undergraduate clinical education programs, discussed in other chapters of this book, also apply to most aspects of the graduate clinical experience. Clinical education at the graduate level requires the same attention to selecting sites, contracting for facilities, assigning faculty advisors and clinical supervisors, developing objectives, and evaluating performance that is necessary in managing undergraduate clinical education. However, additional factors in the graduate situation require special attention and handling by those providing clinical experiences for graduate students. These special requirements are best illustrated by examining the differences between graduate and undergraduate clinical experiences.

Undergraduate clinical education

The purpose of the clinical education components of allied health training programs at the undergraduate or preprofessional level can be stated simply: Undergraduate clinical education is generally intended to provide students with experiences that help them develop minimal levels of competency in the essential skills of their professions. Basic competency in these skills is one of the requirements students must meet to qualify for certification or licensing. The objectives for most undergraduate clinical experiences are, therefore, easily determined, because they are basically the same as the standards of preparation the various professional organizations require for certification of their members.

Graduate clinical education

The most important difference between graduate and undergraduate clinical education is obvious from the purpose of each. Graduate clinical experiences are not offered for the purpose of developing minimal professional skills competencies. The assumption is made that graduate students who have qualified for practice and have at least two or three years of practical experience, as is required by most institutions, do not need to be taught basic professional skills. The purpose of the graduate clinical experience is to give students the opportunity to refine and update their basic skills and add new ones through advanced or specialized skills training. The level of performance required of students in graduate clinical education is not merely competency but proved proficiency as skilled practitioners. Students who are seeking advanced degrees in their allied health profession should be able to demonstrate their ability to function fully as professionals in the clinical setting.

A further difference between graduate and undergraduate clinical education requires special consideration by those providing graduate clinical experiences. Clinical education at the graduate level, since its nature is not confined to the requirements for professional certification, can be an essential factor in increasing student opportunities for career mobility. The type of clinical experiences that faculty advisors and clinical supervisors make available to students can influence their ability to specialize in skills that will help them build their careers. Most graduate students return to school for a more definite purpose than that of getting an advanced degree. They are generally seeking the credentials and skills for a particular type of position. Institutions that provide graduate clinical education, therefore, should provide students every possible opportunity to prepare for careers in the areas they have chosen.

Providing graduate clinical education

A discussion of the methods for managing graduate level clinical education must begin with stress on the importance of developing stated objectives for each student's experience. A systematic approach to providing clinical education is essential; merely hoping that students will gain the experiences they need is wishful thinking. Every clinical experience must be based on objectives that state exactly what the student is expected to accomplish. Since most objectives for each profession are dictated by the requirements for certification and thus are the same for every student in a class, this is less of a problem at the undergraduate level. In graduate clinical education, however, each student's experience may be different. This makes it essential that every graduate student's clinical education be handled on an individual basis and that a statement of objectives be developed specifically for each experience.

The responsibility of the faculty advisor for maintaining the quality of a student's clinical education is far greater at the graduate than the undergraduate level. A graduate advisor must consider two goals of equal importance in providing students with opportunities for clinical experience:

1. Each clinical experience must be structured and managed in such a way that the student is required to demonstrate both competency as a professional and proficiency in advanced skills or in a clinical specialty.

2. At the same time, a clinical experience must not be so rigidly defined in stereotypical terms that it defeats the student's individual goal of increased career mobility.

To provide clinical experiences that satisfy both goals, a faculty advisor must make a consistent effort to develop individualized clinical education for each graduate student.

The key to individualizing clinical education at the graduate level is an approach that allows for flexibility in the statement of objectives for each student's experience. Ideally, this flexibility allows for a realistic balance between the requirements of graduate work in allied health and the career needs of the student. Such a balance is possible in structuring clinical education through an approach that allows students to participate in the development of the objectives for their own experiences. If graduate students are given the opportunity to work with their faculty advisor in picking the site, the objectives, and even the supervisor for their clinical experiences, the clinical experience should be suited to the individual. Such individualized clinical education is more meaningful because it gives graduate students a personal incentive to accomplish the objectives they have helped formulate for their experience.

The graduate faculty advisor has an additional responsibility concerning the objectives for a student's participation in a clinical experience. To simply develop an individual statement of objectives for each student is insufficient; the objectives must be clearly communicated to all involved in structuring and managing the student's experience. This communication is particularly important in graduate clinical education since the objectives in even the same location can vary from student to student. Having the kind of communication that will make the members of a clinic staff aware of the objectives for an individual student's clinical experience is not, however, a simple matter, as anyone who has been around a busy clinic knows.

McBride,[3] an experienced faculty coordinator for graduate students in psychiatric clinics, recommends a series of discussions involving the student, key members of the clinic staff, and the graduate advisor as a way to keep open lines of communication concerning the objectives for the student's presence in the clinic. These meetings, which should be held before and during each clinical experience, help the clinic staff understand the importance of each student's individual objectives and make them more aware of their own role in the student's training. A discussion reflecting on the objectives for an experience while it is in progress also helps impress on a student that those same objectives will be used as the criteria for evaluating performance.

The methods outlined for structuring and managing graduate clinical education all seem to lead to more work for the faculty advisor. There is, however, no substitute for an approach that includes the development of individualized objectives for each student's clinical experience and frequent communication about them to all concerned. A systematic approach to clinical education at the graduate level constantly reminds those providing clinical experience that their purpose is to develop new professionals who can uphold the standards of the allied health professions. This makes it essential that every effort be made to give graduate students preparation of the highest quality possible.

TEACHING PRACTICUM IN ALLIED HEALTH EDUCATOR PREPARATION

Exact figures are not available, but it seems apparent that most of the allied health graduate degrees conferred in the past five years have been in teacher preparation. The increasing importance of these degree programs in the allied health education system necessitates a discussion of the teaching practicum that is generally a part of the educator training curriculum. All types of allied health training programs give students the experience in actual clinical settings to develop whatever skills they must demonstrate to be certified for practice. Although it is not normally required for certification, students training to be allied health educators need practical experience as teachers to become competent at the basic teaching skills. Providing students with opportunities for supervised teaching experience is essential to adequately prepare students in the graduate or 2 + 2 allied health educator training programs.

ADVISING ALLIED HEALTH STUDENTS ABOUT GRADUATE DEGREES

Any allied health professional who considers returning to school to pursue an advanced degree should weigh carefully the advantages of an educator preparation program before reaching a decision. Programs offering educator training degrees are not only more readily available but are also more practical in most cases than a basic science or advanced skills degree, because the majority of allied health professionals are asked to teach at some time during their careers. In addition, an allied health education or administration degree represents a more general background than do the specific advanced skills and basic science degrees. As such, it gives the professional more flexibility to compete for a variety of careers.

In the preface to *A Review of Allied Health Education*, Hamburg, Mase, and Perry[2] point to a lack of communication as one of the most serious problems in the allied health education system. Communication among institutions with allied health programs is still a problem, particularly in the area of graduate education. Many of the schools that offer advanced allied health degrees seem to be generally unaware or uninformed about programs at other schools. This situation can limit the career mobility of allied health professionals who are seeking a particular kind of preparation for advancement.

The allied health field is rapidly becoming more sophisticated. Education in the allied health professions is no longer a local affair, with practitioners trained in nearby schools and hospitals and tending to remain there to work. The specialization of skills within the various professions has resulted in many allied health schools specializing in the specific disciplines in which they have expertise. This trend is especially evident at the graduate level, where an allied health professional will often have to move to another region in order to pursue a particular advanced degree. In such a situation, an individual's career mobility may well depend on the amount of accurate information about degree offerings that is being communicated throughout the nation's allied health education system.

At present, the most effective source of information on allied health graduate programs is probably word of mouth. The two standard directories of institutions with allied health training programs—*The Health Occupations Training Programs Director*, consisting of two volumes published in 1973 by the U.S. Department of Health, Education, and Welfare, and *The Allied Medical Education Directory*, issued yearly by the American Medical Association—do not list graduate degree programs. One source that provides a partial listing of U.S. institutions that have allied health graduate programs is the report on *Instructor Preparation Programs* issued by the Council on Medical Education of the American Medical Association. The *Instructor Preparation Programs* bulletin was last published in 1973, and there are currently no plans to update it. It represents one of the few attempts at providing a general directory of graduate programs in allied health. In 1975, as part of a larger effort, Strong[5] reviewed ten programs at both graduate and undergraduate levels.

The best sources for information on institutions that offer graduate degrees in particular professions are the allied health professional organizations. The American Physical Therapy Association compiles a list of graduate programs in physical therapy that is published bimonthly in its journal. The Subcommittee on Graduate Education of the American Society of Medical Technology also periodically compiles an extensive directory of graduate programs in medical technology. Other allied health professional organizations also occasionally release lists of graduate programs offered in their area, such as the one sent to its members recently by the American Dental Hygienist Association. Most of the professional organizations only give the names and addresses of the schools with graduate programs in their professions. Further information must be obtained from the schools.

SUMMARY

Graduate work in allied health is increasingly one of the most important training grounds for leaders in the allied health professions. Advanced degrees are being more frequently recognized and sought as the credentials for advancement to positions of influence and responsibility in allied health education, administration, and practice. For that reason, if no other, it is essential that clinical education at the graduate level in allied health be approached systematically and conscientiously. Those who rise to leadership positions, in which they can help determine the future of the allied health field, must be the best trained among those in the professions they lead.

REFERENCES

1. *Education for the Allied Health Professions and Services.* Report of the Allied Health Professions Education Subcommittee of the National Advisory Health Council. Washington, D.C.: U.S. Department of Health, Education, and Welfare, 1967.

   This influencial report, prepared at the request of Surgeon General William H. Stewart, reviews problems of meeting U.S. needs for health manpower and recommends development of a strengthened educational system for the preparation of allied health personnel.

2. Hamburg, J., Mase, D., and Perry, J. W. (Eds.) A *Review of Allied Health Education.* Vol. 1. Lexington, Ky.: University of Kentucky Press, 1974.

   The first volume of a projected series designed to improve communication in the allied health field by giving a better understanding of the health care team, promoting the exchange of ideas, and stimulating new thought.

3. McBride, M. A. B. Facilitating a master's program clinical experience. *Nursing Outlook, 16* (November), 1971, 42-44.

   "A faculty coordinator describes how improving communication and confutation within a psychiatric clinical facility aids graduate students' learning." This article also discusses the importance of objectives in all aspects of the clinical experience.

4. Rosenfeld, M. H. Organizing for allied health educational institutions, in E. McTernan and R. Hawkins, Jr. (Eds.), *Educating Personnel for the Allied Health Professions and Services: Administrative Considerations.* St. Louis: C. V. Mosby, 1972.

   A discussion of growth in the allied health professions, educational needs in those professions, and various institutions with allied health training programs. This chapter includes suggestions for organizing schools of allied health professions.

5. Strong, M. E., Lambert, R., and Franken, M. E. *Health Occupations Teacher Education Planning.* Madison, Wis.: University of Wisconsin, Center for Studies in Vocational and Technical Education, 1975.

   A project report of a study undertaken to evaluate the need for a health occupation teacher education program for Wisconsin. It reviews national trends as well as the curricula of ten programs.

8

CLINICAL FACULTY DEVELOPMENT

David M. Irby

A frequently asked question by persons in the health sciences is, "How can I teach students most effectively in a clinical setting?" Concern for this question is raised most vocally by students who complain that particular clinical teachers are not accessible, do not allow them to perform skills already mastered, do not demonstrate up-to-date procedures, and rarely give them feedback. Academic faculty who do not teach in the clinic but hear these complaints wonder what the preceptors or clinical supervisors are doing. Clinical supervisors sometimes grumble: "What am I supposed to do with these students? How can I continue providing patient care and teach students at the same time? I was trained to be a clinician, not an educator. I wonder what good clinical teachers do that I don't do?"

Questions such as these emerge wherever thoughtful clinical supervisors, faculty members, and students in health sciences education programs congregate. Clinical teachers, like their classroom counterparts, continually ask if there is not a better way to teach students so that learning is enhanced and teachers feel better about the process.

A partial answer to these questions about the characteristics of effective clinical teaching can be found in the research on classroom and clinical teaching. The major findings of this research are reviewed here in relation to seven dimensions of clinical teacher effectiveness. Suggestions for improving clinical teaching are also presented.

RESEARCH ON TEACHER EFFECTIVENESS

The study of what constitutes effective teaching is not new. Research in the field of teacher effectiveness has resulted in over 10,000 published studies.[8] This review of the literature, however, is more restricted in nature. It focuses on classroom and clinical teacher effectiveness research in postsecondary institutions.

Many researchers have identified basic components, dimensions, or scales of effective teaching by sorting into related groups the indivudual items that describe aspects of effective teaching. These groups have been determined by subjective examination of items or by factor analysis, which mathematically establishes the tendency of response to the various items to cluster. The number of scales reported ranges from two to fourteen, with four to five particular scales appearing rather consistently even though their terminology differs. The scales for classroom instruction that are also common to clinical teaching tend to reflect instructor: (1) presentation, (2) enthusiasm, (3) knowledge, and (4) relations with students.[12] The scales unique to clinical instruction involve instructor: (5) clinical supervision, (6) clinical competence, and (7) modeling of professional standards and values.[13]

A variety of research methodologies has been employed to develop constructs or dimensions related to effectiveness in teaching. These have included factor analysis, observa-

Table 7

Apparent similarities of dimensions found in sixteen factor analyses of instructor ratings

Studies	Dimensions					
	Organization/ clarity	Enthusiasm/ stimulation	Instructor knowledge	Group instructional skill	Clinical supervision	Other
Classroom						
Isaacson et al. (1964)	Structure	Skill		Rapport		+3 other factors
Solomon, Rosenberg, and Bezdik (1964)	Clarity, expressiveness vs. obscurity, vagueness	Energy vs. lethargy		Lecturing vs. encouragement of student participation		+4 other factors
Solomon (1966)	Precision/organization vs. informality, obscurity; difficulty of presentation vs. clarity	Energy, facility of communication vs. lethargy, vagueness	Control, factual emphasis vs. permissiveness	Warmth, approval vs. coldness; lecturing vs. encouragement of broad, expressive student participation		+3 other factors
Deshpande, Webb, and Marks (1970)	Cognitive merit	Stimulation		Affective merit		+1 other factor
Turner (1970)	Penetrating, clear, focused	Exciting, humorous, stimulating	Prepared, probing, demanding	Approachable, warm, cheerful		+2 other factors
Hildebrand, Wilson, and Dienst (1971)	Organization/ clarity	Dynamism/ enthusiasm	Analytic/synthetic approach	Instructor/ group interaction		+1 other factor
Frey (1973)	Organization/ clarity	Teacher's presentation		Teacher accessibility		+3 other factors
McKeachie and Lin (1973)	Structure	Skill		Group interaction		+1 other factor

Table 7

Apparent similarities of dimensions found in sixteen factor analyses of instructor ratings

Studies	Dimensions					
	Organization/ clarity	Enthusiasm/ stimulation	Instructor knowledge	Group instructional skill	Clinical supervision	Other
Blazek (1974)	Instructor clarity	Instructor knowledge/enthusiasm	Instructor knowledge/enthusiasm	Instructor openness		+3 other factors
Pohlmann (1975)	Organized in presenting material	Increases student's appreciation of subject matter				+2 other factors
Rugg and Norris (1975)	Structure and guidance	Stimulating teaching	Subject matter expertise; research methods expertise	Interpersonal rapport, respect for students		+4 other factors
Clinical						
Cotsonas and Kaiser (1963)		Teaching factor	Teacher knowledge	Attitude factor		
Greenwood et al. (1974)	Facilitation of learning	Voice communication	Obsolescence of presentation; currency of knowledge	Rapport; openness	Commitment to teaching (accessibility); evaluation	
Stritter, Hain, and Grimes (1975)		Preceptor attitude toward teaching	Emphasis on references and research	Active student participation; humanistic orientation	Student-centered instructional strategy	
Dixon and Koerner (1976)			Systematic theoretical orientation		Individualized prescriptive approach	
Irby (1977)	Organization/ clarity	Enthusiasm/ stimulation	Instructor knowledge	Group instructional skill	Clinical supervision	+1 other factor

tional analysis, correlational studies, and use of the critical incident technique. Factor analysis is the most prominent method among studies that deal with students' perceptions of teachers. Table 7 lists five apparently similar dimensions of teaching gleaned from sixteen factor analytic studies of instructor ratings: organization/clarity, enthusiasm/stimulation, instructor knowledge, group instructional skill, and clinical supervision. Research is presented in relationship to each of these factors. Studies related to two additional dimensions of clinical teaching—instructor clinical competence and modeling of professional characteristics—are also reported.

Organization/clarity

Effective teaching in the classroom and clinic is based on the ability to present information clearly and in a well-organized manner. Teacher behaviors associated with this factor were identified in six studies of clinical teaching and nineteen studies of classroom instruction.

One of the most comprehensive studies of university classroom teaching was conducted at the University of California, Berkeley.[12] Students were asked to describe the teaching of those they identified as their best and worst instructors. A list of 158 teacher behaviors was generated and returned to the original sample group to determine whether the characteristics were descriptive of their best and worst teachers. Items that discriminated best from worst instructors were retained and used in a validation study. That study involved 1,015 students, who described their best and worst instructors. Five scales resulted from factor analyzing the data for best teachers. One of these scales, "organization and clarity of presentation," was composed of items such as: makes self clear, states objectives, summarizes major points, presents material in organized manner, and provides emphasis.

The importance of organization and clarity of presentation was reported by Solomon and coworkers[28] who not only isolated eight factors of teaching effectiveness but also correlated teacher behaviors with learning. The factors "clarity/expressiveness" and "ten-

dency to lecture" were related to gains in factual information. Both of these factors related to the efficiency with which the teacher communicates factual information in the course. Solomon[27] later replicated this study on a larger sample of adult learners at five universities and found similar results. These and other studies reflect a common dimension of effective teaching—the clear and organized presentation of ideas.

Enthusiasm/stimulation

An enthusiastic and dynamic teacher is one who is energetic, uses movement, humor, and vocal inflection and is generally characterized as having charisma. Faculty members possessing such a quality are usually highly rated by students. Twenty-six studies—eight from clinical settings and eighteen from classroom settings—have identified this quality as a dimension of teacher effectiveness.

This factor relates to the flair and infectious enthusiasm of the faculty member that comes with confidence, excitement about the subject, and pleasure in teaching. Hildebrand and others[12] term this factor "dynamism/enthusiasm" and includes items related to dynamism and energy, an interesting style of presentation, enjoyment of teaching, enthusiasm, self-confidence, and a sense of humor.

Even in individualized, research-oriented learning experiences involving faculty supervision, stimulating teaching is a significant factor.[25] This factor reflects the supervisor's apparent enjoyment of teaching and supervising students as well as the ability to stimulate further student thinking.

Using correlational analyses, Pohlmann[21] found that the effective instructor is perceived as increasing students' appreciation for the subject. This is similar to what Reichsman and coworkers[23] observed in undergraduate clinical teaching in medicine: the effective clinical teacher successfully encourages students to acquire new knowledge. The ability to stimulate students is a critical teaching behavior in nursing and dentistry as well.[2,31]

Another series of studies examines the role of the "Dr. Fox effect"—the experimental manipulation of teacher seductiveness and charisma. Naftaline and coworkers[20] found that an actor taught to give a nonsubstantive lecture using double-talk and contradictory statements received quite favorable ratings from three separate samples of mental health and education professionals. In a later study, Ware and Williams[32,33] reported that high seductiveness is related to high test performance when content coverage is controlled, in addition to being related to student satisfaction ratings. Their study supports the hypothesis that students who hear lectures by highly enthusiastic lecturers may learn more. The authors, however, caution that enthusiastic lecturers can give little information and still receive high student ratings. Thus the most effective lecturer is one who combines an enthusiastic presentation with a high level of information giving.[14]

These findings are supported by Solomon and others,[28] who found that energy and flamboyance are highly correlated with student learning gains in comprehension. Faculty members who are enthusiastic about their topic and are dynamic and energetic persons seem to stimulate student interest and learning.

Instructor knowledge

Faculty members who exhibit a breadth of knowledge, are up-to-date in their specialty, and can analyze concepts effectively are perceived to be effective teachers. Instructor knowledge is reflected in nine clinical and ten classroom studies.

In a study of teaching effectiveness in nursing, Dixon and Koerner[7] found two factors, one of which they entitled "systematic theoretical orientation." Demonstrating logical thinking, sharing one's thinking, and relating theory to practice are indicators of this orientation toward the theoretical and reflective. Items referring to highlighting significant concepts, systematic presentation, and discussion of current developments all manifest an ability to present knowledge in a systematic manner. Emphasizing the conceptual ability to use knowledge, Hildebrand and others[12] titled this factor "analytic/synthetic approach." It relates to scholarship, with emphasis on breadth, analytic ability, and conceptual understanding.

Several studies point to the importance of correlating clinical medicine with the basic sciences and with the use of scientific principles.[22,23] Knowledge has also been inferred from the teacher's ability to discuss current developments in the field, direct students to useful literature, and discuss points of view other than his or her own. These characteristics emphasize not only the importance of a solid foundation of knowledge as a basis of teaching, but also the analytical use of that information for student learning.

Group instructional skill

Effective clinical and classroom teachers interact with students in a skillful manner. They can establish rapport with the class, create a climate of mutual respect, be sensitive to student response, and stimulate active class participation. Twenty-eight studies—sixteen in the classroom and twelve in clinical settings—identified group instructional skill as a dimension of effective teaching.

More than half of these studies used factor analysis to empirically derive this dimension of teaching. "Instructor-group interaction" was the label given by Hildebrand and others[12] to refer to the teacher's sensitivity to class response, encouragement of student participation, and welcoming of questions and discussion. A closely related, although separate factor, was termed "instructor-individual interaction." This dimension describes the relationship between the instructor and individual student as one of mutual respect and rapport. Both factors portray the importance of the teacher's ability to relate well to students (either individually or as a group) and to stimulate their active involvement in learning.

In the field of nursing education, Jacobson[15] labeled one of six categories "teaching practices in classroom and clinical areas." Teacher behaviors reflective of this dimension were derived from critical incidents supplied by nursing students in five universities. Examples of the seventeen behaviors subsumed under this heading include: skill in group discussion, creating a relaxed atmosphere and making learning enjoyable, and encouraging individuality and creativity.

Using a somewhat similar approach, Walker[31] asked dental students to describe the characteristics of the best and worst teachers they had encountered in dental school. Four factors were subjectively defined. One of these, "Teacher-student interaction," included traits such as being accessible to students, being interested in and understanding of students, offering constructive criticism, and being approachable.

These studies point to the importance of establishing rapport within a class, skillfully interacting with students, and being sensitive to class response.

To summarize, there appear to be four factors of effective teaching that are common to both classroom and clinical teaching:

1. Organization and clarity of presentation
2. Enthusiasm and stimulation
3. Instructor knowledge
4. Group instructional skill

While these factors appeared with greatest regularity, others were present as well. Two other frequently identified factors relate to fairness in evaluation and feedback and the level of course difficulty or overload. These concepts and teacher behaviors are partially subsumed under the dimension of clinical supervision, which is presented next. The other factors unique to clinical teaching include instructor clinical competence and modeling of professional characteristics.

Clinical supervision

Clinical supervision involves the assignment of students and/or residents to an experienced clinician for the purpose of helping them to master professional skills and abilities in a patient care setting. A wide variety of teacher behaviors is included in clinical supervision: (1) being accessible; (2) observing, giving feedback on, and evaluating student performance; (3) guiding students, providing practice opportunities, and promoting problem-solving skill development; (4) giving case-specific comments; and (5) offering profes-

sional support and encouragement. Fourteen studies describe one or more of these aspects of clinical supervision.

Instructor availability is an important part of clinical supervision. The amount of time the clinical instructor spends supervising students determines in large measure the amount of instruction, evaluation, and support that can be provided. Being available, approachable, and accessible are behaviors that appeared in several studies.[16,29] Rugg and Norris titled one of their factors "supervisor accessibility": "Not only is available faculty time important, but also willingness to help when needed. Again, interest in the individual is related, and is probably linked, to willingness to help" (p. 47).[25]

A second component of clinical supervision involves observing student performance, evaluating it, and providing feedback. In clinical teaching, evaluation information is derived primarily from observations of students providing patient care.

In the field of nursing, Dixon and Koerner[7] labeled one of two factors "individualized prescriptive approach." Teachers scoring high on this factor were viewed as responding to students as individuals and basing such responses on evaluation data. Items that loaded highest on this factor are: evaluates the student in a variety of ways, keeps students appraised of progress, identifies strengths, and guides development.

In addition to the important function of evaluation and feedback, specific guidance and direction need to be given by the clinical supervisor. "Structure and guidance" was the label given by Rugg and Norris: "This factor reflected the amount of structured supervision and guidance given to the student which was oriented toward promoting student progress in areas of student interest and concern" (p. 45).[25]

In teaching the diagnostic process in medicine, Elstein and coworkers[9] suggest that one task of clinical supervision is to teach the novice how to engage in diagnosis. This can best be done, the authors suggest, by helping the student develop the critical capacities of observation and hypothesis generation, which lead to a storage of valid information about human behavior. The diagnostic process appears to depend on having a large mental library of cases against which a case currently under examination can be compared.

In an extensive field study of clinical teaching in physical therapy, Scully[26] selected several categories around which to organize observational data. According to her study, some important teacher behaviors associated with clinical supervision are: questioning, coaching, pacing (diagnosing student readiness, selecting appropriate clinical problems, supervising, and evaluating), ensuring minimal risk to the patient, as well as evaluating and enforcing institutional rules. Most faculty members viewed supervision as a process of pacing students to professional competence. Thus the provision of structured guidance and practice opportunities is another aspect of the clinical supervisor's role.

A fourth aspect of supervision involves presenting information relevant to a specific clinical case. After observing psychotherapy supervision of residents, Goin and Kline[11] found that certain types of didactic exchanges are associated with superior supervision. Two "outstanding" supervisors were compared with three "good" supervisors, as rated by residents. Videotapes of the supervisory sessions were evaluated by the participants and by a separate group of two psychiatrists and a psychologist. From the videotapes, sixteen types of supervisor statements were recorded and scored as either case-specific or general. The outstanding supervisors made more didactic comments that were case-specific than did the good supervisors. Thus the supervisor's ability to relate basic science and theoretical concepts specifically to the case under consideration increased resident ratings of teaching effectiveness.

The final area of clinical supervision to be reviewed relates to the student's need for encouragement and support. Several studies suggest the importance of a supportive supervisory relationship to trainee learning. From the field of counselor supervision, trainees who received empathy, warmth, genuineness, and unconditional regard from their su-

pervisors became significantly more open to their own experiences and succeeded better at instilling these characteristics in themselves. Supervisors who were unsupportive (i.e., evaluative or didactic, emphasizing the negative aspects of counselor trainee performance with a client) caused the trainee to shift the focus of concern away from the client and toward self. This was in part a result of trainee feelings of inadequacy and fears of evaluation.

The supportive affective stance of the supervisor provided the necessary conditions for personal change: freedom from fear, empathy, warmth, and genuineness.[24] Such a supportive supervisory relationship was one of the most critical variables in counselor learning and may have a similar impact on student and resident learning in the health sciences.

Several important functions of clinical supervision emerge from these studies. Clinical instructors rated most highly are those who willingly remain accessible to students, provide objective evaluation and frequent feedback, give structured guidance and opportunities for practice, relate comments to the clinical case at hand, and provide professional support and encouragement.

Instructor clinical competence

A health sciences educator must not only be knowledgeable but clinically competent as well. Instructor clinical competence includes the following specific skills: objectively identifying and analyzing patient problems, effectively performing procedures, establishing rapport with patients, and working effectively with health care team members. Eight studies have identified the dimension "instructor clinical competence."

While descriptions of clinical competence vary by health profession, several common characteristics have been identified. The teacher should have a full command of the procedure being taught and demonstrate how to function effectively in a real patient care setting.[6,22] The teacher should also be able to demonstrate psychomotor and interpersonal skills with expertise.[7]

In a systematic examination of the relationship between clinical competence and personal characteristics, Liske and coworkers[17] found that doctors rated highly by their colleagues in providing comprehensive care tended to define problems with a high level of objectivity and self-criticism. Physicians less highly rated tended to define problems in terms of the attributes and limitations of the patients. This difference in attitude on the part of the two groups of doctors suggested that more effective clinical performance is associated with greater humanitarian concern and acceptance of responsibility. Less effective performance appeared to be coupled with an impersonal relationship to patients and with expectations of receiving recognition and attention from them. The study identified several key aspects of effective clinical performance: concern for patients, acceptance of responsibility, objective definition of patient problems, and a high level of self-criticism. These characteristics combined with such others as effectively performing clinical procedures, gathering data, working effectively with the health care team, synthesizing patient problems, and establishing rapport with patients provide some behavioral descriptions of clinical competence.

Modeling of professional characteristics

Throughout the entire length of clinical training, students are able to observe experienced staff members making decisions, performing procedures, and interacting with patients, as well as working with other members of the health care team. These opportunities provide students with ample observations from which to imitate the role of the more experienced health care provider. Such modeling is a powerful teaching technique and one especially well-suited to the apprenticeship system of instruction in the health sciences.[1] Modeling of professional standards and values, the final dimension to be reviewed, was identified in eight studies of clinical teaching.

The role of modeling in psychiatric education is described by Muslin and Thurnblad: "The trainee learns to approach data with the supervisor's eyes, ears, and sensitivities. This *is* the learning mechanism involved, an attempt to approach the supervisor's cognitive and empathetic styles . . . Ideally, the student takes from the supervisory process not only certain knowledge and understanding but certain partial identifications" (p. 168).[19] This analysis of the supervisory process highlights the importance of clinical teachers demonstrating high professional standards.

As stated in the preceding section, two characteristics of highly rated physicians are acceptance of responsibility and self-criticism. These are two professional behaviors that reflect professional standards and values. Other professional characteristics include: (1) being honest with data and one's own limitations and (2) displaying self-confidence and demonstrating skills, attitudes, and values to be developed by the student.

In a study of individualized, research-oriented supervision, one factor relevant to modeling was found.[25] The investigators termed this factor, which was derived from three items (unethical versus ethical, tense versus relaxed, and inexperienced versus experienced), "faculty maturity."

Modeling of professional standards appears to be a dimension of clinical teaching although it is less well represented in the literature. Some of the characteristics to be modeled are: being self-confident, being self-critical, taking responsibility, not appearing arrogant, recognizing one's limitations, and showing respect for others.

A survey of the literature on effective teacher behaviors in postsecondary classroom and clinical settings points to an emerging consensus on the most important factors of teaching. The apparent similarities include:

1. Organization and clarity of presentation
2. Enthusiasm and stimulation
3. Instructor knowledge
4. Group instructional skill
5. Clinical supervision
6. Instructor clinical competence
7. Modeling of professional characteristics

This review of the literature provides a partial

answer to the question: What constitutes effective clinical teaching?

In a separate study, these seven factors together discriminated best from worst clinical teachers in medicine (as perceived by medical school faculty, residents, and students).[13] The most highly discriminating factors were, in order, enthusiasm/stimulation, organization/clarity, group instructional skill, and clinical supervision. The first two factors represent abilities at presenting ideas, while the second two factors reflect skill at interacting with and guiding students and residents. The worst clinical teachers not only lacked these skills, but were characterized by several negative personal attributes (e.g., arrogance, inaccessibility, lack of self-confidence, authoritarianism and dogmatism, insensitivity to others, tendency to belittle students).

FACULTY DEVELOPMENT

This body of educational research provides a basis for designing improvement strategies for clinical teaching. The instructional skills of best clinical teachers can be taught to faculty members who desire to increase their abilities in these areas. The distracting personal qualities of the worst are useful to know in order to reduce these behaviors where possible.

Workshops and inservice education programs can be vehicles for presenting this information to clinical faculty members and for developing the relevant instructional skills.

Another improvement strategy involves individualized educational consultation and self-assessment. A clinical teacher or department can request consultative services on teaching improvement. Before meeting with a consultant, the clinical teacher or department can fill out a Self-Assessment Inventory for Clinical Teaching in Medicine (see Appendix A, pp. 106 to 108). At a mutually agreed time, the consultant can then observe the teaching in question and provide feedback on the instructional process. This can be followed by a review of the completed self-assessment inventory, with focus on the teaching behaviors receiving the highest and lowest ratings. A specific action plan for improvement can also be developed for each problem area. As

the discussion of alternative teaching strategies ensues, the conversation frequently may broaden to include learning theory and educational research. Sometimes, the identified problem areas can be related to poor scheduling, changing student demands, lack of role definitions, and other variables outside of the direct control of the clinical instructor. Follow-up consultations can be negotiated at this time. Faculty reaction to this approach has been positive.

EVALUATION OF CLINICAL TEACHING

Another implication of this educational research is that evaluation of clinical teaching should be based on the major factors already identified. While the list of fifty-four teacher behaviors found in the self-assessment inventory is too long for everyday use in student ratings, single items can be written for each major factor. This will yield seven to ten items. One example of such a student rating form is found in Appendix B, pp. 109 and 110. It was developed for the Department of Medicine at the University of Washington, but could be easily adapted to other departments and health professions as well. One interesting aspect of this evaluation form is the dual focus on teacher behaviors and student achievement of course goals. These emphases provide insight into both the educational process and perceived learning outcomes.

Any evaluation process for determining the effectiveness of clinical teaching should be established to collect useful information to serve multiple purposes. For the clinical instructor, specific items can provide diagnostic data to identify strengths and limitations for self-improvement purposes. For program directors and academic appointment and promotions committees, global items are adequate to determine the overall quality of instruction provided by clinical instructors. If student ratings and peer assessment forms are well constructed, they should serve the needs for self-improvement, administrative decision making, and academic promotions.

To achieve optimal positive changes in clinical teaching, institutional rewards should be used to promote good teaching. If the hospital recognizes technical competence, staff supervision, and seniority as the only parameters for pay increases, change in teaching performance may be difficult to effect. Likewise, if a university rewards research but not teaching, clinical teachers who devote much time to improving their teaching competencies will do so at their own peril.

A wide variety of rewards should be tied to good ratings and efforts expended on self-improvement. Financial reward is the most obvious but not the only means. Academic advancement, recognition, titles, awards, special privileges, travel, release time, space, support for personal development, more challenging work assignments, and other sources of reward should be creatively explored.

SUMMARY

The task of improving clinical teaching will always be an ongoing process. New clinical teachers will need to learn the basic skills of clinical instruction while their more experienced colleagues seek to refine already established abilities. This improvement process will be successful if the faculty and/or clinical supervisors are able to see institutional commitment to excellence in clinical teaching, are told specifically what is expected of them, are rewarded for good performance, and derive personal benefit and satisfaction from the process. The seven dimensions of clinical teacher effectiveness provide useful guideposts for assessing and improving clinical instruction in the health professions.

REFERENCES*

1. Bandura, A. *Principles of Behavior Modification.* New York: Holt, Rinehart and Winston, 1969.
2. Barham, V. Z. Identifying effective behavior of the nursing instructor through critical incidents. *Nursing Research, 14* (Winter) 1965, 65-69.
3. Blazek, H. D. Student perceptions of college teaching effectiveness. *Dissertation Abstracts, 35,* 12-A, 1974, 7764.
4. Cotsonas, N. J., and Kaiser, H. F. Student evaluation and clinical teaching. *Journal of Medical Education, 38,* 1963, 742-745.
5. Deshpande, A. S.; Webb, S. C.; and Marx, E. Student perceptions of engineering instructor behaviors and their relationships to the evaluation of instructors and courses. *American Educational Research Journal, 7* (May) 1970, 289-305.
6. Bolender, C. L., and Guild, R. E. Description of an effective clinical faculty member. *Mentalis, 2,* 1, 1971-1972, 34-35.
7. Dixon, J. K., and Koerner, B. Faculty and student perceptions of effective classroom teaching in nursing. *Journal of Nursing Research, 25* (July-August) 1976, 300-305.
8. Dunkin, M. J., and Biddle, B. J. *The Study of Teaching.* New York: Holt, Rinehart and Winston, 1974.
9. Elstein, A. S.; Kagan, N.; Shulman, L. S.; and others: Methods and theory in the study of medical inquiry. *Journal of Medical Education, 47,* 1972, 85-92.
10. Frey, P. W. Student ratings of teaching: validity of several rating factors. *Science, 182,* 1973, 83-85.
11. Goin, M. K., and Kline, F. M.: Supervision observed. *Journal of Nervous and Mental Disorders, 158,* 1974, 208-213.
12. Hildebrand, M., Wilson, R. C., and Dienst, E. R. *Evaluating University Teaching.* Berkeley, Calif.: University of California, Berkeley Center for Research and Development in Higher Education, 1971.
13. Irby, D. *Clinical Teacher Effectiveness in Medicine as Perceived by Faculty, Residents and Students.* Unpublished doctoral dissertation, University of Washington, 1977.
14. Irby, D.; DeMers, J.; Scher, M.; and Matthews, D. A model for the improvement of medical faculty lecturing. *Journal of Medical Education, 51* (May) 1976, 403-409.
15. Jacobson, M. D. Effective and ineffective behavior of teachers of nursing as determined by their students. *Nursing Research, 15* (Summer) 1966, 218-224.
16. Kiker, M.: Characteristics of the effective teacher, *Nursing Outlook, 21* (November) 1973, 721-723.
17. Liske, R. E.; Ort, R. S.; and Ford, A. B.: Clinical performance and related traits of medical students and faculty physicians. *Journal of Medical Education, 39,* 1964, 69-80.
18. McKeachie, W. J., and Lin, Y. G.: Multiple discrimination analysis of student ratings of college teachers. Unpublished. University of Michigan, 1973.
19. Muslin, H. L., and Thurnblad, R. J. Supervision as an evaluative mechanism. In H. L. Muslin, R. J. Thurnblad, B. Templeton, and C. H. McGuire (Eds.), *Evaluative Methods in Psychiatric Education.* Washington, D. C.: American Psychiatric Association, 1974.
20. Naftaline, D. H.; Ware, J. E.; and Donnelly, F. A. The Dr. Fox lecture: A paradigm of educational seduction. *Journal of Medical Education, 48,* 1973, 630-635.
21. Pohlmann, J. T. A description of teaching effectiveness as measured by student ratings. *Journal of Educational Measurement, 12* (Spring) 1975, 49-54.

---

*Because of the length of this reference list, no annotation is provided. For additional information, see the Bibliography, p. 217, by Ford and Irby.

22. Rauen, K. C. The clinical instructor as role model. *The Journal of Nursing Education, 13,* (August) 1974, 33-40.

23. Reichsman, F.; Browning, F. E.; and Hinshaw, J. R.: Observations of undergraduate clinical teaching in action. *Journal of Medical Education, 39* (February) 1964, 147-163.

24. Rogers, C. R.: The necessary and sufficient conditions of therapeutic personality change. *Journal of Consulting Psychology, 21,* 1957, 95-103.

25. Rugg, E. A., and Norris, R. C.: Student ratings of individualized faculty supervision: Description and Evaluation. *American Educational Research Journal, 12* (Winter) 1975, 41-53.

26. Scully, R. M.: Clinical teaching of physical therapy students in clinical education. *Dissertation Abstracts, 35,* 02-A, 1974, 853.

27. Solomon, D. Teacher behavior dimensions, course characteristics and student evaluations of teachers. *American Educational Research Journal, 3,* 1966, 35-47.

28. Solomon, D.; Rosenberg, L., and Bezdik, W. E.: Teacher behavior and student learning. *Journal of Educational Psychology, 55,* 1964, 23-30.

29. Stritter, F. T.; Hain, J. D., and Grimes, D. A. Clinical teaching reexamined, *Journal of Medical Education, 50* (September) 1975, 877-882.

30. Turner, R. L. Good teaching and its contexts. *Phi Delta Kappan, 52,* 3, 1970, 155-158.

31. Walker, J. D.: Favorable and unfavorable behaviors of the dental faculty as evaluated by dental students, *Journal of Dental Education, 35* (October) 1971, 625-631.

32. Ware, J. E., and Williams, R. G. The Dr. Fox effect: A study of lecturer effectiveness and ratings of instruction. *Journal of Medical Education, 50* (February) 1975, 149-156.

33. Williams, R. G., and Ware, J. E. Validity of Student Ratings of Instruction under Different Incentive Conditions: A Further Study of the Dr. Fox Effect. Unpublished paper presented at the Annual Convention of American Educational Research Association, Washington, D.C. March 30-April 3, 1975.

Self-Assessment Inventory for Clinical and Classroom Teaching in Medicine*

Part I: Teacher behaviors

Directions: In this inventory there are statements which reflect some of the ways clinical instructors can be described. For *each* statement, circle the number on the scale which indicates how *descriptive* the behavior is of your teaching. The scale ranges from 1 for not at all descriptive to 7 for very descriptive. Check (√) if the behavior is not applicable to the type of teaching you do.

In rating your teaching, respond to each item carefully and thoughtfully. Avoid letting your response to some items influence your responses to others.

Teacher behaviors	Not at all descriptive Very descriptive	Not applicable
A. Organization/clarity		
1. Summarizes major points	1 2 3 4 5 6 7	( )
2. Explains clearly	1 2 3 4 5 6 7	( )
3. Communicates what is expected to be learned	1 2 3 4 5 6 7	( )
4. Presents material in an organized manner	1 2 3 4 5 6 7	( )
5. Emphasizes what is important	1 2 3 4 5 6 7	( )
B. Enthusiasm/stimulation		
6. Stimulates students'/residents' interest in the subject	1 2 3 4 5 6 7	( )
7. Is enthusiastic about the subject	1 2 3 4 5 6 7	( )
8. Seems to enjoy teaching	1 2 3 4 5 6 7	( )
9. Is a dynamic and energetic person	1 2 3 4 5 6 7	( )
10. Has an interesting style of presentation	1 2 3 4 5 6 7	( )
C. Instructor knowledge		
11. Reveals broad reading in his/her medical specialty	1 2 3 4 5 6 7	( )
12. Directs students/residents to useful literature in the field	1 2 3 4 5 6 7	( )
13. Discusses current developments in his/her specialty	1 2 3 4 5 6 7	( )
14. Demonstrates a breadth of knowledge in medicine generally	1 2 3 4 5 6 7	( )
15. Discusses points of view other than his/her own	1 2 3 4 5 6 7	( )
D. Rapport		
16. Provides professional support and encouragement to students/residents	1 2 3 4 5 6 7	( )
17. Establishes rapport with others	1 2 3 4 5 6 7	( )
18. Encourages a climate of mutual respect	1 2 3 4 5 6 7	( )
19. Listens attentively	1 2 3 4 5 6 7	( )
20. Shows a personal interest in students/residents	1 2 3 4 5 6 7	( )
21. Corrects students'/residents' mistakes without belittling them	1 2 3 4 5 6 7	( )
22. Demonstrates sensitivity to the needs of others	1 2 3 4 5 6 7	( )
23. Willingly remains accessible to students/residents	1 2 3 4 5 6 7	( )

Teacher behaviors	Not at all descriptive	Very descriptive	Not applicable

E. Instructional skill
- 24. Encourages active participation in discussion   1 2 3 4 5 6 7   ( )
- 25. Utilizes audiovisual resources effectively   1 2 3 4 5 6 7   ( )
- 26. Gives students/residents positive reinforcement for good contributions, observations, or performance   1 2 3 4 5 6 7   ( )
- 27. Gears instruction to students'/residents' level of readiness   1 2 3 4 5 6 7   ( )
- 28. Quickly grasps what students/residents are asking or telling   1 2 3 4 5 6 7   ( )
- 29. Answers carefully and precisely questions raised by students/residents   1 2 3 4 5 6 7   ( )
- 30. Questions students/residents to elicit underlying reasoning   1 2 3 4 5 6 7   ( )
- 31. Helps students/residents organize their thoughts about patient problems   1 2 3 4 5 6 7   ( )
- 32. Demonstrates clinical procedures and techniques being taught   1 2 3 4 5 6 7   ( )

F. Clinical supervision
- 33. Communicates role expectations to students/residents   1 2 3 4 5 6 7   ( )
- 34. Guides students'/residents' development of clinical skills   1 2 3 4 5 6 7   ( )
- 35. Provides specific practice opportunities   1 2 3 4 5 6 7   ( )
- 36. Prepares students/residents for difficult clinical situations   1 2 3 4 5 6 7   ( )
- 37. Offers special help when difficulties arise   1 2 3 4 5 6 7   ( )
- 38. Observes students'/residents' performance frequently   1 2 3 4 5 6 7   ( )
- 39. Identifies students'/residents' strengths and limitations objectively   1 2 3 4 5 6 7   ( )
- 40. Provides frequent feedback on students'/residents' performance   1 2 3 4 5 6 7   ( )
- 41. Makes specific suggestions for improvement   1 2 3 4 5 6 7   ( )
- 42. Seems well prepared for teaching contacts with students/residents   1 2 3 4 5 6 7   ( )
- 43. Questions students/residents in a nonthreatening manner   1 2 3 4 5 6 7   ( )

G. Clinical competence
- 44. Demonstrates clinical skill and judgment   1 2 3 4 5 6 7   ( )
- 45. Demonstrates skill at data gathering   1 2 3 4 5 6 7   ( )
- 46. Objectively defines patient problems   1 2 3 4 5 6 7   ( )
- 47. Synthesizes patient problems rapidly   1 2 3 4 5 6 7   ( )
- 48. Interprets laboratory data skillfully   1 2 3 4 5 6 7   ( )

H. Professional characteristics
- 49. Takes responsibility for own actions and procedures   1 2 3 4 5 6 7   ( )
- 50. Recognizes own limitations   1 2 3 4 5 6 7   ( )
- 51. Seems to have self-confidence   1 2 3 4 5 6 7   ( )
- 52. Is self-critical   1 2 3 4 5 6 7   ( )
- 53. Is open-minded and nonjudgmental   1 2 3 4 5 6 7   ( )
- 54. Does not appear to be arrogant   1 2 3 4 5 6 7   ( )

Continued.

Part II: Summary and action plan

Directions: On the basis of the preceding ratings, circle the numbers on the scales which indicate how descriptive the dimensions of clinical teaching are of your teaching. Check (√) if the dimension is not applicable to the type of teaching you do.

Dimensions	Not at all descriptive	Very descriptive	Not applicable
A. Organization/clarity	1 2 3 4 5 6 7		( )
B. Enthusiasm/stimulation	1 2 3 4 5 6 7		( )
C. Instructor knowledge	1 2 3 4 5 6 7		( )
D. Rapport	1 2 3 4 5 6 7		( )
E. Instructional skill	1 2 3 4 5 6 7		( )
F. Clinical supervision	1 2 3 4 5 6 7		( )
G. Clinical competence	1 2 3 4 5 6 7		( )
H. Professional characteristics	1 2 3 4 5 6 7		( )

1. List your strengths in teaching.

2. Describe how you can more effectively capitalize on these strengths.

3. List general areas and specific behaviors of your teaching which need improvement.

4. Think about specific situations where the need for improvement was apparent.

5. Outline a plan for improving your teaching:
   A. Teaching behavior: _____

      1. New approach:

      2. Assessment procedure:

      3. Summary of results:

   B. Teaching behavior: _____

      1. New approach:

      2. Assessment procedure:

      3. Summary of results:

*© David M. Irby, 1977.

APPENDIX B

Teaching evaluation form*

Instructor _____ Location _____

(attending, resident, preceptor)   (name of hospital or clinic)

Course _____ Date _____

Directions: Please complete a separate form for each clinical instructor you have encountered in this course. When you have completed the form, return it to the Course Committee Chairperson.

Your class: Medical Student: ☐ Year 1   ☐ Year 2   ☐ Year 3   ☐ Year 4
              Resident: ☐ Year 1   ☐ Year 2   ☐ Year 3   ☐ Year 4
              Other:

Teaching setting: ☐ Inpatient   ☐ Outpatient clinic

Primary type of teaching: ☐ Lecture (grand rounds, specialty conferences, and planned presentations)
                            ☐ Group discussion (seminars, tutorials)
                            ☐ Clinical teaching (ward rounds, informal teaching, patient management)

IMPORTANT: In rating this instructor and course, respond to each item carefully and thoughtfully. Avoid letting your responses to some items influence your responses to others. Keep the purpose of each section in mind as you rate the instructor and course.

E—excellent
VG—very good
G—good
F—fair
P—poor
VP—very poor
N—not observed or
   not applicable

SECTION A: To provide a general evaluation

1. The course or rotation as a whole was: E VG G F P VP
2. The instructor's contribution to the course or rotation was: E VG G F P VP
3. The instructor's effectiveness in teaching was: E VG G F P VP

SECTION B: To provide diagnostic feedback to the instructor

4. Clarity and organization of ideas presented were: E VG G F P VP N
5. Enthusiasm and stimulation of interest in the subject were: E VG G F P VP N
6. Breadth of knowledge in medicine was: E VG G F P VP N
7. Rapport with others was: E VG G F P VP N
8. Clinical skills were: E VG G F P VP N
9. Clinical judgment was: E VG G F P VP N
10. Professional characteristics (e.g., self-confidence, openness, lack of arrogance, responsibility) were: E VG G F P VP N
11. Encouragement of active student/resident participation was: E VG G F P VP N
12. Responsiveness to learners' questions and reactions was: E VG G F P VP N
13. Use of questions was: E VG G F P VP N
14. Guidance (e.g., practice opportunities, feedback, assistance) in development of clinical skills was: E VG G F P VP N

---

*As proposed for use by the Department of Medicine, University of Washington   *Continued.*

Teaching evaluation form—cont'd

SECTION C: To assess the extent to which the instructor helped you achieve course objectives

16. Learning factual knowledge, concepts, and/or theories: E VG G F P VP N
17. Developing data collection skills (e.g., H_x, P.E., lab, X-ray):   E VG G F P VP N
18. Learning to interpret and synthesize data: E VG G F P VP N
19. Increasing skill at developing patient management plans: E VG G F P VP N
20. Enhancing technical skills in diagnostic and therapeutic procedures: E VG G F P VP N
21. Improving interpersonal relations with patient and family: E VG G F P VP N
22. Developing clarity and precision in *oral* communication about patients: E VG G F P VP N
23. Developing clarity and precision in *written* communication about patients: E VG G F P VP N
24. Developing professional characteristics, attitudes, and values of a physician: E VG G F P VP N

SECTION D: To provide specific feedback to the instructor

25. What aspects of the teaching do you feel were especially good?

26. What changes could be made to improve the teaching?

part three DEVELOPING AND IMPLEMENTING PROGRAMS

9
INTEGRATING DIDACTIC AND CLINICAL EDUCATION—HIGH PATIENT CONTACT

Craig L. Scanlan

By themselves, proper facilities and sound curriculum content in no way guarantee effective or efficient educational programs. Integration of the clinical and didactic components of an educational program is an essential element in the design and implementation of relevant learning experiences for allied health students.

Such integration promotes the thorough and efficient organization of learning experiences. It motivates learners by providing them with opportunities to analyze and react to various aspects of their total experience until the elements form a meaningful whole. It facilitates the transfer of conceptual knowledge and comprehension to the professional reality of application, synthesis, and problem solving. Without such an integrative framework, learning results in discrete and unrelated episodes of little immediate value to the student or future worth to the clinical practitioner.[3,18] And, of most significance to future practitioners, an integrated academic environment fosters later integrative behavior in the individual.[4] Those who are conscious of the relationships between essential concepts and their application can readily adapt to future change within their profession.

Integration need not occur haphazardly. Systematic planning and evaluation promote the articulation of program, curriculum, and course elements that ultimately resolves the dichotomy of theory and practice so characteristic of professional education.

The integration of didactic and clinical learning experiences must be achieved at three levels of program organization: (1) administrative integration of program components, (2) curriculum integration, and (3) course integration. The successful application of an integrated framework is contingent upon the educator's ability to implement change and evaluate outcomes at all three levels. To do so, the educator will:

- Identify and apply the historical, social, and psychological antecedents of integration to program planning
- Describe and implement administrative, curriculum, and course strategies that promote integration of clinical and didactic program components
- Systematically evaluate and revise existing or planned integrative strategies

INTEGRATION IN PERSPECTIVE

Most allied health occupations exhibit an educational evolution not unlike that of the nursing profession, whose earliest and most rudimentary training was based on a modified apprenticeship system in which students learned entirely at the bedside from a more experienced practitioner. No disparity existed between theory and practice. Under supervision, students provided services at increasing levels of difficulty. Repetitive practice and skills development were emphasized, and what few theoretical concepts were developed were directly correlated with patient care. The success of these early apprenticeships was the result of affiliations with hospitals offering both the number and variety of patients needed for an adequate depth and breadth of learning experiences. Early in the evolution of the apprenticeship system, however, the following deficiencies became apparent[18]:

- Little attention was paid to educational goals because the primary purpose of such systems was to provide improved service.
- Insufficient time was provided for the development of skills prior to their application to patients.
- Insufficient opportunity was provided for gaining the necessary conceptual basis to apply theory to practice.
- The learning of skills was limited to what could be transferred from one practitioner to another.

The institution of supportive didactic instruction heralded a second phase in the evolution of health professions education. Large groups of students could be efficiently presented with theoretical concepts and practical demonstrations in an easily controlled and manipulated environment; concurrently, designated personnel were selected to perform *clinical teaching* based on the educational goals of the school or program, *not* necessarily the service needs of the care-giving institution. Naturally, as old problems were solved, new ones were created[18]:

- Students' motivation in learning waned as the personalized approach to patient care was lost.
- Correlations between the patient and the physiology and pathology described in class were more difficult to perceive.
- The classroom and clinic became dichotomous entities representing, respectively, the ideal and real.
- Poor communication between the didactic and clinical instructors resulted in a loss of interest in educational support by clinical practitioners.
- A discrepancy between didactic and clinical instruction arose as the clinical instructors became less aware of what was being taught in class.

Such problems have more recently been compounded by the increasing tendency of care-giving agencies to rightfully relinquish the administrative responsibilities of allied health programs to educational institutions. At a time when the knowledge explosion and accompanying specialization in medical science are placing greater demands on the integrative behavior of the clinical practitioner, a duality of influence has been created. Without attention, the bifurcation of clinical and didactic learning experiences could become more pronounced.

PRACTICAL BASES FOR INTEGRATION

In traditional, subject-centered curricula, didactic content determines the appropriateness and selection of clinical experiences. Such a methodology is indeed expedient, but of dubious relevance for prospective practitioners. Relevant learning experiences are those that facilitate effective performances by students in their subsequent professional roles. *Competency-based instruction* identifies the professional roles students will assume upon completion of their program *and* determines exactly what constitutes effective performance within these roles.[19] Such behaviors serve as the basis for relevant program goals and meaningful curriculum objectives. In competency-based programs, then, priority must be placed upon the development and refinement of the knowledge, skills, and attitudes that constitute effective *clinical performance*. Didactic instruction thus becomes a contributory factor rather than a determinant in accomplishment of this goal.

Educators planning integrative strategies must be aware of such emphasis. The effective integration of administrative, curriculum, and course elements into a meaningful whole of lasting value and application to the future practitioner is contingent upon placing the horse *in front of* the carriage.

Administrative strategies

The function and purpose of program administration are to facilitate and support the teaching/learning process.[10] The delineation of administrative responsibilities in allied health programs reflects the changing roles care-giving agencies and educational institutions are assuming in meeting the needs for competent delivery of health care. Neither hospitals nor colleges alone can produce the numbers and kinds of personnel necessary to deliver optimal patient care; agency collaboration and administrative strategies promoting integration are prerequisites to the successful development and implementation of allied health programs. The alternative to institutional integration is irrelevant educational preparation, inadequately trained personnel, expensive job turnovers, and high attrition rates.[8]

Regardless of whether the program is centered at a college or hospital, final administrative responsibility must, however, be that of *one* institution. In the case of clinical affiliations, administrative responsibility remains with the educational institution; with academic affiliations, administrative control rests with the hospital. In either case, a written contract facilitates interagency communications by clearly delineating individual roles and responsibilities. Such affiliation agreements must be jointly developed with legal counsel and include the specification of schedules, facilities, communications, academic considerations, student considerations, faculty and staff considerations, and fiscal arrangements.[11,12]

Those administrative responsibilities that facilitate the organization and articulation of program components may be subsumed under three basic principles.

Institutional philosophy and operational goals. The philosophy and operational goals of the program must be determined by the sponsoring institution. Such goals must be rationally derived and compatible with the relevant needs and characteristics of the learners, the availability of resources, and the demands of applicable interest groups and society as a whole. Goals based on identified competencies are the key to successful program integration. However, clinical competencies, though of paramount importance, need not be the *sole* determinants of relevant objectives. Contributing goals may include (1) personal growth and development, (2) communicative skills, (3) professional development, (4) human relations skills, (5) social conscience and consciousness, (6) management and administrative competencies, and (7) personal and community health.[1] The achievement of such goals depends on providing students with well-organized clinical and didactic learning opportunities.

The ability of graduates to actually assume their professional roles can be assessed by carefully designed follow-up. Proper follow-up studies survey both the agencies employing graduates and the graduates themselves[9]; survey questionnaires *must* be based on the delineated goals of the program. Disparities discovered by follow-up may represent either deficiencies in the integration of program content or unrealistic operational goals; both must be amenable to revision and change.

Clinical and didactic instructional components. The majority of degree-granting allied health programs are presently centered in academic institutions. Thus a significant administrative responsibility of such institutions is the selection and evaluation of clinical education facilities.

No single aspect of program planning and implementation is as consequential or potentially difficult as clinical site selection; all subsequent administrative, curriculum, and course integrative strategies are contingent upon development of effective clinical affiliations.

Site selection based on expediency can only result in disintegrative and irrelevant learning. Selection of clinical facilities must be based on a careful investigation of four major concerns: (1) the degree and type of administrative support of the clinical affiliate, (2) patient and equipment resources available at the clinical affiliate, (3) qualifications and characteristics of the clinical affiliate, and (4) the availability and variety of learning experiences at the clinical affiliate.[13]

Such generalizations can be translated into workable criteria to be used for the selection and evaluation of clinical affiliates. Twenty such standards have been developed by the American Physical Therapy Association[13]; a modified listing of that organization's criteria for the evaluation and selection of clinical education sites appears in Appendix A, p. 130. Evaluation forms may be generated from such a criteria list.

The educator can use the forms to rationally and systematically evaluate the strengths, weaknesses, adequacies, and inadequacies of proposed or existing clinical affiliates. If a clinical site meets all or most of the established criteria, the administrative integration of clinical and didactic program components is greatly facilitated.

The effective administrative integration of didactic and clinical components is additionally influenced by both the number and proximity of selected clinical learning centers. A single clinical center should be used only if (1) the affiliate meets the above criteria, and (2) the operational goals of the program can, indeed, be fully achieved in conjunction with that affiliate alone.

The single-center approach to clinical education offers the following significant integrative advantages[14]:

- Extended contact between students and faculty provides supervisors with better knowledge and understanding of each student's needs and abilities.
- Unnecessary duplication of supervised clinical practice is eliminated.
- Student transfer of knowledge into clinical application can be more closely scrutinized.
- Consistent supervision can be provided.

Changing patterns of health care delivery, however, make it unlikely that a single clinical center can provide the full breadth of experiences necessary to meet the operational goals of a program. The educator must perceive the broad spectrum of present and future roles the student is likely to encounter on the job. Such roles and competencies must be reflected in *both* the operational goals of the program and the selection of clinical learning experiences. If most graduates will be working in community hospitals of fewer than 200 beds, it makes little sense to limit students' clinical exposure to a 1,000-bed university medical center. If home care or health maintenance represents an identified professional competency, then public and community health agencies must be enlisted as supplemental clinical resources. Such secondary affiliates are chosen for their ability to provide the specialized experiences necessary to fulfill both the program goals and the reality of professional competence; they need not meet the criteria for the variety of clinical learning experiences required of primary affiliates.

The selection of primary and secondary clinical affiliates must also be based on the proximity of the various centers to the educational institution. Integration is facilitated with ease of communication and interagency mobility of students and staff [2]; geographically isolated clinical facilities often become educationally isolated learning centers.

Although both unique and semiautonomous in their function, health care agencies and educational institutions probably exhibit more similarities in administrative operation than differences. Common goals, therefore, should enhance the establishment of administrative and educational liaisons. *Liaison committees*, with representatives in decision-making capacities from both the educational institution and clinical agencies can be organized; the resultant problem solving of shared issues reinforces collaborative roles and promotes the integration of clinical and didactic program components. *Advisory committees*, representing a larger body of both internal and external interest groups, can serve a similar function but are generally not responsible for actual policy.

Personnel resources. Integration is an active process implemented by an interested and capable faculty. The distribution, responsibilities, functions, and characteristics of program faculty members will ultimately determine the success or failure of integrative strategies.

The tradition-bound, stereotyped, quasi-specialized faculty model, expediently appropriated from medical education, is notoriously inefficient and unsuccessful in promoting integration. More often than not, instructors designated as experts have not had sufficient educational background to operate as specialists in their field; those with highly sophisticated and specialized education and experience lack the pedagogical knowledge and ability necessary to model integrative behavior and communicate holistically.[18] The result is usually failure to develop an integrative approach to learning, to health care, and to the behavior of the prospective health professional.

Careful administrative planning in designating and developing the role and function of faculty resources will promote the integration of didactic and clinical education. Three strategies are particularly effective: (1) utilization of a coordinator of clinical education, (2) rotation of clinical and didactic faculty assignments, and (3) establishment of staff and faculty development programs.

The *coordinator of clinical education* (CCE) is indisputably the individual most responsible for developing and implementing integrative strategies at all three program levels (administrative, curriculum, and course). The CCE is delegated responsibilities in five interelated areas, including:

1. Organization, direction, supervision, and integration of clinical education into the total curriculum
2. Development of clinical affiliates and clinical faculty members
3. Development of students through guidance and counseling
4. Participation as an academic faculty member
5. Administration of integrated instructional effort

A detailed listing of these responsibilities, based on a summary of job descriptions for the academic coordinator of clinical education in twenty-five physical therapy educational programs[13] appears in Appendix B, p. 131.

Such a broad scope of responsibilities requires an individual of remarkable professional characteristics and personal attributes.

The CCE must possess skills in interpersonal relations, counseling and guidance, administration and supervision, systematic planning and evaluation, and listening. Such an individual must additionally be interested and enthusiastic, possess in-depth understanding of the program and problems involved, and most importantly, have the institutional status necessary to actually perform the designated responsibilities. The CCE should also have had experience as a clinical instructor; have an advanced degree with preparation in education, counseling, administration, and interpersonal communications; and maintain clinical skills and awareness of current trends in the given discipline.

The role model established by the CCE's close clinical relationship with students will have both immediate practical consequences and lasting significance to the students' later professional behavior; CCEs must themselves develop and display integrated behavior if they expect their students to do likewise.

Administratively, the CCE should have coequal status with the educational director. Such role delineation recognizes the significance of clinical competence in determining desired program outcomes and facilitates cooperative planning and communication. Evaluation of the CCE must be based on an objective analysis of desired performance, rated by observers (administrators *and* students) who are using the delineated responsibilities (see Appendix B) as criteria.

The selection and scheduling of faculty assignments are taking on new importance as increasing technological sophistication demands specialization. The effect of specialization on undergraduate allied health education can be disastrous if integrative strategies are poorly planned. The research physiologist with little conception of pathological alterations and their clinical management is unlikely to be able to assist students in seeing the relationships between normal and abnormal function. Didactic instructor/specialists reviewing principles of basic therapeutics will have difficulty describing the nuances of clinical application unless they themselves are involved in clinical activities. A delicate balance can, however, be achieved. Thoughtful administrators encourage the continued professional growth of the faculty within their individual specialties and concomitantly insist on providing students with the holistic perspective necessary for entry level as a clinical practitioner. This is best accomplished by generating faculty teaching schedules that have every full-time faculty member responsible for some portion of the clinical learning experience and ensure that faculty members rotate course assignments on a regular basis. These strategies encourage faculty members to perceive interrelationships between clinical and didactic learning experiences, to maintain a comprehensive view of their discipline, and to better understand the need and mechanism for implementing integration.

Once the roles and functions of faculty members have been designated and once the rotation of clinical and didactic assignments is scheduled, staff and faculty development can begin. It must reach not only the full-time faculty of the educational institution, but also those contracted as part-time clinical instructors and those identified as supervisors at the various clinical agencies. The latter individuals, whose commitment to the program is secondary, are often the ones with whom the students have most contact; it is, therefore, not enough that their role in the program be clearly recognized and described; their participation can make or break the successful integration of program components. In order to ensure that their participation is active and enthusiastic, program directors and administrators must continually seek and provide faculty and staff development programs of relevance to both the academic and clinical needs of the individuals involved. Such programs should be organized jointly by the academic institution and clinical agency and based on the sound principles of adult and continuing education.[13] The underlying assumption is that the improvement both of faculty skills and of the working relationships between the various resource personnel of the program creates a more efficient and orderly educational process; that is, integration of the program components.

Curriculum strategies

Administrative strategies promoting integration set the stage for the development, planning, and implementation of a well-organized curriculum. An integrated curriculum provides the opportunity and environment in which concepts can be perceived in relationship to one another and as part of a whole.[3] The systematic planning, selection, and evaluation of curriculum is based on the Tyler model,[20] in which the educator identifies desired educational goals, determines the available educational experiences, modifies the educational goals in accordance with available resources, organizes educational experiences to achieve those goals, evaluates the achievement of the desired outcomes, and, if necessary, revises the goals or methodology according to evaluated need (see Fig. 6). This approach is similar to suggestions Ford makes in the Prologue.

In competency-based curricula, the factors that influence the formulation of both general goals and specific objectives include the actual professional performance exhibited by practitioners; the nature and extent of learning resources; the characteristics of the learners themselves; and the demands of professional organizations, private and governmental regulatory agencies, and society as a whole. Generating an accurate and reliable description of actual professional performance is, therefore, the first step toward developing an integrated curriculum of relevance to the learner.

Once the goals appropriately match the availability of learning resources, specific objectives can be identified and described. Objectives foster integration if (1) they contribute to the satisfaction of a learner need; (2) the relationship between enabling objectives and the general goals is made clear; (3) overspecificity is avoided; and (4) integration of learning experiences is itself revealed as an objective.[15]

Learning activities that are most appropriate for the desired outcomes must be selected and arranged. In most allied health programs three curriculum components are utilized: large group meetings (didactic instruction), a clinical laboratory, and a practice laboratory.

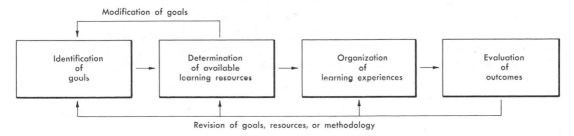

Fig. 6

A systematic model for curriculum planning, development and implementation.

Less traditional institutions are beginning to use other effective modes of learning that emphasize more flexible scheduling and individual responsibility. Even in these programs, however, the three basic components persist. Their integration depends on an understanding of their functions, advantages, and limitations.

Large group meetings, or lectures, have several advantages. They provide a frame of reference for learning and effectively transmitting information. They allow substantial amounts of information to be presented to large numbers of people in short periods of time with little cost or delay. They facilitate the presentation of up-to-date information not otherwise available. Unfortunately, didactic methods based solely on lecture provide a low level of stimulation, limit student participation, and neglect differences in level or style of learning.[19]

The clinical laboratory represents *any* environment in which the learner comes into contact with patients for the purpose of acquiring, developing, and refining the knowledge, skills, and attitudes characteristic of professional performance.[6] The uniqueness of the clinical laboratory as a curriculum component cannot be overemphasized. The proper integration of clinical observation, learning, reinforcement, and practice within the program provides students with the unparalleled opportunity to translate basic theoretical knowledge into the diversity of intellectual and psychomotor skills necessary to provide patient care. The knowledge, skills, and attitudes synonymous with professional competence can be developed *only* in conjunction with the clinical laboratory experience.

Systematically planned and flexible clinical learning experiences are the keystone to competency-based allied health programs. Clinical education is, however, costly and difficult to effectively organize. It should be planned and implemented only when it furnishes the very best or only method of achieving student competencies.

The third curriculum component designed to assist students in achieving professional competencies is the practice, or skills, laboratory. Having evolved from the classical science laboratory, in which theoretical concepts are verified by observational research and controlled experimentation, the allied health practice laboratory represents a unique and essential aspect of curriculum planning and design. Such a facility assists students in verifying theory by practical application and in demonstrating competence during supervised performances. The use of practice laboratories is based on the premise that it is less wasteful of time and more advantageous to learning to practice the parts of a complex behavior before applying the learning to actual patients.[6] Practice laboratories are thus designed to facilitate the acquisition and mastery of concepts and skills by providing association with concrete reference stimuli and opportunities for equivalent or analogous practice behavior.[17]

The only element missing from such a facility is, of course, the patient. The practice laboratory can neither supplant any portion of the clinical experience requiring direct patient contact, nor can it alone verify the achievement of professional competence.

How, then, are these three diverse elements to be unified into a workable, relevant curriculum? The basis for such organization is systematic *curriculum design*. Successful curriculum design is an active and ongoing process whereby an integrative pattern, framework, or structural organization of the various curriculum elements is planned, developed, implemented, evaluated, and revised. Successful curriculum design defines the scope and sequence of learning experiences. It designates the breadth, variety, type, placement, and function of such experiences within a unified whole.[21]

Such a systematic design requires the educator to develop a three-dimensional perspective of the curriculum and its components in which the integration, continuity, and sequence of elements determines the efficacy of the learning process (see Fig. 7). *Integration* organizes learning experiences to provide for horizontal relationships between curriculum elements. It provides opportunities for students to assess and synthesize the various aspects of the total experience into a meaningful whole. *Continuity* establishes a vertical relationship between different levels of the same skills or subject matter. It provides sustained

and recurrent opportunities for practice and reinforcement. *Sequence* organizes learning experiences in order to progressively develop knowledge and skills at successively higher levels of understanding—broadening, deepening, and extending the learner's ability to apply skills in more diverse situations under less controlled circumstances.[18] The ideal result of such carefully organized curriculum elements is a professional competence that is continually expansive, flexible, and adaptive.

Curriculum strategies that assist the educator in planning and implementing such a framework should thus provide *both* vertical and horizontal organizing threads of concepts, skills, and values, as well as opportunities for students to actively pursue goal-directed activities. The organizing elements themselves should also be internally consistent (i.e., not in conflict with one another) and of long-range utility to the learner.

Integrating strategies that meet these criteria and facilitate the articulation of clinical and didactic learning experiences include (1) the use of a practice, or skills, laboratory; (2) the

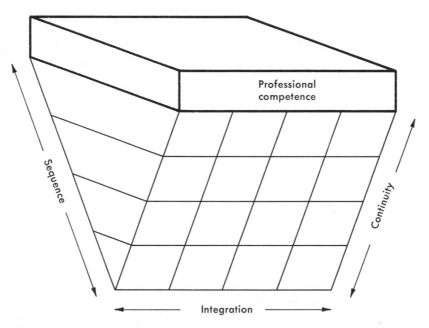

Fig. 7
A three-dimension perspective of curriculum organization.

patterning of clinical, didactic, and laboratory instruction; and (3) the use of organizing centers.

Practice laboratory. The practice laboratory represents more than a physical structure of workbenches and equipment. Properly planned and designed, the laboratory becomes an integral part of a dynamic curriculum, *not* just a supplemental aid for demonstrations or an expedient tool for summative evaluations. The systematic integration of a practice, or skills, laboratory with the didactic and clinical curriculum components requires careful identification of those skills and concepts considered prerequisite to clinical problem solving. It also requires delineation of those learning activities that might be enhanced by joint exposure to both environments.

The practice laboratory functions as an intermediary between the theoretical base of didactic instruction and the application of concepts and skills at the patient's bedside[17] (see Fig. 8). Those theories and concepts proposed in class are tested for validity or mastered in the laboratory; manual skills are developed,

practiced, refined, and evaluated prior to clinical application. As learners advance through the curriculum, the laboratory additionally provides opportunities for independent problem solving and research.

In order to accommodate individual styles and aptitudes for learning, a practice laboratory must not confine learners to arbitrary schedules or mandate that everyone accomplish the same specified objectives in the same time. Successful learning experiences should be provided whenever and to whatever extent the learner perceives them necessary. Such open scheduling has the following significant advantages over traditionally scheduled learning experiences:

- Reinforcement of key principles is adjustable according to the needs of the individual.
- Worthwhile information is presented only when the learner is receptive and alert.
- Experiments requiring specialized or expensive equipment, normally prohibitive under traditional scheduling, can be included because equipment use is distrib-

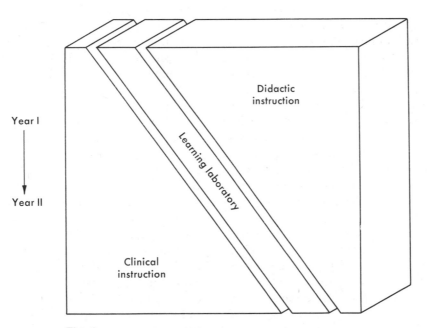

Fig. 8
The articulation of curricular components.

-uted over a greater timespan, and fewer such items are required.[16]

The open-scheduled practice laboratory supports and makes feasible the flexible clinical scheduling necessary in competency-based curricula.

The design of the physical environment is equally important. The more analogous the laboratory is to the actual conditions under which the prospective graduates will indeed perform their professional functions, the more likely association and transfer will occur. Creative instructors can devise laboratory simulations to assist students in mastering complex behaviors and to evaluate their problem-solving processes. Such simulations can provide students with immediate feedback and reinforcement with less anxiety than supervised applications at the patient's bedside, thereby improving both the efficacy of clinical instruction itself and the confidence of the learners.

The full implementation of an open-scheduled practice laboratory further depends on the availability, proximity, and articulation of multimedia learning resources. Organized into a meaningful combination with the three classic curriculum components, educational media no longer supplement learning, but become the very core of an instructional program. Left to be used without some systematic arrangement, however, multimedia materials often suffer from disuse or misuse, leading to piecemeal learning and *dis*integrative behavior. The optimal combination of tutoring, goal-directed laboratory activities, and properly selected media can produce a synergistic learning environment in which students actively seek out and identify relationships between course and curriculum components. The achievement of this goal can be evaluated only by assessment of the process itself (i.e., the participants' opinions of the value and effectiveness of the various activities in reaching the objectives). A student evaluation form used to assess the integrative strategies of a program, curriculum, or course is shown in Appendix D, p. 133.

The educator planning to implement the practice laboratory as an integrative strategy must be acquainted with the following misconceptions and/or limitations:

1. *The learning laboratory is not, and should not be, a substitute for clinical experience.* It is only a vehicle that facilitates transfer of concepts, skills, and problem solving to the clinical setting.[17]

2. *The elegance of the facility and the amount or cost of equipment in no way guarantee relevant, meaningful, or successful learning experiences.* Careful delineation of professional competencies and specification of objectives are necessary prerequisites to development. Thorough and efficient education is not purchased.[17]

3. *The laboratory must not be considered an autonomous learning environment.* Learning in isolation lacks transfer.[17]

4. *The freedom of open scheduling and individualized instruction can result in poor attendance and organizational dilemmas.* Initially, students should have a portion of their time scheduled, with transition to true open scheduling being gradual.[16]

5. *The particular performance of skills or behaviors should be given less emphasis than the understanding and mastery of underlying principles.* Technical skills should not be emphasized at the expense of meaning. Principles can be easily transferred to new environments; necessary skills in a profession are often transient.[6]

Patterning of instruction. Two basic patterns of curriculum organization are usually employed: nonconcurrent and concurrent. In the nonconcurrent curriculum, clinical and didactic learning experiences are separate entities: students engaged full-time in a clinical setting have no didactic responsibilities; students participating in formally scheduled classes or academic learning activities have no clinical involvement. Such a design is practical, easy to schedule, and expedient. The discontinuity of experiences characteristic of nonconcurrent curricula is, however, both educationally unsound and personally unfair to learners; it contradicts the basic psychological principles of association and contiguity and fails to provide the initial exposure essential in achieving affective objectives and learner motivation. How fair is it for a student to sit through as many as four years of class instruction before gaining any clinical exposure?

In the concurrent curriculum a portion of each day or week is devoted to didactic instruction matched with a related clinical component. Four common types of concurrent organization are employed[13]:

1. A concurrent pattern throughout the curriculum, with all clinical education occurring concomitantly with didactic instruction and with no full-time clinical assignments
2. A concurrent pattern with a full-time clinical assignment at the end of the curriculum
3. A concurrent pattern with a full-time clinical assignment in the middle of the curriculum
4. Concurrent patterns interspersed with multiple, full-time clinical assignments throughout the curriculum

The optimal arrangement appears to be weekly clinical experiences throughout the curriculum, culminating in a full-time clinical assignment scheduled near the end of the program. This organization serves the multiple purposes of facilitating the transfer of learning between curriculum components; providing frequent practice and reinforcement for skills development and mastery; maintaining and promoting the students' interest in learning; and providing integration, continuity, and sequence among and within curriculum components.[13] These occur in three identifiable, but not exclusive, stages: initial exposure and observation, learning and reinforcement, and minimally supervised performance.

Initial exposure and observation. The observational phase must occur as early as possible in the curriculum. Besides having motivational and affective influences on the student, this early phase of clinical exposure can introduce the student to the commonalities among allied health professions: astute observation and data collection, professional-client interaction, and basic nursing and emergency life-support skills. This phase may be part of a professional orientation course or integrated within a health care curriculum. In the latter case, the team approach to health care delivery can be presented and applied.

Learning and reinforcement. The learning and reinforcement phase is of variable duration and must be flexible enough to accommodate learners with prior clinical experience or exposure at different entry levels, as well as individual differences in learning styles or aptitudes. The temporal and content contiguity of didactic and clinical laboratory experiences must be maintained throughout this phase: appropriate behaviors are identified and described in class, demonstrated and tried in the practice laboratory, and then, and only then, applied at the patient's bedside. In this manner, the identified clinical competence is established at the apex of a hierarchy of knowledge, skills, and attitudes. Enabling objectives at the lower cognitive levels are best mastered by using traditional didactic or mediated instruction. The higher levels of application, evaluation, and problem solving are achieved in the practice laboratory, the precursor of clinical application. Synthesis can only be achieved in the clinical context within which practitioners actually perform their professional responsibilities.

Minimally supervised performance. The final, minimally supervised performance phase is essential in those occupations in which entry into the profession occurs simultaneously with completion of the formal educational program. It is during this phase that a significant alteration in integrating strategies must occur. Until this phase, the integrating agent has been the instructor. Learners nearing completion of their formal educational program must, however, become their own integrating agents, capable of perceiving and developing relationships among diversified components of the whole (i.e., capable of adaptive and flexible behavior in a changing professional and societal milieu).

Organizing centers. The final curriculum integrative strategy the educator may employ is the identification, development, and implementation of organizing centers. An organizing center is a unifying theme or motif that pervades all curriculum components and transcends much of the factual detail so often emphasized in professional education. Organizing centers are designed to promote the application of learning to a variety of problems at different levels and in different contexts. Characteristically, an organizing center[3]:

> Is broad enough to provide learners with numerous opportunities to identify problems, ideas, and concepts and to move them about within the curriculum.
>
> Has significance for the learner (i.e., suggests learning activities that are interesting, relevant, and worthwhile for students)
>
> Provides easy access to learning resources
>
> Demonstrates sufficient breadth and scope to meet the demands of the variety of interests and capabilities characteristic of a group of learners, accommodating their many learning styles
>
> Ties together cognitive, psychomotor, and affective behaviors
>
> Displays continuity, sequence, and integration
>
> Encourages learners to identify new and worthwhile experiences for themselves
>
> Requires solving of patient-related problems in a variety of clinical situations

A portion of a typical organizing center used in a respiratory therapy curriculum is demonstrated in Appendix C, p. 132. Such a conceptual theme is based on an essential clinical competency (i.e., maintaining tissue oxygenation) that pervades all professional courses throughout the typical two-year curriculum. Horizontal integration is developed among the three professional curriculum components. In addition, the supportive content of the basic sciences is also listed. The vertical continuity and sequence take the learner from physiological knowledge and comprehension, through technological application, to supportive management in increasingly difficult and complex patient-related problems. Well-designed organizing centers enhance opportunities for integration and synthesis of learning experiences. Evaluation of the efficacy of organizing centers in achieving this goal is best accomplished by graduate follow-up and the student process questionnaire (See Appendix D, p. 133).

Course strategies

Once the coordination of administrative components is a reality and the various elements of the curriculum have been articulated, the perceptive educator is bound to ask for practical integrative strategies that can be readily employed within the framework of an organized course. Such strategies include unit organization of content, flexible clinical scheduling, team teaching, the case or care study, and the seminar.

Successful implementation of the strategies fully depends on the presence of an instructor who realizes which behaviors facilitate integration. An instructor may establish a learning environment conducive to the integration of content *and* the integrative behavior of the learners by[7]:

> Modeling integrative behavior
>
> Organizing behavior around identified student goals
>
> Planning outcomes that are visible, contribute to learner satisfaction, and clarify means/ends relationships
>
> Explicitly revealing integration as an objective
>
> Providing opportunities for learners to associate prior learning
>
> Utilizing readiness experiences to ensure that conceptual levels are appropriate to students' capabilities
>
> Encouraging learner participation
>
> Soliciting learner criticism
>
> Minimizing threatening learning experiences

Within such an environment, instructors often employ organizational components of courses called *units*. A unit is a valid integrative strategy that brings together a number of learning activities into a related whole. Each unit characteristically includes a general directive or goal, the identification and delineation of enabling objectives, a description of appropriate means (learning experiences) necessary to achieve the specific objectives, and methods to evaluate the outcomes of the learning experiences. A unit should relate to other units within the course or curriculum framework, but should not depend on them for its structure.

Units should be designed to facilitate learning rather than expedite teaching. Properly organized units guide students through frequent and successful learning experiences toward readily visible goals. Improperly organized units stand as roadblocks to the meaningful integration of learning experiences. Autonomous and irrelevant units may be avoided by organizing goals and activities around patient-centered professional competencies.

If every professional course is to have a clinical component (as it should) and if educators are to accommodate individual abilities and learning styles (as they must), then the *individualization* of clinical experience becomes imperative. Individualized clinical learning is, however, the specter of allied health education—often seen and heard, but never grasped. Theoretically, it facilitates the integration of diverse clinical experiences by providing the levels of content, paces of learning, and methodologies commensurate with individual learning needs.[18] To put the theory into practice, however, the allied health educator must be fully aware of the prerequisites, essential elements, and conditions inherent in individualized clinical learning.

Clinical education designed to meet individual levels of ability requires instructors who can objectively diagnose and measure student learning needs, students who are indeed willing to assume the responsibility for learning, and a modification of the traditional instructor's role from that of a primary learning resource to that of a learning manager or facilitator.[18]

Implicit in the application of individualized clinical education is the continual diagnosis of student progress and provisions for multiple avenues of learning. Student progress cannot be assessed and alternate pathways cannot be proposed unless *measurable* competencies for each level of progression and each learning objective are clearly specified. If a program is competency based, such identified behaviors already exist; instructors then need only compare each learner's existing competencies with those they seek to develop in the learner.

Under such conditions, progress from one clinical area to another is contingent only on mastery of the specified behaviors, *not* on an arbitrary time requirement. Prerequisite to such competency-based progression is the provision of *flexible scheduling* whereby the duration, nature, and type of learning situations can be altered to meet the needs of the students.

Flexible scheduling can be achieved only if ample time and opportunities are provided for the learner to review and practice complex behaviors before applying them to patients or to go beyond specified core objectives to areas of individual interest. Both can be accomplished in the practice laboratory, without which individualized clinical education would be difficult, if not impossible.

Team teaching is a third strategy allied health educators often use to promote the integration of clinical and didactic instruction. Team teaching is the coordinated and cooperative planning, teaching, supervision, and evaluation of a group of learners by two or more instructors, each having special competencies and knowledge. The assumption, however, that two heads are indeed better than one can often be fallacious. Poorly planned team teaching can subvert integrative strategies by overemphasis on specialization, arbitrary divisions of factual knowledge, and needless repetition. It is probably less important that the instructors involved be complementary specialists than that they be cooperative and communicative allies jointly responsible for development of the objectives, choice of instructional methodologies, and evaluation.

Learners can be encouraged to develop and refine high-order cognitive skills by implementing two interrelated strategies: the *case study* and the *seminar*. A case study is a problem-solving activity in which a student undertakes a comprehensive review and assessment of a patient management problem—proposing, planning, implementing, and evaluating appropriate interactions based on the sound application of previously mastered knowledge and skills. The integrative benefits are obvious: students are required to organize their thinking and establish meaningful relationships between otherwise discrete elements of theory and practice. Educators employing the case study as an integrative course strategy should adhere to the following guidelines if they expect successful outcomes[18]:

> The patient management problem should be within the realm of comprehension and abilities of the individual students, yet not limit their potential development of new knowledge, skills, or attitudes.
>
> Sufficient time must be provided for the student to pursue the study simultaneously with actual patient care.
>
> Guidelines for the format and content of the case study should be limited to basic instructions.
>
> Case studies should be employed flexibly, when and where the needs exist, as an integral part of the total curriculum and should not be arbitrarily assigned.
>
> Case studies should be presented orally to peer groups for constructive critique, analysis, and review.

The final guideline is most noteworthy. The critique and analysis of a patient-centered case study by a small group of well-informed and highly motivated learners, each with a unique perspective and potential contribution, provide an unparalleled opportunity to integrate otherwise disparate elements of classroom theory and clinical practice into a meaningful whole. Group interaction, discussion, and analysis are conditions of learning that facilitate problem solving.[5] Such problem solving under guidance is appropriately called the *seminar*.

The effectiveness of the seminar approach as an integrative strategy depends on the[18]:

1. Ability of the instructor to facilitate and meaningfully direct the group process
2. Instructor's expert knowledge of the problem selected
3. Students' ability to employ systematic evaluation and problem solving
4. Students' ability to effectively utilize group discussion techniques

The seminar need not be limited to a critique and analysis of the case study. Depending on the general goals of the program and specified objectives of the curriculum, other problems may be appropriately identified and analyzed in order to facilitate and encourage a well-rounded perspective on the individual discipline itself and on society as a whole. Examples of pertinent and contemporary problems that make excellent seminar topics are the cost of health care delivery, medical ethics and euthanasia, and health maintenance organizations. Such topics can challenge students to synthesize didactic knowledge, clinical experience, and social consciousness into meaningful relationships of personal, professional, and social significance.

EVALUATION OF INTEGRATIVE STRATEGIES

Regardless of the program level at which they are implemented (administrative, curriculum, or course), all integrative strategies share a common goal: They increase the likelihood that students will perceive significant relationships among otherwise diverse learning experiences. The systematic application of any learning strategy also demands a realistic assessment of whether the desired goals have been achieved.

Unfortunately, the variety and complexity of learning conditions and the dearth of basic or applied research in allied health education have engendered an immature evaluative methodology, often lacking sufficiently valid or reliable criteria for assessing outcomes. The integrative strategies described in this chapter have grown *not* out of experimental design, but out of practical application. Descriptive studies and survey research indicate that the methods so derived are increasingly employed with variable success.

The wary allied health educator will, however, stop to ask the following pointed questions: What measures of success can I use to assess integrative strategies? Even if I deem the strategies a success under the specified conditions, can I hope to achieve the same results under different circumstances? All of the answers are not available now, nor will they be in the future; this is, in part, the challenge of allied health education.

The allied health educator need not, however, flounder in despair. Systems theory makes the educational process both amenable and responsive to change. Educators, therefore, need not depend solely on basic research for innovation. The applicability and efficacy of an integrative strategy can be readily assessed within a functioning curriculum by both process and product evaluations. Although the results of such assessments may not be generalizable to larger or different populations, they can yield sufficient internal data to make informed decisions possible.

Evaluating integrative processes requires assessments made by the learners themselves. Students engaged in the learning process are in the best position to perceive the effect of organizational patterns and curriculum strategies on their ability to establish meaningful relationships among diverse learning experiences. The sample student questionnaire (Appendix D, p. 133) provides an approach to the assessment of integrative strategies. The actual structure of such a questionnaire depends on the nature of the integrative strategies used.

The process questionnaire provided appraises the contribution administrative, curriculum, and course strategies make in providing integrated experiences. The effect of such organizational patterns on the latter *integrating* behavior of the individual is, however, harder to evaluate. Such a valid product assessment would require trained observers and measurable criteria specifying exactly what constitutes integrating behavior. Practical questions can, however, be generated and included in follow-up studies of program graduates. Pertinent questions directed to supervisors observing graduate performance may include the following: Do graduates (employees):

1. Find it easy to adapt to new procedures?
2. Demonstrate enthusiasm in identifying similarities in principles?
3. Readily apply theory to application?
4. Have a narrow view of their occupation?
5. Need assistance in recognizing parallel situations?
6. Like to piece information together for themselves?

7. Easily identify relationships among areas of practice?
8. Synthesize diverse concepts with difficulty?

The list is by no means inclusive; it is not intended to be. Integrating behavior is a difficult goal to specify, precisely because it is a difficult construct to objectively describe—difficult, but not impossible. As educators grow in their knowledge of the learning process, its product, and the methodology of evaluation, they can expect to measure outcomes with increased precision and thereby more rationally effect change. If they are to expect such change, allied health educators must continue to develop evaluative competencies *and* never hesitate to implement innovative strategies based on informed decisions.

SUMMARY

The systematic planning, organization, implementation, and evaluation of allied health programs require educators to recognize three basic premises:

1. Continual changes in the roles and functions of allied health personnel must be expected and planned for.
2. Formal educational processes can no longer impart all the necessary knowledge, skills, and attitudes characteristic of present or future professional competency.
3. Teaching must be responsive and relevant to the needs of students.

The integration of clinical and didactic program components is one strategy that recognizes the significance of such premises and accommodates their intent. By providing frequently planned and well-organized experiences that enable students to transfer theoretical knowledge into practical application, allied health educators increase the likelihood that students can establish meaningful *and* lasting relationships among otherwise discrete elements of the learning process. Environments that provide opportunities for *integrated* experiences can encourage learners to develop and apply *integrating* behavior. The individual who is cognizant *and* capable of such behavior can more readily adapt to those professional and social changes not yet even envisioned.

REFERENCES

1. Callahan, M. E.; Addoms, E. C.; and Schulz, B. F. Objectives of basic physical therapy education. *Physical Therapy Review*, 41 (November) 1961, 795-797

   An article that presents five major categories of educational objectives for physical therapy that can be used to identify and describe general goals applicable to allied health curricula.

2. Cogland, S.: A method of clinical education—Simmons College. *American Physical Therapy Association Newsletter* (Spring) 1966, 43-44.

   A case report of one school's experience in maintaining the continuity of clinical instruction. A single faculty teaches in both didactic and clinical environments at clinical affiliates located near the college; classes are small and instruction is individualized.

3. Conely, V. C. *Curriculum and Instruction in Nursing*, Boston, Mass.: Little, Brown and Company, 1973.

   A scholarly, comprehensive examination and review of the nature, development, and basic issues of curriculum that transcend nursing education. The author describes sources of curriculum decisions; the design, structure, and evaluation of curriculum components; the nature, variety, and utility of various instructional modes; and strategies for systematic curriculum change.

4. Dressel, P. L. The meaning and significance of integration. In N. B. Henry (Ed.), *The Integration of Educational Experiences*, Fifty-seventh Yearbook of the National Society for the Study of Education, Part 3. Chicago: University of Chicago Press, 1958.

   An overview of the interrelationship between integration and education that differentiates between integrated experiences and integrating behavior. The author describes various concepts of integration in curriculum planning and delineates a rational approach to integration in selecting and organizing educational experiences.

5. Gagné, R. M. *The Conditions of Learning.* 2nd ed. New York: Holt, Rinehart and Winston, 1970.

   An identification and description of eight types of learning and their conditions. The author delineates the principles and practical application of a learning hierarchy based on preconditions and learning levels that range from simple to complex.

6. Infante, M. S. *The Clinical Laboratory in Nursing Education.* New York: John Wiley and Sons, 1975.

   A systematic identification of the essential elements of clinical laboratory education and their effective use in baccalaureate nursing programs. The author provides descriptive research data as a guide for educators in planning clinical laboratory activities.

7. Krathwohl, D. R. The psychological bases for integration. In N. B. Henry (Ed.). *The Integration of Educational Experiences*, Fifty-seventh Yearbook of the National Society for the Study of Education, Part 3. Chicago: University of Chicago Press, 1958.

   A review of the characteristics, levels, and determinants of integrative behavior. The author provides practical guidelines, based on behavioral dynamics, to guide the instructor in facilitating integration in the classroom. He also identifies the applicability and conditions for their implementation.

8. Light, I., and Frey, D. C. Education and the hospital: Dual responsibility for allied manpower training. *Hospitals*, 47 (March) 1973, 85-88.

   A review of the problems confronting educational institutions and hospitals in the training of allied health personnel. The authors recommend collaborative contracts, joint standing committees, academic appointments for clinical faculty, cooperative staff development, rational financial arrangements, and competency-based curricula and evaluation as methods to create meaningful alliances.

9. Love, R. L. Followup. In C. W. Ford and M. K. Morgan (Eds.), *Teaching in the Health Professions.* St. Louis: C. V. Mosby, 1976.

   A succinct description of how various criteria for evaluating program effectiveness may be used to make informed decisions. The author identifies techniques for obtaining follow-up information and the importance of data acquisition in deciding on program continuation or termination.

10. McTernan, E. J. Administration and supervision. In C. W. Ford and M. K. Morgan (Eds.), *Teaching in the Health Professions*, St. Louis: C. V. Mosby, 1976.

    A useful overview of the potential contribution of administration and supervision in allied health programs. The author identifies leadership and planning functions, sources and methods of funding, and coordinated organizational structure; describes the need for and utility of systematic evaluation; and reviews a rational approach to accountability.

11. McTernan, E. J. Clinical instruction in affiliated or cooperating institutions. In A. S. Knowles (Ed.), *Handbook of College and University Administration.* New York: McGraw-Hill Book Company, 1970.

    A description of the necessary prerequisites for administrative integration of interinstitutional allied health programs. The author identifies responsibilities, communicative routes, and methods of policy formulation and reviews the content of written affiliation agreements or contracts.

12. Moore, M. L.; Parker, M. M.; and Nourse, E. S. *Form and Function of Written Agreements in the Clinical Education of Health Professionals.* Thorofare, N. J.; C. B. Slack, 1972.

    An identification and clear description of the rationale and need for mutual philosophies of contractual or written agreements between educational institutions and clinical facilities.

13. Moore, M. L., and Perry, J. F. *Clinical Education in Physical Therapy: Present Status/Future Needs.* Final Report of the Project on Clinical Education in Physical Therapy. Washington, D.C.: American Physican Therapy Association, 1976.

Guidelines and standards, based on descriptive research data, on the selection and use of clinical facilities, selection and roles of clinical faculty, the process of clinical education, and the evaluation process in clinical education in physical therapy. This book is of significance to all allied health professionals.

14. Myers, C.; Shanon, P. P.; and Sunderstrom, C. Strategies in clinical teaching. *American Journal of Occupational Therapy,* 23 (January-February) 1969, 30-34.

An article on the educational concepts, teaching strategies, and advantages encountered in using a single-center approach to clinical education.

15. Pace, C. R. Educational objectives. In N. B. Henry (Ed.), *The Integration of Educational Experiences,* Fifty-seventh Yearbook of the National Society for the Study of Education, Part 3. Chicago: University of Chicago Press, 1958.

An identification of the characteristics and value of integrative objectives, conditions affecting their potency, and methods to translate them into effective organization.

16. Postlethwait, S. N.; Novak, J. D.; and Murray, H. T., Jr. *The Audio-Tutorial Approach to Learning— Through Independent Study and Integrated Experiences.* 3rd ed. Minneapolis: Burgess Publishing Company, 1972.

A description of the course structure, physical facilities, and operational aspects of a multisensory individualized approach to learning in a college botany course, including examples of study units and materials.

17. Scanlan, C. L., and Clark, D. W. A respiratory therapy learning laboratory. *Respiratory Care, 19* (May) 1974, 347-353.

Details on the necessary prerequisites, theoretical basis, and application of an open learning laboratory as an integrated part of a respiratory therapy curriculum in a community college.

18. Schweer, J. E., and Gebbie, K. M. *Creative Teaching in Clinical Nursing.* 3rd ed. St. Louis: C. V. Mosby, 1976.

A review and application of the various methodology for the selection, planning, design, organization, and evaluation of clinical learning experiences to meet varying levels of student ability and achievement.

19. Segall, A. J.; Vanderschmidt, H.; Burglass, R.; and Frostman, T. *Systematic Course Design for the Health Fields.* New York: John Wiley and Sons, 1975.

A seminal work in allied health education. This book provides an overview of a competency-based course model and details implementation problems and methods to facilitate application. A succinct guidance system provides step-by-step procedures and expectations for the identified phases of course development. The author includes a finished example of a single unit of instruction.

20. Tyler, R. W. *Basic Principles of Curriculum and Instruction.* Chicago: University of Chicago Press, 1950.

An identification of the systematic development of curriculum strategies based on four fundamental educational questions. Emphasis is on evaluation of specific outcomes to assess achievement of desired goals.

21. Tyler, R. W. Curriculum organization. In N. B. Henry (Ed.), *The Integration of Educational Experiences,* Fifty-seventh Yearbook of the National Society for the Study of Education, Part 3. Chicago: University of Chicago Press, 1958.

A review of the meaning, purpose, and dimensions of curriculum organization. The author describes the identification of basic elements, organizing principles, and structure that facilitate integration of learning experiences.

APPENDIX A

Criteria for evaluation and selection of clinical affiliates*

1. The clinical agency's philosophy and objectives for patient care and education must be similar to and compatible with those of the educational institution.
2. The clinical agency must demonstrate support of and interest in the educational program(s).
3. Communication within the clinical agency itself should be effective and positive.
4. The affiliate service department should provide an active, stimulating environment appropriate for the learning needs of the student.
5. The affiliate service department should have an active and viable process of internal evaluation of its own affairs and should be receptive to procedures of review approved by approximate external agencies.
6. Consumers should be satisfied that their needs for the designated service are being met.
7. Selected support services should be available to affiliating students.
8. Adequate space for study, conferences, and patient treatment should be available to affiliating students.
9. Programs for affiliating students should be planned to meet the specific objectives of the curriculum and the student.
10. The clinical agencies must have a sufficient variety of learning experiences available to affiliating students.
11. The staff of the clinical agency must maintain ethical standards of practice.
12. The roles of the various affiliate departmental personnel must be clearly defined and distinguished from one another.
13. There should be an active staff development program for the clinical agency.
14. The staff of the affiliate service department should be interested and active in professional associations.
15. The staff of the affiliate service department must possess the expertise to provide quality patient care and, where required, be of adequate size to provide appropriate supervision/instruction.
16. One staff member of the affiliate service department should be designated to coordinate the activities of the students at the clinical agency.
17. Selection of clinical instructor/supervisors must be based on specific criteria.
18. Clinical instructor/supervisors must be able to apply the basic principles of education to clinical learning.
19. The special expertise of the various clinical agency staff members should be shared with the affiliating students.
20. The clinical agency must be committed to the principles of equal opportunity and affirmative action as required by federal legislation.

*Adapted from Moore, M. L., and Perry, J. F. *Clinical Education in Physical Therapy: Present Status/Future Needs*. Washington, D.C.: American Physical Therapy Association, 1976.

Responsibilities of the coordinator of clinical education*

1. Organizes, directs, supervises, and coordinates the clinical education program of the curriculum:
   a. Establishes procedures, guidelines, and manuals for the clinical education component of the curriculum
   b. Schedules students for clinical education and coordinates schedules among affiliates.
   c. Serves as liaison between the academic and the clinical faculty:
      (1) Assists the clinical faculty in planning student learning experiences
      (2) Relates curriculum objectives to the clinical affiliates in order to make clinical education relevant and coordinated
      (3) Maintains communication with the affiliates in the interest of the students
   d. Coordinates and participates in an ongoing evaluation program for the clinical education experience:
      (1) Evaluates student performance by developing valid and reliable evaluation devices and feedback mechanisms
      (2) Grades students
      (3) Evaluates the clinical education experience (the clinical faculty and the facility) by developing evaluation devices and feedback mechanisms
   e. Works cooperatively with clinical coordinators in other health disciplines
2. Develops the clinical affiliates and clinical faculty members:
   a. Develops new clinical affiliates by various means
   b. Maintains optimal functioning of clinical facilities in regard to clinical education through:
      (1) Rapport with administrators, physicians, and service department staff
      (2) Frequent visits to the clinical affiliates in the interest of development and maintenance of working relationships
      (3) Feedback from the evaluation of the clinical faculty members and supervisors
   c. Works to secure college and university recognition and appointment and privileges for clinical faculty members
   d. Assists the clinical faculty members in developing and perfecting their teaching, education, and communication skills
3. Develops students through guidance and counseling:
   a. Counsels students on an interactive personal basis
   b. Assists students in understanding and benefiting from evaluation of their clinical performance
   c. Assists students with career needs and job placement
   d. Conducts seminars for students on topics relevant to their clinical experiences
4. Functions as a didactic teacher and a faculty member:
   a. Teaches in the basic didactic curriculum
   b. Develops and evaluates learning materials, including audiovisual and other educational media
   c. Plans and teaches in continuing education programs of benefit to faculty, staff, students, clinical faculty, and the allied health community (may serve as chairperson of the department's committee on continuing education)
   d. Plans and teaches in the in-service education program of the academic institution and clinical affiliates
5. Participates as a member of allied health and institutional faculty in appropriate ways:
   a. Performs administrative roles as requested or necessary:
      (1) Assists with the writing of grant proposals
      (2) Assists with the preparation of the proposed departmental meetings
   b. Attends and participates in required departmental meetings
   c. Serves as liaison between the allied health program and the professional community
   d. Serves on and participates in the affairs of departmental committees

*Adapted from Moore, M. L., and Perry, J. F. *Clinical Education in Physical Therapy: Present Status/Future Needs.* Washington, D.C.: American Physical Therapy Association, 1976.

APPENDIX C
ORGANIZING CENTER: MAINTAINING TISSUE OXYGENATION

Professional didactic	Support didactic	Learning laboratory	Clinical experience
Applied characteristics of oxygen	*Chemistry*—molecular structure, molecular weight, physical properties *Physics*—thermal conductivity	Principles of gas analysis: Katharometer Electrochemical reduction Paramagnetism	Safety precautions in oxygen administration Measurement of F_IO_2's
Physiological need for oxygen	*Physiology*—cellular metabolism	Measurement of oxygen consumption—open and closed circuit Measurement of respiratory quotient	*Data review*—hypoxemia as cause of mortality; physiological effects of hypoxia
Oxygen storage and supply	*Chemistry*—change of state, critical temperature, critical pressure *Physics*—adiabatic compression, kinetic molecular theory, expansion cooling, measurement of gas pressures	Cylinder and manifold systems; safety and handling of compressed gases Regulator and flowmeter principles, use and comparison	Bulk oxygen delivery systems, zone valves, alarms, compressed gas storage facilities
Oxygen therapy modalities	*Physics*—fluid dynamics Bernoulli theorem Venturi application	Practice set up, application, use of assorted therapeutic apparatus; quantify their effects	Observation of therapeutic modalities in clinical usage; overview of general problems in oxygen administration
Treatment of patients with hypoxemia due to hypoventilation	*Physiology*—relationship between ventilation and oxygenation *Pathology*—causes of alveolar hypoventilation	End expired gas analysis: hyperventilation, breathholding, hypoventilation	Assisted ventilation in the management of hypoventilation: drug overdose, CNS depressing, severe obesity
Treatment of patients with hypoxemia due to diffusion limitation	*Physiology*—limitations to diffusion *Pathology*—causes of diffusion impairments	Methods of delivering high partial pressures of oxygen Measurement of diffusing capacity	Oxygen therapy in the management of diffusion limitation: fibrosis, pulmonary edema
Treatment of patients with hypoxemia due to ventilation-perfusion inequalities	*Physiology*—distribution of ventilation and perfusion *Pathology*—maldistribution of gases in obstruction, abnormalities of the pulmonary circulation	Measurement of physiological deadspace (Bohr method) Estimates of shunt fraction	Oxygen therapy in the management of ventilation-perfusion inequalities: COPD, asthma

APPENDIX D

Student process questionnaire

Course _____ Date _____

Students are an important part of the evaluation process in education. We continually need your assistance in refining, revising, and improving instruction. Please be frank and honest in reacting to the following statements. *SA* means you strongly agree; *A* means you agree; *U* means you are uncertain; *D* means you disagree; and *SD* means you strongly disagree.

Circle the response you believe is most appropriate. Comment, if you like, on any of the responses at the end of the questionnaire.

1. Everyone at the clinical affiliates knows what is expected of us.   SA A U D SD
2. The objectives for this course are too detailed.   SA A U D SD
3. The instructors are always demonstrating how things relate to one another.   SA A U D SD
4. I think the learning laboratory is a waste of time.   SA A U D SD
5. I have plenty of opportunities in this course to do the things I want.   SA A U D SD
6. I think the clinical instructors should go to class once in a while.   SA A U D SD
7. Even when they are used as a test, I learn a great deal from the simulations.   SA A U D SD
8. I don't see any relationship between this course and any other I've taken.   SA A U D SD
9. I always feel well prepared before I go for clinical instruction.   SA A U D SD
10. Case studies are basically busywork.   SA A U D SD
11. I see a close relationship between what we do in class and what we do in the clinical affiliates.   SA A U D SD
12. The class instructor should spend more time in the hospital.   SA A U D SD
13. I am always made aware of exactly what the goals are for each section of instruction.   SA A U D SD
14. I can't wait until all this theory is done, so we can actually get involved in what we're supposed to be doing.   SA A U D SD
15. We need more problem-solving situations and fewer facts.   SA A U D SD
16. I really sense that everything is starting to fit together for me.   SA A U D SD
17. The learning laboratory helps me understand what is expected of me in the clinical setting.   SA A U D SD
18. The instructors should practice what they preach about relating different aspects of the program.   SA A U D SD
19. I think the seminar really helps me understand the clinical application of classroom theory.   SA A U D SD
20. The clinical scheduling is too inflexible.   SA A U D SD

10

INTEGRATING DIDACTIC AND CLINICAL EDUCATION—LOW PATIENT CONTACT

Patricia J. Pierce
Shirley A. Eichenwald

The designers of clinical education for a low patient contact profession would do well to read the previous chapter, which focuses on high patient contact professions. The history, philosophy, and general concepts covered in Chapter 9 can be applied to all allied health education and so are not repeated here. This chapter addresses only the particular needs and problems that the allied health educator in a low patient contact profession may encounter in integrating didactic and clinical components in a course.

Low patient contact professions are specifically those allied health professions that do not focus on direct patient contact but rather involve the establishment and maintenance of support systems for direct patient care providers. Medical record administrators, for example, design, maintain, and control an information support system. Medical technologists assume responsibility for the performance and control of laboratory analyses designed to detect the presence, course, and extent of pathological conditions.

Although direct patient care is not a function of all allied health professionals, Osler's quote in the Preface of this book has equal applicability to the support professions and might be restated as:

To study disease without books is to sail an uncharted course, but to study books without the re-

ality of the patient care setting is not to go to sea at all.

For those with a more analytical mind, the quote has been numerically expressed in the formula $P - P = 0$: Principles without Practice equals Zero.

It is the dynamics of the patient care environment (clinical setting) that legitimately exposes any allied health student to the interrelationship of knowledge and practice. So, it is in that setting that the student's level of professional competence can be best developed and evaluated.

This chapter focuses on how clinical exposure, beginning with the first year of the educational program, can be more effectively integrated with classroom theory. The model presented is one approach to the design and implementation of such a plan. Although it has not been fully evaluated, the model has merit on the basis of extant research.

DEFINITION OF INTEGRATED CLINICAL EXPERIENCE

In this chapter, *integrated clinical experience* is defined as the component of clinical education in which classroom theory and associated clinical experiences are drawn together in the same time frame. This means that the specially designed clinical activities that complement theoretical instruction are carried out not only *during* the span of time covered by the course, but also *as soon as possible* after the presentations of related theory. This definition adds a new dimension to the traditional block affiliation (period of time ranging from weeks to months, quarters, or semesters).

The concept of integrated didactic and clinical experiences has been interpreted in a traditional manner as the integration in a short or extended clinical experience of all the concepts and skills learned in the classroom or simulation laboratory prior to the clinical experience. In this way, students have an opportunity to obtain a clearer picture of how the various parts blend into a whole and how those parts blend in different ways in different settings into an acceptable procedure or total operation. This interpretation of the integration concept is valid and necessary to the learning process. Although this interpretation is well accepted and, indeed, is already applied in allied health educational programs, it is not addressed in detail here because local circumstances (e.g., number of clinical facilities, number of students, program philosophy) make it difficult to produce a universally acceptable model.

The concept of integrating theory and clinical education as presented in this chapter has as its objective the immediate reinforcement of classroom learning by application in the clinical setting. It is, therefore, a technique for increasing the effectiveness of learning. Although teachers like to believe they are lighting lamps of knowledge, nothing becomes real until it is experienced. The closer the experience is to the acquisition of knowledge, the more effectively it contributes to the learning process. The reality of the clinical setting clarifies the student's image, born of didactic instruction, of how things are or may be.

SURVEY OF INTEGRATION PRACTICE

To what extent has the practice of integrating clinical and didactic instruction permeated allied health education? Our survey of medical record programs sheds light on this subject. Though the survey reflects the responses of only one allied health field, it provides insights into the general effectiveness of this process that may benefit other allied health educators who are seeking ways to enhance clinical components of their programs.

Of the 100 existing accredited medical record programs, 61% responded to the survey. Of the respondents 60% reported some integration of clinical experience with classroom instruction. The responses imply positive support for the concept from program faculty. Especially gratifying is the general enthusiasm reported by students for this approach to clinical education. Additional references to this survey are made as they relate to specific topics.

INTRODUCTION TO AN INTEGRATION MODEL

An integration model was developed by faculty members and clinical consultants in conjunction with the implementation of a totally revised curriculum in medical record administration at the College of St. Scholastica in Duluth, Minnesota. The model is not presented as a unique approach to clinical integration, but rather as an example of a systematic method of assuring such integration within a curriculum.

Premises for model design

The model design incorporates three specific premises that serve as its structural framework. These premises are briefly described here to set the stage for discussion of the model itself.

Premise 1. Not every knowledge area requires accompanying skill-building activities. Moreover, in those areas where skill building or practical application is desired, activities can often best be designed, performed, and evaluated in simulated laboratory settings rather than in the clinical facility. Therefore, it is a basic premise of this model that activities defined for clinical exposure be only those which in the judgment of the course instructor are best carried out in the clinical setting (i.e., when an essential objective of the activity cannot be adequately met in a simulated laboratory setting or a needed resource is not available in the simulated setting).

Premise 2. Learning is more effective when activities designed for application of knowledge are closely aligned with the actual didactic presentation. Those activities defined for clinical settings should be scheduled to occur immediately after the didactic presentation of related material, and they should be structured in such a way as to focus specifically on application of classroom theory.

Premise 3. The clinical instructor defines the experience, but an academic faculty member designated as clinical coordinator is necessary to manage activities. These activities include scheduling of experiences desired by different instructors and making frequent determinations of the reactions, evaluations, and problems of the clinical supervisors. In short, the clinical coordinator needs to ensure a balance between the needs of the educational institution and the clinical facility. Such a balance maximizes satisfaction while minimizing conflicts and changes in scheduling. The tendency of the clinical supervisor who has little contact with the coordinator may be to adapt the student's experience to the situation that exists on any given day rather than to follow the prescribed schedule. This is often done with the best of intentions and motivation but generally defeats the objectives of the particular learning experience.

This premise assumes that the clinical experience is supervised by professional personnel from the clinical facility. This supposition was substantiated in the survey by 100% of those who use several sites.

THE MODEL

The very base of an integration model must be a clear definition of the course objectives and activities that are needed for developing and evaluating desired student behaviors. Each faculty member is responsible for ensuring the strength of this base. Therefore, an integral part of the definition of each course is the instructor's specification of learning activities appropriate to each unit of material and the designation of those activities best carried out in the clinical setting. Careful consideration must also be given to the use of simulation techniques in the classroom or in laboratory sessions. If simulation techniques would help the student meet the desired objectives, then placing the student in the clinical setting is placing an unnecessary burden on the time of clinical instructors and on the space in clinical facilities.

Clinical activity plan

Once the decision is firmly made that a clinical activity is what is needed, the clinical activity can be outlined in considerable detail. Appendix A (p. 141) is a sample of a clinical activity planning outline that has been completed by the course instructor. The instructor should complete a separate outline for each clinical activity identified. Through documentation of each item (i.e., course title, unit number, learning objectives, etc.), the instructor can define the activity sufficiently to guarantee its relevance to the course objectives and to establish an appropriate evaluation methodology for it.

Survey findings revealed that in those programs that are integrating clinical experiences, the faculty member who designs the course assumes responsibility for identifying the objectives, designating the required hours of clinical practice, timing the clinical activities in relation to classroom schedules, and determining the method of clinical evaluation.

This model may be used to send any number of students to only one or two clinical sites. However, the health care system in a given locale generally offers a variety of facilities that in the aggregate utilize each type of allied health professional. Fully realizing that professionals may function somewhat differently in each facility, program faculty often specifically elect to use several clinical sites for each activity, with only a small number of students going to each site. A significant advantage of using a variety of sites for clinical activities is the opportunity for providing exposure to a diversity of systems and procedures that students can share and compare with one another in classroom discussion or seminar. In addition, exposure to a variety of facilities broadens the students' view of future job opportunities.

Indeed, survey findings showed that 78% of the medical record education programs attempting an integrated clinical component send students out in pairs or singly for these activities, and 86% use from three to fifty-five sites.

While the use of a variety of sites also reduces some of the time and space pressures on individual facilities and facilitates the accomplishment of an activity for the entire class within a short time span, it does increase the need for effective communication and coordination of effort between program and clinical facilities, simply because of the increased number of people involved as clinical faculty. Items addressed on the clinical activity planning outline (e.g., estimates of number of students, hours of student contact, approximate dates the activity will occur, etc.) are important items to have available when presenting the total clinical activity proposal to the sites for their consideration. The planning outline also effects complete and consistent communication and understanding of the intent of each activity between the program faculty and clinical faculty.

Clinical activity grid

When the instructor has completed the clinical activity planning outline, the clinical coordinator can chart each activity on a clinical activity grid. Appendix B (p. 142) is a sample of the clinical activity grid for one quarter. The activity outlined in Appendix A is incorporated into the grid and is shown in relation to other clinical activities scheduled for the students at all levels within the program during the same quarter (semester). The grid is extremely helpful in pinpointing potential overloading of clinical facilities during specific periods of time during the quarter (semester). As it is analyzed by both program and clinical faculty, areas for scheduling adjustments can be recognized and appropriate changes made to assure even distribution of students in the clinical facility over the quarter (semester).

A major premise of this integration model is that clinical activities are scheduled as soon as possible after the presentation of preparatory

theoretical material in the classroom. Therefore, any readjustment in the scheduling of clinical activities must be reflected in the timing of the presentation of related classroom material. Therefore, the course instructor and the clinical coordinator must have a close working relationship with opportunity for frequent communication.

Statement of projected time commitment

At this point in the process, the clinical coordinator also develops a total projected time commitment for integrated clinical activities specific to each clinical site. The potential exists for considerable variability in the number of integrated activities planned for each facility. The specification of total hours of instructional commitment for each facility is an essential consideration at the point of contract negotiation.

Establishing the clinical relationship

With the completion of these three steps (i.e., preparation of a clinical activity planning outline for each course, completion of a clinical activity grid for each quarter or semester, and development of a total projected time commitment for each clinical site), the clinical coordinator must take action to establish the desired relationships with identified potential clinical sites. Practicing professionals selected as clinical instructors in these facilities should be introduced by the clinical coordinator to the integration concept and given an opportunity to review those clinical activity planning outlines specified for their facility and to analyze the clinical activity grid for each quarter (semester) in which their involvement is desired. Whether this is done on an individual basis with each practitioner or in a group session is a decision based primarily on local preference. In any case, the clinical coordinator must recognize that this initial contact is crucial to establish acceptance of the concept and commitment for participation by the clinical instructor.

For a long-term affiliation, a formal contract with the clinical facility is generally necessary. Likewise, to establish stability in the operation of this model, a signed, ongoing clinical agreement is best negotiated with each facility, even though the contact with that facility may be for only one or two activities each year. This agreement can be an addendum to an already existing agreement for block clinical experiences or a single agreement negotiated with a site that is utilized solely for one or more clinical activities. A sample agreement is presented in Appendix C (p. 143). Because the total number of projected instructional hours per facility is incorporated into the agreement, any significant change in hours necessitates renegotiation of the agreement. (See Appendix D, p. 144.)

The next step in establishing the clinical relationship is confirmation of the procedure to be used by the clinical coordinator in establishing the specific schedule for each activity each quarter (semester). Covered by this procedure must be the name of the person to be contacted for each activity at the facility, a minimum notification time required for making each arrangement, the mechanism for confirming dates and/or times and the names of students assigned to the site for each activity, and a provision for emergency cancellation and rescheduling of activities. The procedure can be standardized to a great degree; however, allowances for individual facility preferences should be made.

Each instructor has the following continuing responsibilities:

1. To notify the clinical coordinator as early as possible in the quarter (semester) of the specific time frame in which each clinical activity needs to occur in order to be integrated with related classroom presentation(s). This notification initiates the procedure(s) as described previously.

2. To present the activity descriptions and all materials to be given to students to the clinical coordinator for dissemination and discussion with the clinical faculty.

With all of these items in hand, it is desirable for the clinical coordinator to meet with the clinical instructors individually or in a group to clarify the intent of each activity.

When the activity schedule has been finalized with the clinical sites, the clinical coordinator communicates these to the instructor, who in turn presents the activity description (i.e., objectives, methods of evaluation) along with related references, guide sheets, and/or special instructions to the class. Students are given the opportunity to sign for the facility, date, and time of their choice. The clinical coordinator finishes the arrangements by presenting to the clinical instructor the names of students scheduled for each site.

Evaluation

The final phase of the integration model is the establishment of a feedback loop for the system. The clinical coordinator needs to collect and process information from the students, program faculty, and clinical faculty on the value of each activity. Once this information is in, the clinical coordinator can join other program and clinical faculty members in analyzing it.

The first step in evaluation can be accomplished on a one-to-one basis (clinical coordinator with clinical instructor) at the conclusion of the activity. This should be followed by a combined program faculty and clinical faculty evaluation at the end of the quarter (semester). Student evaluation can be conducted on an activity reaction sheet immediately following the clinical activity and/or in conjunction with the full course evaluation. If, at any point, evaluation indicates low satisfaction with a clinical activity, the reasons must be closely analyzed and the activity revised or deleted to bring it into line with student and faculty needs and expectations.

CHALLENGES FOR IMPLEMENTATION OF THE MODEL

As with all new models, potential flaws may be detected in this model by the discerning educator. These flaws must be viewed as problems that challenge allied health educators to seek practical and creative resolutions. A few of the challenges awaiting the users of this model are already evident.

The cooperation of the clinical instructor in arranging and conducting a short-term experience directed toward a specific objective is essential. This requires close communication between the clinical instructor and clinical coordinator in the planning of such activities. In addition, the clinical instructor must agree with the basic philosophy or concept of integrated education. It is up to the program director (who, according to the survey results, often doubles as clinical coordinator) to assure this cooperation.

The number of clinical sites available close to the academic setting, the number of other academic sites close to the clinical site, and the number of students in each educational program tend to affect the ease with which integrated education is implemented. To avoid overloading any one site, it would be well for the program to seek out nontraditional settings that would be appropriate for a single short-term experience as defined by the established objectives (e.g., industrial labs).

Because of the limited clinical possibilities, an experience related to a specialized area such as psychiatry presents a greater than usual problem in integration. However, the clinical experience can be divided into many smaller parts, some of which will be the same whether or not they are encountered in a mental health facility. Some parts can, therefore, be conducted in a more general environment, (e.g., an acute care facility), and the student can make the necessary assimilation in longer clinical affiliation experiences in a mental health facility. The integration model demonstrated can turn this forced division of clinical activities into very short, specific experiences leading to successful, integrated learning. The clinical coordinator, therefore, can attack a seemingly impossible task of this nature by questioning whether the experience desired actually is *many* activities which, considered separately, can be made workable through the integration model.

Flexibility on the part of both program and clinical faculty in establishing specific dates and times for accomplishing clinical activities is certainly a paramount consideration. The clinical coordinator should assure such flexibility through the establishment of good rapport between the program and the clinical facility. Early planning and notification of clinical needs with clinical facilities are essential to flexibility in scheduling.

Postclinical evaluation by the clinical coordinator and constant feedback to both clinical and program faculty are absolute necessities to the ongoing improvement of clinical activities. Continued cooperation of the clinical instructors directly affects the smooth functioning of the system. This cooperation is assured by clinical instructors' satisfaction with the system.

Problems encountered by those who responded to the survey included the following:

1. Variations in clinical resources and practices that could not be resolved by faculty-student discussion in the academic setting
2. Poor communication between program and clinical personnel
3. Scheduling problems brought about by personnel absences at the clinical site
4. Changes made at the clinical site to include experiences involving principles or skills the student had not yet learned
5. Timing problems
6. Difficulty in getting the same experience for all students at the same time
7. Exploitation of students and the lack of college control at the clinical site

These problems are all related to the challenges delineated and can be resolved chiefly through the efforts of an effective clinical coordinator. Significantly, the survey indicated that 47% of the respondents did not have clinical coordinators.

As indicated in the Prologue, the ideal is not always possible because of human limitations. But the ideal should still be the goal. In those instances in which continuous efforts to cooperate in establishing and maintaining quality clinical experiences are not meeting with success, they should be abandoned. More constructive efforts should be directed toward establishing new relationships at new sites.

SUMMARY

Integration of the didactic and clinical components occurs when classroom theory and associated clinical experience occur at the same time. The objective of such integration is the immediate reinforcement of classroom learning by application in the clinical setting. These integrated experiences are not meant to replace traditional block clinical affiliations but rather to complement them.

A model approach to integration is suggested. Three underlying premises of the model design and implementation are discussed:

1. Only those experiences that can better be learned in the clinical setting than in simulated laboratory settings should be included.
2. Well-defined clinical activities should occur frequently for short periods of time and immediately follow the didactic presentation.
3. A clinical coordinator has a vital role in maintaining satisfaction on the part of the instructors in both the classroom and clinical settings.

Problems in integrating classroom and clinical learning are recognized, but are seen as challenges that can be met without sacrificing the overall goal of establishing and maintaining quality education for students.

APPENDIX A

Clinical activity planning outline*

To be used by instructor and clinical coordinator in planning for clinical experience

Title of course: Storage and Retrieval Systems for Health Information
Course number: HIA 233
Unit: I and II

Objectives for clinical experience

At the end of the clinical experience, the student will be able to:
1. List the advantages and disadvantages of straight numeric and terminal digit filing.
2. Describe the filing controls utilized at the clinical site to control misfiles.
3. Determine space and equipment needs for a medical record file area if given information regarding variables.

Student activity preparation

1. Resources prepared by instructor (e.g., structured questionnaire):
   The student will be given guidelines for observation of the physical layout of a file area and filing/retrieval system in a medical record department.
2. Duties of clinical coordinator:
   a. Needs to make arrangements for student activities?
      Yes
   b. Needs to accompany students?
      No. This visit should involve primarily observation of physical equipment and will require minimal involvement of hospital or clinical personnel.

Sites

1. Types of health care facilities or agencies in which students can gain this experience: Hospital or large clinic
2. When during the quarter the clinical experience is needed: Early (week 3-4 of quarter)
3. Estimated number of hours needed for the clinical experience at each site: 2 hours
4. Approximate size of group at each site: 4 persons

Method of evaluation

The class will be divided into groups of four to five participants, each of which will observe file systems at different sites. The group will reconvene to discuss the systems and will be assigned a group project relating to Objective 3. Evaluation will be based on the report of the group.

*As used by the College of St. Scholastica, Duluth, MN.

APPENDIX B

Clinical activity grid*

Year: 1976-1977
Quarter: Spring
Months: April-May

Week of the quarter

Unit	1	2	3	4	5	6	7	8	9	10
HIA 233 Units I and II		Hospital and/or clinic → Filing systems								
HIA 233 Unit IV							Hospital and/or nursing home → Disease index			
HIA 313 Unit II				Hospital and/or nursing home → Utilization review						
HIA 313 Unit III	Hospital, clinic, and/or nursing home → Patient care audit									

*As used by the College of St. Scholastica, Duluth, MN.

APPENDIX C

Agreement for clinical education experience*

I. It is agreed that ____(name of clinical site)____ will participate in the clinical education for ____(name of program)____ from ____(name of college/university)____ .

II. It is agreed that the clinical education shall provide learning experiences that will give the student the opportunity to:
   A. Practice professional behavior by presenting a professional appearance and conducting himself or herself in a professional manner.
   B. Gain direct experience in establishing appropriate interpersonnel relationships in the professional environment.
   C. Observe the role of the medical record administrator or health care professional in the clinical setting.
   D. Apply medical record principles appropriately in intra- and interdepartmental medical record functions.

III. It is agreed that the ____(name of program)____ , ____(name of college/university)____ , will assume responsibility for:
   A. Preparation of the students through classroom instruction for clinical experience and for scheduling of students to the facility.
   B. Discipline of the students in the event of a misdemeanor, unethical conduct, and/or unbecoming conduct while assigned to ____(name of clinical site)____ .
   C. Provide the services of the clinical coordinator, ____(name of program)____ , ____(name of college/university)____ , as liaison between the College and ____(name of clinical site)____ .

IV. It is agreed that ____(name of clinical site)____ will, in turn, assume responsibility for:
   A. The supervision of the students by a qualified professional.
   B. Executing meaningful and appropriate learning experiences aimed at the stated objectives.
   C. Notify the college immediately in the event of any emergency or problems that may threaten the students' successful completion of the assignment(s).

V. It is agreed that the students in the ____(name of program)____ of the ____(name of college/university)____ , while on the assignment at ____(name of clinical site)____ , will assume responsibility for:
   A. Any living expenses during the assignment.
   B. Abiding by all facility rules and regulations regarding appearance and conduct, as explained to them.

VI. It is agreed that the ____(name of college/university)____ will provide liability insurance for the students during the assigned hours of clinical experience.

VII. This agreement will be reviewed annually and may be changed, amended, or revised by mutual agreement in writing.

VIII. This agreement may be terminated by either part upon notice, provided such notice is received before the end of the academic year preceding the one in which the termination is to become effective.

_____   _____
President   Administrator
(Name of college/university)   (Name of clinical facility)
Date _____   Date _____

_____   _____
Chairman of the Department   Director of Medical Record Services
(Name of college/university)   (Name of clinical facility)
Date _____   Date _____

*As used by the College of St. Scholastica, Duluth, MN.

APPENDIX D

Specific statement of responsibilities for other than full time directed practice*

_____(Name of clinical site)_____ agrees to provide facilities and materials for observation of select activities during the sophomore, junior, and senior years and to provide a person at a supervisory level for limited guidance and instruction in these select activities. Arrangements will be made through the department head for a time acceptable to both parties, but the actual responsibility for the student(s) may be delegated to a departmental supervisor.

The _____(name of college/university)_____ agrees to send sophomore, junior, and senior _____(name of program)_____ students to _____(name of clinical site)_____ during the academic school year in order to observe and/or participate in selected clinical experiences throughout the health facility. All experiences shall be arranged at a time convenient to both parties. In no instance shall more than four (4) students be present at one time, unless otherwise arranged, and there shall not be more than ____ educational instructional hours.

_____   _____

Clinical coordinator   Director of Medical Record Services
(Name of college/university)   (Name of clinical facility)

Date _____   Date _____

---

*This form is not applicable to full-time directed practice and affiliation experience. It is used by the College of St. Scholastica, Duluth, MN.

11

SIMULATION: A TECHNIQUE FOR INSTRUCTION AND EVALUATION

J. Dennis Hoban
John P. Casbergue

The health professions have taken great strides in the past ten to fifteen years to upgrade educational practices. Health educators have attempted to be responsive to students and faculty in terms of such issues as educational processes, curriculum structures, and evaluation methodologies. Many of the offices of educational development (or similar title) found in professional schools today were noticeably absent fifteen years ago.

Unfortunately, not all of the increased attention to education has been for the better. Rather, there remain many old ideas in the guise of new gimmicks. In a word, many promises have been made and few fulfilled. Jason laments this unfortunate situation and offers some suggestions:

The basic issue is that the automatic response of many medical educators has been the accommodation of conventional instruction to available technology. The pressing need is for continuous study and modification of the instructional process itself, with adaptation of technology to the needs of that instruction.

The conventional uses of technology have tended to reinforce the conventional approach to medical instruction: that is, the primary preoccupation has been with the transmission of information. One of the major changes now taking place in medical education is the growing awareness that in the domain of information-learning, acquisition is merely the first of three necessary steps. Simple acquisition of information at some point in time is of no value if the conditions have not been arranged for effective retention of that information and for its availability for transfer to a variety of different settings. A companion recognition is that retention and transfer are optimized by having the original acquisition occur in a setting that is maximally like the setting in which this knowledge will later be applied (pp. 739-740).[12]

Jason further points out that increased attention is being given to complex intellectual skills such as problem solving and decision making as well as interpersonal skills. Again, he argues that the student should be given opportunities to engage in the application of these skills in settings as realistic as possible.

A technique suggested by Jason, which offers an approximation of the real-life setting, is simulation. This technique is gaining wide acceptance in schools and in-service training programs in medicine, nursing, denistry, and the allied health fields. In the education of health professionals, simulation refers to the act of closely approximating and controlling some aspects of the practical realities of health care for purposes of accomplishing specific instructional objectives or evaluating specific performance competencies. These two uses of simulation technology are discussed in detail in this chapter.

Simulation technology attempts to bridge the gap between the abstract and the concrete. When used properly, it minimizes the complexity of real experiences by deleting details that distract the student from the task being learned or evaluated. At the same time, it maximizes retention of knowledge, transfer of training to actual settings, and the availability of numerous clinical experiences.

TYPES OF SIMULATION

In a recent study of simulation technology in medical education (including medical, dental, nursing, and allied health education) conducted by Maatsch and coworkers[16] five types of simulation used in health professionals education are identified.

Written simulations

Written simulations are usually presented in a paper-and-pencil format. A problem is presented and the student is asked to respond to a number of alternatives. After selecting a response alternative, the student receives feedback on the consequence of that action or is referred to another decision point. The flow of the problem follows the actual order of events, and the information and consequences are abstracted from actual events.

Example. Patient management problems described by McGuire and Solomon[19] are clinical problems constructed to simulate a clinical situation as closely as possible. Their format is that of a programmed tutorial. Problems are introduced with a patient complaint similar to that elicited from a patient or an accompanying friend or relative. A list of interventions or strategies to be employed follows the complaint. For example, in the problem the student needs to make decisions about the need for requesting further history, physical examination results, laboratory data, or to propose immediate therapy and the like. After making each decision, the student receives feedback regarding the decision and directions for proceeding through the problem. At the conclusion of each problem, the student receives explanatory comments and a consultant's advice on the workup and management of the patient.

Simulated patients

Some simulations involve real people trained to represent patients and their prob-
lems. These people are sometimes referred to as programmed patients or models. Such a person may have a detectable clinical problem or be an actor or fellow student trained to exhibit certain clinical symptoms. The simulated patient may be used to simulate a medical history including an emotional problem or to give feedback to students about pain or relief from specific physical techniques such as manipulations and physical examination maneuvers.

Example. Simulated patients are often trained to provide the student with feedback on interviewing skills. The simulated patient memorizes pertinent historical information and nonverbal behaviors. The patient then acts out a role in an interview with a student. This encounter is normally videotaped and played back. The simulated patient provides feedback to the student in terms of the appropriateness of the questions asked, the empathy expressed, the nonverbal behaviors exhibited, the degree of ease felt by the patient, and so forth. An independent observer is often present at such interviewing sessions to provide objective feedback on the inclusion or exclusion of student interviewing behaviors.

Computer simulations

Computer simulations usually present a complete patient case accessible by means of a remote terminal that uses natural language or codes. The student plays the role of a physician or nurse, while the computer presents patient information in response to the student's inquiries or orders.

Example. The Computer-Aided Simulations of the Clinical Encounter (CASE) was developed under the leadership of Harless.[6] A patient is presented via a printout, and the student is required to make decisions about acquiring additional history, getting data from a physical examination, requesting laboratory work, and making a therapeutic intervention. The student assumes the role of a practicing physician and uses everyday language to interact with the computer in order to elicit data and prescribe treatment. Based on the student's decision and command, the computer provides the information requested and asks the student to continue to engage in the problem-solving exercise. After the student completes the problem, feedback provided in the form of an ideal diagnosis and treatment of the case with which the student's handling of the case can be compared.

Audiovisual simulations

An audiovisual simulation presents a case, task, or problem that uses a single medium or multiple media (slides, videotape, film, etc.) to represent some aspects of reality. Visual and/or auditory cues generally represent the class of stimuli to which the student is expected to respond and about which the student will receive concrete feedback on appropriateness and consequences.

Example (single medium). Enelow and associates[5] describe an audiovisual simulation used to teach interviewing skills. In this simulation, patients are trained to present an interviewer with verbal and nonverbal information while being videotaped. Once made, the taped interview can be interrupted so that the viewer can be asked to choose between a number of possible actions the interviewer could take. Each action is shown on tape. The viewer records the action that seems most appropriate. Then the patient's response to each of the interviewer's actions is shown and a narrator comments on the appropriateness of each action. The taped interview concludes with a short exposition of the principles and techniques used to meet the instructional goals of that interview.

Example (multimedia). Problem boxes developed by Barrows and Mitchell[2] and patient games developed by Maatsch[17] are designed with a mixture of materials and aids students need to solve clinical problems. In the case of Maatsch's patient games, a physician plays the role of the patient, instructor, nurse, consultant, and information giver. The student plays the role of a physician. The game starts with a statement of the context and the patient's chief complaint. The student then elicits a history, followed by an interpretation of laboratory and physical examination data. Much of the data is presented via still pictures, videotape, 8 mm film, etc. Specially designed contingency reactions of the patient that might occur after inappropriate procedures or treatment are also available for the instructor to use.

When the patient game is completed, the physician critiques and evaluates the student's performance against key instructional objectives central to the simulation playing the patient and/or instuctor role.

The use of the health professional allows for flexibility not found in computer and written simulations. It also helps the student have access to the various media used to present information.

Mannequins

Another type of simulation is the use of lifelike models of some part of the body. Such simulations are designed to teach or evaluate a specific clinical skill. In many simulations of this type, interchangeable parts are used to introduce different pathological conditions or bodily functions. One of the main advantages of a mannequin simulator is that the student can practice a clinical skill as often as necessary for mastery with no risk of harm to a real patient.

Example. The IV Arm is a reproduction of an adult arm made of spongelike foam plastic and covered by flesh-colored latex. It is designed to help the student learn venipuncture. Two major surface veins are represented by rubber tubes molded into place. An innocuous fluid can be injected into the vein. Students receive feedback on their ability to perform venipuncture by observing whether or not the fluid comes out the tube at the end of the model.

USES OF SIMULATION

Two major educational functions of simulation are teaching and evaluation.

An instructional method

Instruction is mainly concerned with providing information and facilitating concept formation, skill learning, attitudinal change, and problem solving. As a method of clinical instruction, simulation can be used to facilitate (1) learning and retention, (2) transfer of training, (3) understanding, (4) attitude formation, and (5) motivation. These are best accomplished when the simulation incorporates the following four properties:

1. The student should respond sensitively to the stimulus in the simulation. For example, the learner interacting with a mannequin such as Gynny (the pelvic exam device) is expected to palpate the ovaries.

2. The spatial, tactile, chromatic, mobile, auditory, and/or temporal relationships found in the simulation should be analogous to real life. For example, a simulation such as the ophthalmoscopic model developed by Colenbrander[4] prepares students to use the ophthalmoscope. The model is made of styrofoam in the shape of a normal face with a nose, eyes, and a mouth. The eyes are proportioned realistically to allow students to use the ophthalmoscope to detect types of fundus pathology, which are represented by 35 mm slides placed behind the eye in the model.

Similarly, temporal relationships are illustrated in the simulation of ectopic pregnancy developed by Holzman (see Maatsch and others[16]). In this simulation the student is expected to take certain actions based on the fact that the patient's blood pressure is going down during a specified time span. If the student does not start an IV within a given amount of time, information is provided that indicates that the patient is deteriorating.

3. The fidelity of the critical properties and actual sequence of the activities in the simulation should be sufficient enough to assure that the activity being practiced transfers to real situations. For instance, Recording Resusci-Anne, an advanced cardiopulmonary resuscitation (CPR) simulation incorporates all essential diagnostic properties. Two critical properties found in this simulation device are a palpable carotid pulse and pupils that dilate and constrict. These two features are critical so that the rescuer can determine which emergency activity to perform. It is important in the training of basic life support first aid to recognize respiratory and cardiac arrest and to start the proper application of cardiopulmonary resuscitation. The prescribed sequence of events described in a

Journal of the American Medical Association supplement[11] is the ABC method to be used with unmonitored patients and witnessed cardiac arrests. The ABC method calls for opening the Airway, checking to see if the patient is Breathing (ventilate if not), and checking carotid pulse for Circulation (absence of pulse indicates the need to start artificial circulation by means of external cardiac compression).

4. Feedback to the students should provide them with information about the consequences of their actions. One form of feedback is sensory. Students can hear, touch, see, or smell something that allows them to judge the appropriateness of their actions. For example, the pelvic model, Gynny, has ovaries that can be placed in the model to simulate various conditions of health. By touching the ovary, students receive feedback about their ability to locate an ovary and to differentiate one state from another.

A second form of feedback is direct instructional intervention. An instructor, programmed patient, or mediated instructional package can provide information about the appropriateness of an action taken by the student. For instance, a female simulated patient who trains students to conduct a pelvic examination may use the following verbal feedback as students proceed with their examinations: "To the left" or "That's too hard" or "Warm the damn thing up."

A third form of feedback is a critique. This is conducted at the end of a simulation and may be oral or written or both. The critique provides the student with an opportunity to review what has been done correctly and incorrectly and to ask specific questions prompted by engaging in the simulation.

These four properties (student response, realism, fidelity of the critical properties, and feedback) represent variables that should be present to some degree for a simulation to be of instructional value to the student.

In implementing a simulation, the instructor needs to consider four important implementation procedures:

1. Specify the learning outcomes desired relevant to the health care area.
2. Determine if the simulation is applica-

ble to the specific educational context in which the instructor is teaching.

3. Plan for an evaluation of learning (i.e., the performance and/or attitudinal outcomes expected of the student participating in the simulation).

4. If applicable, assess the value of the simulation compared to other teaching methods formerly applied by the instructor.

Effectiveness of simulation as a teaching method. Simulation as an instructional method has been acknowledged to be a powerful learning tool. It is difficult, however, to judge whether or not simulation is cost beneficial without knowing the value of the learning outcome. It is worth noting that many of the dollar costs for simulations are hidden (i.e., space required, accessories, lighting, temperature and acoustical control, amortization of development costs, instructional time, and personnel costs). It is also worth remembering that most education has a high cost to effectiveness ratio.

A number of recent studies demonstrate the effectiveness of simulation as an instructional method in the health fields. Kretzschmar,[14] Johnson and associates,[13] and Holzman and coworkers[8] found that programmed simulated patients are as effective and in some areas more effective than traditional methods of teaching pelvic examination skills. Abrahamson and coworkers[1] demonstrated that SIM I, a computer-controlled patient (mannequin) simulator, is an effective method for training anesthesiology residents in the skill of endotracheal intubation. The two main advantages of SIM I are savings of time in training personnel and a decrease in threat to the patient's safety.

Penta and Kofman[20] show that simulators are effective in teaching certain physical examination skills. These authors conclude that a critical amount of practice time is needed for some simulators to increase student learning.

Other studies that lend support for simulation as an effective teaching method for accomplishing specific objectives in health professions education are reported by Enelow and coworkers[5] (interviewing), Helfer and associates,[7] (interviewing) and Tinning[21] (simulated patients).

An evaluation method

Irby and Dohner[9] point out that evaluation of clinical performance is one of the most complex areas of the learning process in the health professions. The use of simulations for improving the evaluation of clinical skills and attitudes has been increasing in the health professions (see Maatsch and Gordon[15] and Irby and Morgan[10]).

During use of a simulation for clinical evaluation purposes, the following principles should be applied:

1. The performance (knowledge, skill, or attitude) that is expected of the student at the end of training should be specified along with the minimal acceptable level of performance the student is required to demonstrate. For example, in a simulation designed to assess a student dietitian's ability to function as a therapist, the following specifications might be appropriate:

   a. Given a (simulated) patient, the student dietitian will be able to explain a dietary plan without error.

   b. Given a (simulated) patient, the student dietitian will be able to assess without error a dietary plan constructed by the patient.

   c. Given a (simulated) patient, the student dietitian will be able to explain without error necessary changes needed in the patient's constructed diet plan.

2. The simulation should represent reality with enough fidelity to assure face validity of the test of the student's performance. For instance, suppose students are being evaluated on their ability to indirectly examine the larynx. Further suppose that a simulation device such as the Laryngeal Model, consisting of a head and neck mounted on a wooden base and having a retractable tongue, is being used to assess this skill. The simulation should provide a realistic gag reflex that would impede the examination if the pharynx is touched by one of the examinees. If such a gag reflex is not built into the simulation, the assessment of a

student's ability to perform such an examination is questionable.

3. The simulation being used to evaluate student performance should be standardized: the simulation should produce the same kind of responses from a variety of students and provide the same feedback to students when they engage in similar activities. This principle is especially important when simulated patients are being used for assessment. For example, assume different simulated patients are being used to assess different students' abilities to open an interview with a compliant patient. Each patient should be trained to give similar responses to those behaviors being performed by the student interviewer and to portray similar relevant patient characteristics so as not to elicit dissimilar student behaviors. A simulated patient should exhibit the characteristic of compliance and not characteristics found in hostile, passive, or reluctant patients. Likewise, the simulated patients should respond to verbal and nonverbal student behaviors in similar ways, so that the simulations are about the same for each student. If the student greets the simulated patient with an authentic smile, each patient should react in the same manner to the smile so that the conditions for each student are about the same. If done, the final assessment of opening an interview with a compliant patient can be reliably assessed for all students and not be contaminated by a role shift by a simulated patient.

4. Decisions regarding the purpose of the evaluation should be made before a simulation is used. Maatsch,[17] in discussing simulation as an evaluation tool, makes a distinction between two forms: formative and summative.

Formative evaluation is an in-depth individualized assessment of clinical knowledge and skills, generally used for diagnostic evaluation. The postsimulation critique can be viewed as this type of evaluation, and assignments can be made to students to correct deficiencies uncovered by it.

Summative evaluation (e.g., final grades and certifying examinations) is also an in-depth appraisal of clinical skills. The primary emphasis in this form of evaluation is, however, in-depth appraisal against specified standards for the purpose of grading or certifying a student.

While the processes for formative and summative evaluations may be the same, the purposes are distinctly different. Because of the difference in purposes, the attitudes of the instructor and student are also different. In the former, the attitude of the instructor is supportive; in the latter, it is judgmental. Hence the instructor must decide on the purpose of the evaluation before using a simulation.

ADVANTAGES, BENEFITS, AND DISADVANTAGES
Advantages

Simulation as a method for clinical instruction and evaluation has a number of clear advantages over other instructional/evaluational methods.

Perhaps the most important advantage is the low risk it presents to students and patients. By using simulation, an instructor can free students from concern that they may make a sick patient uncomfortable while they learn a skill or procedure. By using a simulation for instructional purposes, students can practice over and over again until the skill or procedure is perfected without subjecting a patient to needless abuse or errors.

A second advantage simulation provides is relevancy. In nearly all health-related fields, a frequent lament of students is that little clinical contact is available in early stages of the curriculum. By utilizing simulations, clinical skills can become part of early training at least on a limited basis. Newly acquired skills and knowledge can be practiced and student motivation and interest can be maintained at a high level.

Another important advantage of simulation in the training of health professionals is the promise that what is learned in the simulation will transfer to real-world situations. For example, the therapeutic skills that the occupational therapist learns and practices by interacting with simulated patients will be the same skills that can be confidently employed with a real patient.

Finally, simulation provides a standard against which a student can be evaluated—the simulation itself. Barrows and Abrahamson write that:

[simulation] offers the far more important advantage of guaranteeing that the patient is constant for all students being tested. Thus, faculty may far more easily determine the strengths and weaknesses of the teaching program through a careful analysis of the types of errors made by students. In addition, records of the performance by individual students may be readily analyzed for purposes of further individual instruction and counseling. While it is true that other techniques of measurement of clinical performance may be used similarly, the virtual elimination of the variable of patient behavior seems to make the use of the programmed patient a most effective evaluative tool (p. 805).[3]

Benefits for the learner

Simulation provides an almost optimal opportunity for the learner to move from being a passive recipient of knowledge to being an active participant in the application of knowledge, skill, and/or attitude.

Simulation further requires the learner to apply knowledge and make sense of facts learned in other situations, as well as to ensure that adequate and appropriate facts have been collected, analyzed, and evaluated. The learner has increased opportunity to seek and test alternative solutions for any given situation or circumstance. The reader might contrast these aspects or opportunities with other instructional methods, such as lecture, independent study, and the seminar. This point is not raised to criticize these approaches but rather to critically evaluate the instructional methods that can be used to help students learn.

Simulation provides situations in which success depends on the learner taking certain actions or exhibiting certain attitudes, behaviors, or skills. Successful completion of the simulation provides positive reinforcement of these actions by providing the learner with the opportunity to experience success of accomplishment—not just to receive a "good grade."

Simulation can also prepare students for future roles. An example might be that of providing students in allied health with role-playing experience in health team planning, leadership, and participation. This approach to patient care is evolving slowly, but promises to be a part of future medical care. It may not be available to students in many of the schools of allied health, but rather than omitting the experience or relying only on print material, an instructor can use a role-playing simulation to prepare students for team membership.

Benefits for the instructor

Simulation experiences not only appear to benefit the student, but also can be a way for clinical instructors to increase their own teaching effectiveness. They must make decisions about what is to be learned, what details are most and least important, how the students know whether or not they have done a good job, and how feedback should be provided.

Such a systematic approach to planning educational activities is desirable but seldom taken. Nonetheless, clinical instructors who have designed simulations or used simulations designed by others report considerable enrichment of their planning for other instructional approaches (i.e., lecturing, laboratory, and evaluation).

Another benefit of simulation is the control it provides instructors over complex learning tasks. In other words, instructors can graduate the difficulty of the task by introducing more complexity as students master portions of the task.

Similarly, the use of simulation in early clinical training helps the instructor control the distractions found in the real world. For example, if an instructor is trying to teach a student in a busy hospital or clinic, numerous distractions such as visitors, other patients, and other health professionals may interfere with the student's learning. In such a busy environment, it is difficult for the student to sort out the important from the unimportant and to concentrate on the task of learning a clinical skill.

Simulations also provide a wide range of clinical experiences that may not be available at any given time during an educational program.

Other benefits for instructors obviously exist. Those just mentioned, however, are consistently recognized as major benefits by those writing about simulations in health professions education.

Disadvantages

A number of arguments have been leveled against the use of simulation. Although this chapter is written with a very positive attitude toward simulation, it would be incomplete if some potential disadvantages were not presented. Four disadvantages adapted from Twelker[22] are presented:

1. Generally, the acquisition of facts can be more efficiently learned through use of other instructional methods.

2. The cost of simulation is a disadvantage. Costs can be thought of as materials cost, design cost, and purchase cost. If instructors design a simulation, materials and design time should be costed out and weighed against the potential benefit for the student and budgetary constraints. Purchase costs should also be determined and weighed against budgetary constraints and the demonstrated effectiveness of the simulation under consideration.

3. Simulation may force the instructor to engage in an unfamiliar teaching role. Unfamiliar roles are often looked upon with great suspicion. When using a simulation, the instructor may become a manager of contingencies, such as playing the role of a patient and evaluating a student's performance based on objectives. Some instructors may find this difficult to do.

4. Finally, simulations available commercially often have little data supporting their effectiveness or clear instructions on how to use them. Hence, it is difficult to evaluate or use them.

These disadvantages represent points to consider when trying to decide if a simulation is an appropriate and realistic choice for instructing or evaluating students.

DESIGNING SIMULATIONS
What to simulate

Before addressing the question of how to go about designing a simulation, a designer must first confront the difficult question of what to simulate. This first question involves the process of subtraction, while the second involves abstraction. Maatsch[18] explains that the answer to the *what* question involves an iterative series of trade-offs between practical considerations, instructional objectives, and learning principles. The key element in the trade-off process is the designer's ability to determine how little of the real world can be simulated without materially affecting the specific objectives of instruction before beginning to make trade-offs involving cost, feasibility, and instructional principles. In essence, the designer must identify what can be subtracted from the real-world situation without significantly affecting the student's learning or the predictive validity of the simulation when used as an evaluation tool.

The design of simulations based on a *general* instructional objective such as "the student will be able to draw blood from all patients of different age groups" requires a complex arrangement of components such as needles, simulated patients or mannequins, and so forth, with which the learner must interact and about which the learner must make decisions. On the other hand, if a simulation is designed for a *specific* instructional objective such as "the student will be able to draw blood from an infant's heel," only those aspects of the environment that support the skill being taught or evaluated need be provided. Needless to say, the more specific the instructional objective, the less complicated will be the arrangement of a simulated environment (the greater the portion of reality that can be subtracted).

Once the objectives of the simulation have been determined, half of the what question has been answered. Now, the designer needs to determine what relevant cues will support the student's interaction with those aspects of reality being simulated. For instance, in designing a simulation that allows a student to practice drawing blood from an infant's heel, the designer must decide on the cues needed to help the student attend to that aspect of reality being simulated and assist in the recall and application of relevant knowledge.

Another form of cue to be considered in the design of a simulation is a feedback cue. Such a cue functions to guide students to perceive the consequences of their actions. In the case of the student drawing blood from a simulated foot, the feedback cue could be the observed flow of an innocuous liquid from a tube in the foot into a capillary tube.

Three important questions help the designer to determine what to simulate:

1. What are the instructional/evaluation objectives?
2. What are the critical cues needed to assist the student in interacting with that aspect of reality being simulated in order to teach/evaluate skills relevant to the objective(s)?
3. What feedback cues are necessary to allow the students to perceive the consequences of their actions?

When these questions are answered, the designer is ready to address the question of how to design the simulation.

How to simulate

When deciding how to simulate a real-world environment, problem, or task, the designer must analyze what is being simulated and separate important and critical elements from unimportant and irrelevant elements. Maatsch[18] suggests that three things should be analyzed, namely (1) the setting, (2) the problem or task, and (3) the training plan.

The setting. The setting refers to the physical layout, the tools and equipment needed to accomplish a task or procedure, data necessary for decision making, support personnel, and communications systems necessary to perform the task specified in instructional objectives. Obviously, the more complex the task being simulated, the more difficult will be the analysis of the setting. Similarly, for a complex simulation the recreation of the environment could be prohibitively expensive or inconvenient.

In deciding how to simulate a setting the designer must first analyze those components found in its realistic counter-part. This analysis activity should point out the critical elements of the setting that interact with the task to be performed in it. These critical elements are then separated or abstracted from actual settings and become the basis for the design of the simulated setting. It is crucial that these critical elements be abstracted because without them learning and transfer to real-world settings will not occur.

Maatsch summarizes the principle of simulating the setting by stating: "The critical aspects of the functional environment (setting) can be simulated with the lowest fidelity possible to maintain the critical properties and sequences of the activity to be trained" (p. A-7).[18]

An example of analyzing the setting for purposes of designing a low-fidelity simulation of the critical elements follows:

Assume that the task to be performed in the setting is an interview of a hostile patient in an outpatient clinic. The critical elements found in the setting are the patient, a room, two chairs, and perhaps a uniform or white coat to be worn by the student. Some other elements that could be found in the setting, but which are not critical for either accomplishing the objectives or transferring to a real setting, are a desk, pictures or ornaments on the wall, examining tools and materials, an examining table, and a telephone. Given all the possible elements in an interviewing setting, the designer separates only the critical ones from those which are less important and includes the former in the simulation.

The problem or task. Whereas the setting does not necessarily need to be very realistic, the problem or task must be. Maatsch summarizes a principle governing the simulation of the task or problem by saying that it "should be as realistic as possible . . ." (p. A-11).[18] Furthermore, he states, "Major changes in fidelity should be based on training principles or training objectives. As departures from realism increase beyond these limits in the simulation, the amount of positive transfer can be expected to decrease significantly" (p. A-11).[18]

Analysis of the problem or task being simulated is done in relationship to the instructional/evaluation objectives. It should help the designer to abstract all relevant aspects of the corresponding real clinical task or problem. These aspects should include the actual sequence of events, data, and health care resources normally available in completing the task or solving the problem, and the patient or organism with which the student is to interact. Furthermore, relevant stimuli should be available to cue the participant's responses

necessary to complete the task or solve the problem.

In analyzing the task of intramuscular injection in the gluteus maximus site, some of the components of the task that need to be performed in actual sequence are the following:

1. Identify the greater trochanter.
2. Place thumb on trochanter and extend fingers toward posterior iliac spine.
3. Locate a point between index finger and thumb.
4. Inject the needle on a direct back-to-front route.

If other equipment or personnel are neces-

TRAINING PLAN

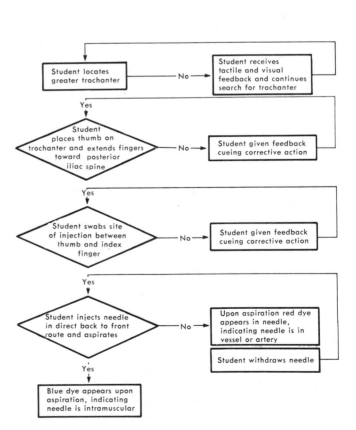

Fig. 9
Example of training plan flow chart.

sary to complete this task, they would also be identified through analysis of the task.

Rather than use an actual person to train the student to perform an intramuscular injection, the designer can abstract only that part of the anatomy relevant to completing the task. At least two such anatomical simulators are available commercially and allow the student to palpate and visualize the reference points for successful injection.

In the design of a simulation, these critical features of the task are separated from the less critical aspects. This example is a rather simple one. The more complex the task or problem, however, the more important and complicated the job of separating the relevant and important features becomes.

The training plan. The training plan is the scheme for arranging the appropriate aspects of the setting and task/problem and scheduling the appropriate temporal flow of action taken to accomplish the task. It is similar to what a playwright does in positioning the actors and setting the sequence of actions to be taken. The key elements in planning are the arrangement of temporal and spatial sequences from the real-world order in such a way that there is a beginning, middle, and end to the simulation exercise. How will the simulation begin? Where will the student and essential equipment and tools be? How will time be dealt with? What will happen if the student does the wrong thing? What is the real-world order of completing the task or solving the problem? These are some of the questions the designer must answer in creating a training plan to go along with the simulation.

One way of dealing with this final analysis stage of deciding how to simulate is to develop a flow chart. An excerpt from such a chart is shown in Fig. 9. The flow chart depicts the sequence of the problem or task as it would occur in the real world. It also shows various contingencies that need to be thought out before the student begins the simulation. Obviously, students could take a number of irrational actions as they proceed through the simulation. It becomes important, therefore, to consider a contingency plan that halts the students from further action.

Finally, when simulating a problem or task that is time dependent, time needs to be considered in the training plan. Of course, time too can be simulated. This can be accomplished by simply telling the student the amount of simulated time that has elapsed (e. g., "two hours have gone by"). When real time is being used, it is important to plan a procedure that allows the student to keep track of time.

SUMMARY

Five types of simulations found in health professions education were presented in this chapter: (1) written simulations, (2) simulated patients, (3) computer simulations, (4) audiovisual simulations, and (5) mannequins. Simulations, as described here, serve two major educational functions: namely, to instruct or to evaluate. Furthermore, the advantages, benefits, and disadvantages of simulation are presented. Finally, design considerations (what and how to simulate) are discussed.

Simulation has many implications and great potential for clinical teaching and evaluation of students in the allied health professions. Clinical faculty members and their institutions are presently stressed by the educational needs and demands of their professions, students, and educational programs. Increasing the quality of learning is a goal of most educational programs. Simulation, coming at a time of limited material resources, limited manpower, and increased demands on health care systems, is one means of meeting educational program needs while improving instruction. Clinical faculty members with sufficient opportunity (inservice education) to effectively design and/or learn to use simulation in clinical education will find simulation an exciting, effective, and rewarding educational tool.

REFERENCES

1. Abrahamson, S.; Denson, J. S.; and Wolf, R. W. The effectiveness of a simulator in training anesthesiology residents *Journal of Medical Education, 44,* (June), 1969, 515-519.

   A discussion of the results of an experiment using a computer-controlled patient simulator (SIM I) for training anethesiology residents in the skill of endotracheal intubation. The major findings were a savings in training time and reduced risk to patient.

2. Barrows, H. S., and Mitchell, D. L. M. An innovative course in undergraduate neuroscience: Experiment in problem-based learning with "problem boxes." *British Journal of Medical Education, 9,* 1975, 223-230.

   A report on the organization and evaluation of an undergraduate course in neurology in which problem boxes are the basic learning resource.

3. Barrows, H. S., and Abrahamson, S. The programmed patient: A technique for appraising student performance in clinical neurology. *Journal of Medical Education, 39,* (August) 1964, 802-805.

   A discussion of uses of simulated patients to evaluate clinical performance. The authors describe problems in using traditional techniques for evaluating clinical competence.

4. Colenbrander, A. A simulation device for ophthalmoscopy. *American Journal of Ophthalmology, 74,* (October) 1972, 738-740.

   A description of a mannequin used for teaching and evaluating clinical ophthalmoscopy.

5. Enelow, A.; Adler, L.; and Wexler, M. Programmed instruction in interviewing: An experiment in medical education. *Journal of American Medical Association, 212,* (June 15) 1970, 1,843-1,846.

   A description of a simulation that uses videotaped interviews to facilitate student learning of interviewing principles. Evaluation of indicated significant student learning.

6. Harless, W. G.: Drennon, G. G.; Marxer, J. J.; Root, J. A.; and Miller, G. E. CASE: A computer-aided simulation of the clinical encounter. *Journal of Medical Education, 46,* (May) 1971, 443-448.

   A description of a computer simulation system developed at the University of Illinois College of Medicine.

7. Helfer, R.; Black, M.; and Helfer, M. Pediatric interviewing skills taught by nonphysicians. *American Journal of Diseases of Children, 129,* (September) 1975, 1,053-1,057.

   A report that mothers trained as simulated patients can teach pediatric interviewing as well as pediatricians.

8. Holzman, G. B.; Singleton, D.; Holmes, T. F.; and Maatsch, J. L. Initial pelvic exam instruction. . .The effectiveness of three contemporary approaches. *American Journal of Obstetrics and Gynecology, 129,* (September) 1977, 124-129.

   A report on a study that demonstrates the effectiveness of using programmed simulated patients to teach beginning students pelvic examination skills (cognitive, psychomotor, and interpersonal).

9. Irby, D. M., and Dohner, C. W. Student clinical performance. In C. W. Ford and M. K. Morgan (Eds.), *Teaching in the Health Professions.* St. Louis: C. V. Mosby Company, 1976.

   A presentation of a conceptual model for constructing and conducting clinical evaluation.

10. Irby, D. M., and Morgan, M. K. (Eds.) *Clinical Evaluations: Alternatives for Health Related Educa-*

tors. Gainesville, Fla.: University of Florida, Center for Allied Health Instructional Personnel, 1974.

   A practical guide to the development of clinical evaluation instruments, this book includes an annotated bibliography on evaluation in nursing.

11. Supplement to JAMA standards for cardiopulmonary resuscitation (CPR) and emergency cardiac care (ECC). *JAMA, 227,* (February 18) 1974, 833-851.

   Explains emergency care and life support techniques.

12. Jason, H. Instructional technology in medical education. In S. G. Tickton (Ed.), *To Improve Learning,* vol. 2. New York: R. R. Bowker Company, 1971.

   The author argues for the use of instructional technolgy in medical education and strongly encourages the use of simulation in the education process.

13. Johnson, G. H.; Brown, T. C.; Stenchever, M. A.; and others. Teaching pelvic examination to second year medical students using programmed patients. *American Journal of Obstetrics and Gynecology, 121,* (March) 1975, 714-717.

   An assessment of the value of using programmed patients to teach pelvic examination. The authors conclude that this method adds realism to the study of obstetrics and gynecology.

14. Kretzschmar, R. M. Teaching pelvic examination to medical students using a professional patient. Newsletter No. 21 of the Steering Committee on Cooperative Teaching in Obstetrics and Gynecology, Department of Obstetrics and Gynecology, University of Utah, College of Medicine, January 1971.

   A discussion of three aspects of a program to teach pelvic examination skills: (1) the teaching of interpersonal skills; (2) the use of a patient-physician rating scale; and (3) the use of a team concept for evaluating student examination skills.

15. Maatsch, J. L., and Gordon, J. J. Simulations in clinical evaluations. In D. M. Irby and M. K. Morgan (Eds.) *Evaluating Clinical Competence in the Health Professions.* St. Louis: C. V. Mosby, 1978.

   A presentation of two different rationales for using simulation for clinical evaluation. The authors discuss concepts, principles, strategies, and types of simulation and provide a selective annotated bibliography.

16. Maatsch, J. L.; Hoban, J. D.; Sprafka, S. A.; and others. *A Study of Simulation Technology in Medical Education.* A Final Report Prepared for the National Library of Medicine. East Lansing, Mich.: Michigan State University, Office of Medical Education Research and Development, 1977.

   A state-of-the-art study of the use of simulation in health sciences education. Significant projects and funding sources are identified and teacher preference for simulation is determined. An extensive annotated bibliography is also included.

17. Maatsch, J. L. *An Introduction to Patient Games; Some Fundamentals of Clinical Instruction.* East Lansing, Mich.: Michigan State University, Office of

Medical Education Research and Development, 1974.

A description of patient games and how to use them. The author explains four basic principles of effective clinical instruction.

18. Maatsch, J. L. Designing cost-effective simulations. East Lansing, Mich.: Michigan State University, Office of Medical Education Research and Development, 1972. Mimeo.

    A description of the principles of designing simulations and a comparison of advantages with conventional classroom instructional techniques.

19. McGuire, C., and Solomon, L. M. (Eds.) *Clinical Simulations: Selected Problems in Patient Management.* New York: Appleton-Century-Crofts, 1971.

    A presentation of twenty written simulations of clinical problems. The introduction provides a useful description of written simulations.

20. Penta, F. B., and Kofman, S. The effectiveness of simulation devices in teaching selected skills of physical diagnosis. *Journal of Medical Education, 48,* (May) 1973, 442-445.

    An evaluation report on four simulations used to teach physical examination. Simulations were (1) Iowa Ophthalmoscopic Model. (2) Strabismus Cover Test Demonstrator, (3) Bartner Eye Model, (4) Heart Sound Simulator. Results were favorable for (1) and (2). For (3) and (4), students who practiced more learned more.

21. Tinning, F. C. *Simulation in Medical Education.* East Lansing, Mich.: Michigan State University, College of Osteopathic Medicine, 1975.

    A presentation of the rationale and empirical justification for use of simulated patients. The author presents results of extensive study of simulated patients in medical education.

22. Twelker, P. A. Designing simulation systems. *Educational Technology,* 9, (October) 1969, 64-70.

    An outline of an approach to designing simulation systems. The author discusses when simulation is appropriate and inappropriate.

12
CLINICAL FACULTY ISSUES

Jennie D. Seaton

Historically, educational programs for allied health professions evolved from training apprenticeships. Initially, qualified practitioners (i.e., clinical instructors) taught clinical skills and techniques to individuals with lesser academic preparation. The basic scientific knowledge imparted was usually limited to the information pertinent to the clinical task being taught. Invariably, the field of practice, as well as the number of skills and techniques used in the clinic kept expanding. The new clinical practitioner became the expert and began teaching others. Programs were then formalized and institutionalized, and the institutional base shifted from the clinic to the collegiate or academic setting. The programs were reviewed by accrediting bodies; practitioners were credentialed. Those who previously taught in a clinical facility were pressed to make the transition to the academic community by undertaking additional training in specialty areas and educational methodologies, and by pursuing advanced degrees in order to satisfy the accrediting bodies. As programs became larger and more institutionalized, the need to shift specific components of the clinical portion back to the real world of the health care delivery facilities became obvious.

While students gain practical clinical experiences and integrate the didactic and clinical segments of their program, they are supervised by clinical instructors. The role of the clinical instructor in this evolutionary process remains appreciably unchanged. Clinical instructors still teach, supervise, and evaluate the student in coordinated, prescribed learning experiences. The changes in their role are primarily in the degree of involvement in a variety of areas: the development of curricula, the selection of the student population, the selection of prescribed learning experiences, the definition of the clinical instructor's role, the lines of responsibility and communication, and the modes of compensation and recognition.

GUIDELINES FOR AFFILIATION AGREEMENTS

In the past decade, the need for formalization of affiliation agreements has been emphasized by a number of organizations, institutions, and associations. Use of clinical resources and affiliation/contractual agreements in allied health education are discussed at length in recent publications.[7-9,11] Many groups have considered the complex interrelationships, cost, and other factors of clinical affiliations; some have developed and circulated specific guidelines. Among these groups are the Administrative Institute of the Association of American Medical Colleges,[14] American Association of Junior Colleges,[1] American Hospital Association,[3] American Physical Therapy Association,[8] American Occupational Therapy Association,[4] and the State Department of Education for the State University of New York System.[12] Documents for specific programs are reviewed as a portion of the accreditation review process.

Areas set forth in the affiliation agreements usually include goals and objectives, definition of the clinical education pattern, time frames, number and selection of the student population, criteria and standards for performance, evaluative techniques, provisions for clinical supervision, and responsibilities of the cooperating institutions and the students. The definition of *clinical education* set forth in *Clinical Education in Physical Therapy: Present Status/Future Needs* is adequate for all allied health professions:

The portion of the students' professional education which involves practice and application of classroom knowledge and skills to on-the-job responsibilities. This occurs at a variety of sites and includes evaluation and patient care, administration, research, teaching and supervision. It is a participatory experience with limited time spent in observation (p. 2).[8]

Other terms used to describe this segment of allied health education programs are clinical training, clinical assignment, practicum, clinical affiliation, field experience, and clinical experience. Basically, clinical education is organized into two patterns: concurrent, in which the student is participating in the didactic and clinical instruction at the same time, or nonconcurrent, in which the student participates in the practice and refinement of skills full-time upon completion of the didactic program or a defined segment of the didactic program. Obviously, the roles of the individuals involved in the planning and supervising of the clinical experience will vary with the clinical education pattern. Scanlan in Chapter 9 and Pierce and Eichenwald in Chapter 10 elaborate on the curriculum models; this chapter concentrates on the role models.

DEFINITION OF ROLE MODELS

This discussion is limited to five basic role models for individuals involved in providing clinical education. The titles assigned are: coordinator of clinical instruction, faculty clinical instructor, hospital/agency coordinator for clinical instruction, hospital/agency clinical instructor, and clinical practitioner/su-

pervisor. The general description of these positions follows.*

Coordinator of clinical instruction

The coordinator of clinical instruction is generally a faculty member employed by the academic institution. The title coordinator of field-work instruction is frequently used in occupational therapy. In some institutions, the term "education" is substituted for "instruction."

The primary role of the coordinator of clinical instruction is to coordinate and administer clinical education programs. The coordinator interacts with the academic faculty and with the staffs or designated individuals of affiliating institutions to plan, coordinate, and evaluate each student's clinical education program, taking into consideration the academic preparation of the student and his or her previous experiences. Additional responsibilities include writing contracts and agreements, developing new and reviewing existing affiliations, orienting students to the clinical facility and experiences, and counseling students in clinical segments of their programs.

Appendix A (p. 168) is the job description used for the coordinator of field-work education by the Department of Occupational Therapy, Virginia Commonwealth University. At that university, the coordinators of clinical instruction of students in physical therapy and in nurse anesthesia have a similar role. The department chairperson assumes these responsibilities for medical technology students at that institution.

Faculty clinical instructor

The faculty clinical instructor is employed by the academic institution as a regular faculty member and is assigned responsibility for di-

---

*These role definitions and general descriptions were generated from a review of the literature, conversations with health practitioners, and personal observations. In developing guidelines for clinical appointments for the School of Allied Health Professions, Virginia Commonwealth University. Information was gathered from a number of four-year institutions that offer health programs affiliated with clinical facilities.

rect instruction and supervision of the clinical experiences of students in the clinical facility. This clinical instructor may or may not participate in the didactic segment of the program.

Colleges of nursing have used this role model extensively. The Departments of Occupational Therapy and Physical Therapy, School of Allied Health Professions, Virginia Commonwealth University, have three individuals in this role at the McGuire Veterans Administration Hospital; the job description used for occupational therapy clinical instructors at Virginia Commonwealth University is given in Appendix B, pp. 169 and 170.

Hospital/agency coordinator for clinical instruction

The hospital/agency coordinator for clinical instruction is employed by the clinical facility to coordinate and arrange the clinical education of students assigned to the facility. This coordinator may function for one or more disciplines; may or may not have other responsibilities; and may or may not have an appointment, title, or a designated role in the educational program or institution.

The Veterans Administration has a long-standing commitment to the education and training of health workers. A variety of role models exists within Veterans Administration Hospitals. Guidelines for developing affiliations and relationships between the staffs of Veterans Administration hospitals and accredited, formalized educational programs are set forth in Part 2 of the Veterans Administration Department of Medicine and Surgery Manual.[13] A position of associate chief, Nursing Service Education, is described in *Education for Nursing Service*. The statement of policy, Section 4.05 (Collaborative Educational Relationships), reads as follows:

(1) The quality of patient care will be enriched by productive interrelationships between the VA Nursing Service staff and faculty from schools of nursing. Resources from schools of nursing and those of the Nursing Service will be carefully integrated to support nursing students using VA facilities for clinical experiences. It is expected that the faculty from schools of nursing will be committed to the improvement of nursing practice, teaching and research programs. Members of the nursing staff who have intellectual abilities and investigative interests similar to those of the university nursing faculty will engage in deliberate teaching and research. There will be joint appointments between University Schools of Nursing and VA Nursing Service.

(2) The Chief, Nursing Service, in collaboration with hospital management, will be responsible to promote inclusion of deans from schools of nursing on a Deans Committee in order to benefit the Nursing Service and the University Schools of Nursing. The development of relationships between the Nursing Service staff and the faculty from schools of nursing will be consistent with the philosophy and procedures outlined in M-3, "Research and Education in Medicine," part II. (p.4-4).[13]

Generally, the associate chief works with a number of institutions of higher education to provide clinical experiences for nursing students and nurse practitioners in Veterans Administration hospitals. The learning experiences for nursing students are cooperatively planned; the students are supervised by the faculty of the educational institution. In some Veterans Administration installations, the associate chief, Nursing Service Education, receives an academic appointment. The policies for Nursing Service Education have been more highly developed than for most other allied health professions. In part, this is because of the recent formalization of most allied health programs in an academic setting, the smaller number of programs, and the low numbers of students enrolled in affiliating programs. Programs with larger enrollments tend to have a better defined organizational structure and established procedures.

In the Veterans Administration Social Work Service, a different role for the hospital/agency coordinator for clinical instruction exists. The position title is social work educator. In addition to maintaining and developing all educational activities for the service, this individual is responsible for undergraduate and graduate field experience for affiliating universities. In this capacity, the social work educator coordinates the selection of students for Veterans Administration assignments and supervises and coordinates all elements of the students' clinical experiences during the training period. Some of the responsibilities for clinical education are delegated to other staff members.

Roles similar to the one described for the social work educator exist in physical therapy, occupational therapy, and the medical laboratory; frequently, chiefs of services assume the role of coordinator of clinical instruction in their service area. This is especially true when small numbers of students are involved.

For some programs, the coordinator's role is assumed by someone designated by the administrative officer. Programs administered in this manner are generally developing ones. The college faculty negotiate with the hospital administration for specific types of clinical experiences; the responsibility for the students' clinical experience is usually delegated. An example is the clinical practicum for students enrolled in a program for human services workers at John Tyler Community College in Chester, Virginia. This program is affiliated with a number of agencies and institutions, each with a designated person serving as a liaison with the program director or college coordinator of clinical instruction. In an affiliated Veterans Administration hospital, the coordinator's role is assumed by the administrative assistant to the chief of staff.

Hospital/agency clinical instructor

The hospital/agency clinical instructor (the title preceptor may be used) is employed by the clinical facility and given a title or clinical appointment at the rank of instructor or higher by the academic institution. This instructor may receive some monetary and/or tangible or intangible benefits from the academic institution. The major responsibility of this position includes the instruction, supervision, and evaluation of the clinical education of the students. These duties may be delegated to another staff person. Individuals in these positions usually work closely with the coordinator of clinical education, director of the educational program, hospital/agency coordinator for clinical instruction, or some designated faculty member in establishing the

elements of the clinical education program. This individual may also participate in the didactic portion of the educational program.

Clinical practitioner/supervisor

The clinical practitioner or clinical supervisor is an individual employed by the clinical facility, who instructs, supervises, and may evaluate students' clinical experiences. This individual may or may not be designated by name, may or may not receive any tangible or intangible benefits, and is not awarded a special title or clinical faculty rank. The responsibilities assumed by this individual may or may not be formalized in written documents.

INVOLVEMENT OF THE FIVE ROLE MODELS

The *coordinator of clinical instruction*, who is a faculty member of the educational program, is involved not only in determining the selection of clinical sites, but also in establishing the content of the affiliation agreement. Generally, this coordinator examines the total academic program, those clinical experiences available, and those provided by the affiliating institution. From this examination, the coordinator either recommends the continuation of an affiliation or the establishment of an alternate affiliation in order to better integrate the academic and clinical experiences deemed necessary for the total educational program. This coordinator also has continuing responsibility for evaluating the clinical experiences at the various affiliation sites and for educating and developing the clinical faculty. This position creates a bridge between the practicing clinician and the faculty members of the educational program.

The *faculty clinical instructor* prescribes the learning experiences to be conducted within the time frame set during negotiations with the clinical facility. The faculty clinical instructor makes recommendations to the general faculty about the adequacy of the clinical facility to provide for the experience needed to augment academic portions of the course.

Generally, clinical supervision is carried

out at the facility by the faculty clinical instructor; this arrangement is the best model for integration of the academic and clinical experience. On occasion, there may be problems with the integration of the teaching program and the service functions. Such problems must be open to negotiation between the staff of the clinical facility and the faculty clinical instructor. Sometimes, however, negotiations may be broader in scope, with a number of individuals from each of the affiliating institutions involved.

If, at some time, the faculty clinical instructor delegates some of the clinical supervision of students to a staff person, the faculty clinical instructor and the staff member must agree on the activities to be carried out by the students and on the procedures for evaluation and review of the clinical education experience.

For these two positions—the coordinator of clinical instruction and the faculty clinical instructor—there is no monetary exchange between institutions. These individuals are compensated by the academic institutions and are eligible for tenure and other benefits provided for regular faculty members. If the hospital or agency receives any benefits, it is from the consultation by the assigned faculty member or other resource persons from the academic institution, from the service rendered by the students and faculty while in the clinical education program, or from the recruitment of employees to staff of the hospital or agency. Indirectly, the staff may benefit by becoming more aware of what is going on in the didactic or academic portion of the program, of changes in health care delivery, and of new developments in the practice of the particular discipline.

The involvement of the *hospital/agency coordinator for clinical instruction* is variable; three distinct models were presented in the previous section. The first is the individual designated by the administration of the facility as the contact person for academic institutions and programs desiring to use the facility as a clinical site. In this case, the coordinator delineates the concerns, restrictions, and assistance that may be provided by the hospital or agency; and directs the individual

seeking to establish the affiliation to the appropriate individuals to develop the specific guidelines of the affiliation agreement. All of these affiliation agreements are developed in accord with basic policies set forth by the administration of the facility. The involvement of the hospital/agency coordinator in prescribing the learning experiences, determining criteria in standards of performance, and evaluating instruction of the students is minimal; however, in most cases the coordinator has some input concerning who provides the clinical supervision. The coordinator is also involved in determining how the teaching programs are integrated with the service functions of the facility. This role is viewed primarily as one of coordination and is necessary to facilitate channeling of representatives of the academic program to the appropriate individuals within the clinical facility.

A second model is the coordinator for clinical instruction in a specific discipline. In this case, the role is somewhat modified. More emphasis is placed on the impact of integrating the teaching program with the service functions of the facility. The coordinator determines who, within the service area, will supervise the students. In some cases there may be a coordinator of clinical instruction from the academic institution and also a faculty clinical instructor. Of course, the role of coordinator in the specific discipline will be somewhat modified with the involvement of these other two individuals; the roles of each will have to be well delineated, and communication will be between the representatives of the academic institution and the hospital/agency coordinator for clinical instruction at the facility. There may be some arrangements whereby this individual is given an appointment, title, and/or a designated role in the education program of the academic institution.

The third possible role is the individual designated as the hospital/agency clinical instructor. In this case, the instructor is generally given a special title, special appointment, and/or clinical rank. This individual usually possesses certification in the area of instruction being considered; clinical instructors should have the same academic preparation as do the academic faculty. This individual is involved in determining the prescribed learning experiences, negotiating for adequate time for the students at the facility, determining criteria in standards of performance, and aiding in evaluation of the students and the program. Special recognition of individuals by clinical rank or clinical title adds status to the individual and to the importance of his or her role. Tenure, however, is generally not offered; titles of special recognition are reviewed at regular, specified intervals. This status adds a needed dimension when joint decisions are made setting forth the guidelines for clinical affiliations. In addition to this title and status and the involvement component of this role model, there may be other kinds of fringe benefits.

The *clinical supervisor* or *clinical practitioner* supervises some prescribed educational experiences for the student. In terms of input to the establishment of guidelines for clinical affiliation, the practitioners determine the length of time they are willing to supervise the student and in which areas they are willing to provide the clinical supervision. Frequently, out of such an arrangement evolves formalization of a provision for a specific title and better defined relationships with members of the academic faculty. When this role evolves to a high level, problems or frustrations may arise because of the lack of recognition and status for the clinical practitioners, who are making a major contribution. Supervision of students serves as a stimulus for the continuing education of the practitioner. Generally, there are no other benefits (at least none stated in a formal document).

GENERAL PROVISIONS FOR CLINICAL FACULTY

Most universities have policy statements on the appointment, promotion, tenure, and separation of faculty members. They may also make provisions for various categories of faculty; clinical, adjunct, lecturer, preceptor, visiting, and research are frequently among the defined titles. If there are provisions for clin-

ical faculty, a definition, list of titles, and conditions for appointment are generally contained in the document.

In policy statements of the Medical College of Virginia, Health Sciences Division, Virginia Commonwealth University (MCV/VCU), the term *clinical* is inserted in the title before the word *professor* or lesser rank in those instances in which the faculty member participates in education in a minor rather than major area of activity. However, there is some variation within the university. The School of Pharmacy designates individuals as *adjunct faculty*. After a period of significant contribution, the individuals are named *clinical instructors*. The Department of Hospital and Health Care Administration designates clinical faculty as *preceptors*. Usually the faculty are not geographically located at the institution, do not receive significant pay from the university, and are reappointed annually.

The School of Allied Health Professions (MCV/VCU) recently approved a policy statement for clinical appointments. It provides that the faculty members of each department will set their criteria for appointments, including the educational qualifications, professional credentials, professional memberships, and experience levels for individuals being recommended. Contractual agreement and mechanisms for evaluation and review are also to be developed.

At the University of Kentucky, a different nomenclature is used. Individuals may receive appointment at *clinical professor* or lesser ranks. In addition, individuals are designated as *voluntary* or *part-time*. If *voluntary* is part of the title, the individual receives no remuneration from the university; if *part-time*, the individual is a faculty or staff member of another department or division of the university and receives payment from the institution for services rendered. In each instance, clinical faculty are listed in the brochures and catalogues of the College of Allied Health Professions, may attend faculty meetings as nonvoting members, and may attend faculty retreats and college social events. At the departmental level, the clinical faculty are involved in decisions relating to changes in curriculum, policies, and evaluative procedures. One university, the State University of New York at Buffalo, grants weighted voting privileges to the clinical faculty in the School of Health Related Professions.

Some institutions pay for the utilization of the clinical facility. There is a variety of arrangements. At one university, funds are transferred to the personnel budget of the clinical area. No individuals are designated as the recipients; theoretically, this provides additional workers to compensate the clinical facility for employee time spent in teaching, supervising, and evaluating students. In other instances, partial or full salaries of designated individuals are paid by the academic program. In still other arrangements, the clinical facility receives students' tuition or a negotiated amount for each student assigned to the facility. This question has been addressed recently by the American Hospital Association.[2] Although the education of health manpower is integral to the treatment and care of patients, the costs of the programs must be identified and allocated to the appropriate parties.

In some areas of the country, namely New York and Pennsylvania, clinical facilities are requesting compensation for providing clinical experiences. This serious question is considered by Brown of the University of Pennsylvania:

Institutions have to carefully consider what they can offer to the clinical facility, such as the use of the computer, the library, the tennis courts, etc. There are any number of service-in-kind exchanges that are feasible (p. 63).[5]

From the perspective of the clinical facility, Martel, vice-president of Northwestern Memorial Hospital, writes*:

If hospitals are going to continue to provide clinical learning experiences (and from all indications, I think we are beyond "going"), then at some point we must give serious consideration to charging fees for such experiences. Hospitals are under the gun

---

*From Martel, G. Clinical perspectives. In M. Boyles (Ed.), *Proceedings: Selected Papers from Health Manpower Conferences, 1974-76.* Washington, D.C. American Association of State Colleges and Universities, 1976, p. 64.

for cost effectiveness, and if the educational process is properly done, it will involve planning time, evaluation time, and clinical instruction time on the part of full-time employees in the clinical setting. And time is money; we all know that! To make joint ventures sound business arrangements (thus allowing educators to set expectations and expect to have those expectations met), it is in our mutual interests to set fees (p. 64).[6]

In order to satisfy the challenge of accountability for the distribution of the cost of health manpower education, the activities, services, and weighted cost must be documented. A true collaborative effort in the educational process should be balanced in terms of assets and liabilities to the cooperating institutions. The balance will include tangible benefits; some of the factors involved will be intangible and difficult to quantitate.

Tangible benefits that have been awarded to some hospital agency clinical instructors include participation in continuing education programs, frequently without charge. Parking privileges at the academic institution; the opportunity to buy tickets, sometimes at a reduced rate, to athletic, special entertainment, or recreation programs; and use of the library and learning resource centers at the academic institution represent other tangible benefits. Some institutions have day-care centers that are open to clinical faculty members. Institutional benefits may also include access to the computer facilities of academic institutions, readily available consultants in numerous areas, and an increased pool of potential health workers.

Pascasio,[10] dean of the School of Health Related Professions at the University of Pittsburgh, describes the reciprocal relationships the school has defined in its contractual affiliation agreements. In recognition of its affiliations, the school offers the following services:

1. Continuing education at no charge to clinicians
2. Access to learning resource center
3. Opportunity to audit regular class offerings
4. Instructional space, equipment, and other resources of the university avail-

able to staffs of clinical facilities and professional organizations

5. Faculty appointments for clinicians for their participation in didactic and clinical segments of educational programs
6. Filling of prescriptions at the university health center pharmacies, often at reduced cost
7. Associate membership in the faculty club
8. Check cashing and notary public services
9. Use of university athletic and recreational facilities
10. Use of university libraries

Each contractual arrangement is somewhat different. Academic institutions and clinical facilities are unique entities; therefore, the balancing of the contributions and responsibilities of the participating institutions will be reflected in the content of the contractual agreements and accepted practices in the conduct of collaborative efforts.

CLINICAL APPOINTMENTS: ADVANTAGES AND DISADVANTAGES
Academic institutions

By making clinical appointments, the academic institution is assured of some continuity in the relationship with the clinical area of the affiliating facility. The appointment provides a constant evaluation of students and review of the clinical affiliation. Information relative to any changes in the clinical practice, policies, staffing, equipment utilized, etc., is readily available to the academic institution. Any questions relative to the scheduling, progress, and performance of students may be directed to designated individuals. Input from active practitioners is provided for review and revision of the academic curriculum. In addition, the development of better evaluation instruments for clinical experience is possible.

The major disadvantage for the academic institution is the lack of control over clinical personnel. If the two affiliating institutions are geographically separated, the distance may contribute to communication problems and prohibit full faculty participation in the educational process.

Individuals remain primarily responsible to their employers. The qualifications of practitioners to serve in these capacities are quite variable. Frequently, the individuals are named because of the position they hold rather than the qualifications they possess. Often the titles are accepted without a true commitment to the responsibilities entailed. Problems arise when the appointed individual does not meet the commitment. In order to preserve access to the clinical facility, the academic appointment is continued with little or no contribution from the designated individual.

Hospital/agency

The advantages for the clinical facility are its ready access to the resources of the academic institution, the stimulation of staff members to remain abreast of new developments in their field of interest, an ensured voice in educational programs, services provided by the students assigned to the facility, and a ready source of in-service and continuing education for other staff members. There is also general acceptance of the notion that the quality of patient care is better in teaching institutions, and quality patient care is the objective of most hospitals and agencies.

The disadvantages for the clinical facility are the increased demand on a designated practitioner's time and the increased use of space, equipment, and supplies. There are additional subtle demands placed on resources by having an officially recognized clinical instructor (e.g., increased telephone usage). All of these increase the expenditures of the clinical facility.

Students

The major advantage to students of formalized appointments is that they are then responsible to someone who has the official sanction of the faculty of the program. Professional qualifications are generally a part of the appointment consideration. This individual usually has a better understanding of the academic background of the student and can make clinical experience more relevant. By having an individual designated, the student may be readily informed about situations or concerns that have been troublesome to other students who have previously been assigned. In addition, student evaluation is more uniform when the responsibility is assumed by one or a limited number of individuals.

The major disadvantage to the student may be the restriction of having to relate to one designated individual. If the student and practitioner are unable to relate, serious problems may arise. In addition, the establishment of relationships with other staff members in the clinical facility may be impaired. All practitioners have special areas of expertise; access to these persons may be limited because only one individual is officially recognized.

SUMMARY

In establishing an affiliation or contractual agreement, the two parties must agree on the role models that will function within the constraints of the agreement. Consideration must be given to the obligations, responsibilities, and benefits that will be afforded the individuals assuming the specific role. When negotiating the agreement, the parties must make specific stipulations that are realistic in terms of the resources of the participating institutions and the abilities and qualifications of the personnel involved.

REFERENCES

1. American Association of Junior Colleges. *Extending Campus Resources: Guide to Using and Selecting Clinical Facilities for Health Technology Programs.* Washington, D.C.: American Association of Junior Colleges, 1968.
   Guidelines and criteria suggested to assist junior college personnel in planning and developing health program clinical affiliations.
2. American Hospital Association. *Health Education: Role and Responsibility of Health Care Institutions.* Chicago: American Hospital Association, 1975.
   Consideration of the role and responsibilities of health care delivery institutions in preparatory education and training and the continuous education of health manpower.
3. American Hospital Association. *Statement on Role and Responsibilities of the Hospital in Providing Clinical Facilities for a Collaborative Program in the*

Health Field. Chicago: American Hospital Association, 1967.
   A discussion of the role of hospitals in providing clinical experience, including considerations for patient services, relationships between the staffs of affiliating institutions, contractual agreements, and shared responsibilities for evaluation.
4. American Occupational Therapy Association, Committee on Basic Professional Education. Standards and guidelines for an occupational therapy affiliation program. *American Journal of Occupational Therapy*, 25, (September) 1975, 314-316.
   Definition of standards applied to the philosophy, function, selection, and evaluation of affiliating clinical facilities.
5. Brown, R. Educational uses of clinical resources. In M. Boyles (Ed.), *Proceedings: Selected Papers from Health Manpower Conferences, 1974-76.* Washington D.C.: American Association of State Colleges and Universities, 1976.
   A discussion of the educational uses of clinical resources, assessment of the clinical facility resources, and contractual agreements between educational institutions and clinical facilities.
6. Martel, G. Clinical perspectives. In M. Boyles (Ed.), *Proceedings: Selected Papers from Health Manpower Conferences, 1974-76.* Washington, D.C.: American Association of State Colleges and Universities, 1976.
   A discussion of the relationships between clinical facilities and educational institutions: administrative, operational, and programmatic considerations.
7. Moore, M. L.; Parker, M. M.; and Nourse, E. S. *Form and Function of Written Agreements for the Clinical Education of Health Professionals.* Thorofare, N.J.: C. B. Slack, 1972.
   Formulation of contractual agreements for use of clinical resources.
8. Moore, M. L., and Perry, J. F. *Clinical Education in Physical Therapy: Present Status/Future Needs.* Washington, D.C.: American Physical Therapy Association, 1976.
   An exploration of the characteristics of clinical sites; characteristics and functions of clinical faculty; and problems of clinical education, the educational process, and evaluation of clinical affiliations and learning experience.
9. Pascasio, A. Clinical facilities. In C. W. Ford and M. K. Morgan (Eds.), *Teaching in the Health Professions.* St. Louis: C. V. Mosby, 1976.
   A discussion of the evaluation of clinical facilities as clinical learning sites, focusing on the development of collaborative arrangements and agreements between clinical and educational institutions.
10. Pascasio, A. Relationships in educational use of clinical resources: Reciprocity/service in-kind. In M. Boyles (Ed.), *Proceedings: Selected Papers from Health Manpower Conferences, 1974-76.* Washing-

ton, D.C.: American Association of State Colleges and Universities, 1976.

A discussion of resource sharing among affiliating institutions.

11. Pascasio, A. Selection, evaluation, and utilization of clinical resources. In E. McTernan and R. Hawkins (Eds.), *Educating Personnel for the Allied Health Professions and Services: Administrative Considerations.* St. Louis: C. V. Mosby, 1972.

Considerations of factors and procedures in the selection and use of clinical resources in allied health education programs.

12. University of the State of New York. *Guide to Selection of Clinical Facilities for an Associate Degree Nursing Program.* Albany, N.Y.: State Education Department, 1966.

A guide to assist college personnel in selecting ap-propriate clinical education facilities by using defined and recommended criteria.

13. Veterans Administration, *Department of Medicine and Surgery Manual, Professional Services M-2 Part V, Nursing Service.* Washington, D.C.: 1975.

A statement of policy for in service education and for educational programs affiliating with the Nursing Service of Veterans Administration hospitals. This manual is revised periodically.

14. Wolf, G. A.; Brown, R. E.; and Bucher, R. M. (Eds.), Medical school–teaching hospital relations: Report of the Second Administrative Institute of the Association of American Medical Colleges. *Journal of Medical Education, 40,* (November) 1965.

A report on costs, complex and interrelated objectives, specification of goals, and evaluation processes considered by representatives of teaching hospitals and medical schools.

APPENDIX A

Job description*

Coordinator, field-work education

Position responsibilities

A. Specific

1. Coordinate, organize, and assist in planning for clinical education programs for all students in the department
2. Schedule all undergraduate and graduate students for clinical affiliations and practicums
3. Manage correspondence relative to affiliations
4. Maintain up-to-date files on all clinical affiliations
5. Orient students to their responsibilities toward the affiliation center and to the university during affiliations
6. Write and conclude written contracts and letters of agreement between affiliation centers and the university
7. Promote communication between centers, the university, and affiliation students; visit centers and students as often as practical
8. Act as liaison between center and school to assist with student problems and provide consultation
9. Promote and assist with the development of new affiliation programs
10. Review and evaluate present centers against standards for continued use
11. Engage in certain teaching responsibilities in area of specialty, as necessary
12. Receive certification examination applications of candidates and submit in proper form to AOTA education director
13. Act as advisor to certain undergraduate and graduate students (number and level to be determined by department chairperson) in regard to academic progress and continuance in school, advance registration, etc.
14. Act as advisor to clinical affiliates in regard to registration and performance progress in the affiliation
15. Participate on these committees
16. Assist school's council chairperson in arranging annual meetings

B. General

1. Participate in Occupational Therapy Department committees and university committees
2. Participate in departmental administrative functions
3. Be involved in professional associations
4. Be involved in activities for self-improvement and continuing education

*This job description is used by the Department of Occupational Therapy, Virginia Commonwealth University.

APPENDIX B

Job description*

Clinical instructor

 I. Qualifications

    A. Education

Completion of both the didactic and clinical requirements and graduation from an approved program in occupational therapy (approved by the Council on Medical Education of the American Occupational Therapy Association in collaboration with the American Medical Association) followed by successful completion of the national certification examination, and registration with the American Occupational Therapy Association.

    B. Experience/special skills

A master's degree, or one or more years of clinical experience. Should be skilled practitioner who has demonstrated ability for administration and working with others. Should be competent in the area of educational processes and procedures and capable of maintaining an educational program concerned with the growth and development of students.

II. General guidelines for duties and responsibilities

    A. Develops, administers and coordinates a comprehensive clinical education program

    B. Supervises and teaches assigned students

    C. Evaluates programming, plans for immediate and long-term needs, and interprets these to grant project coordinator

    D. Prepares budgets, estimates program needs, and communicates these to grant project coordinator

    E. Establishes and maintains effective working relationships with administration and staffs of VA and VCU Occupational Therapy Departments, other professional staffs, and the community

    F. May provide in-service education and continuing education

III. Specific duties

    A. Development of the clinical training faculty

        1. Examines and evaluates existing facilities and procedures of the VA hospital to assure maximum utilization of these programs in student training and patient rehabilitation

        2. Works with the VCU faculty, VA personnel, and VA grant coordinator in designing clinical education programs and clinical education facilities

        3. Requisitions equipment and supplies to permit students to experience a variety of evaluative and treatment techniques as they apply to the patient population of the VA hospital

    B. Maintenance of program

        1. Provides quality treatment to VA hospital patients referred by physicians of the hospital; maintains an adequate census to provide field-work experience as required by the school

        2. In coordination with VCU faculty, provides occupational therapy students with formal instruction, guidance, demonstration of skills, and supervision in the evaluation and treatment of hospital patients in the occupational therapy clinic

        3. Incorporates into the program a variety of individual and group techniques, such as: evaluation and facilitation techniques, analysis of activities, adapted devices, splints, ADL, prevocational training, etc.

        4. Schedules demonstration programs with other departments within the VA hospital system, such as physical therapy, corrective therapy, speech therapy, dialysis, prosthetics, orthotics, etc., pertinent to the didactic portions of the curriculum

*This job description is used by the Department of Occupational Therapy, Virginia Commonwealth University.

Continued.

Job description—cont'd

     5. Maintains records as they apply to the VA hospital and VCU Department of Occupational Therapy for the management of patient treatment and evaluation of students' performance

     6. Creates an educational climate, utilizing TV, films, library, lectures, etc., for training of students, staff, and patients

     7. Attends clinics, rounds, and staff meetings for effective communication and integration into the overall program of the hospital

  C. Coordination of program

     1. Keeps abreast of the basic preparation of the occupational therapy students enrolled in the revised curriculum, based on a developmental model, and adjusts program as needed

     2. Schedules field-work assignments to the advantage of students' time and clinic operation

     3. Collaborates with chiefs of other units within the VA hospital to coordinate development and training of students and hospital personnel as related to student supervision

IV. Supervision

  The instructor receives primary supervision from the Occupational Therapy Department chairperson, Virginia Commonwealth University. In addition, the instructor cooperates with the project coordinator and the VA chiefs of services.

part four **ASSESSING OUTCOMES**

13
THE CLINICAL EDUCATION GUIDE

Charles W. Ford

A problem in addressing the issues of clinical education is the diversity of disciplines and the concomitant diversity of clinical experiences. What may be appropriate in an acute care hospital may not fit a physician's office. What is suitable for a distant clinical experience in physical therapy may not fit a self-contained, independent clinical experience in a dental hygiene laboratory operated by an educational institution. Nevertheless, commonalities of problems and solutions are posited by various persons in this book.

One problem that is evident in *all* clinical education settings is the need for communication and coordination.

A DHEW report[1] notes the following common deficiencies in communication and coordination:

Health care institutions that affiliate are not clear about what is expected from them in terms of type and extent of student exposure and facilities and equipment to be provided.

Insufficient information about the content and curricula are (sic) given to the health care institution to assist its personnel in planning and maximizing their support of the student experience.

Sponsoring institutions provide limited information on the experiences received by the students before they begin the clinical education phase (p. 123).[1]

The clinical education guide is one simple, effective method for improving communication and coordination.

The meaning of the words "clinical education guide" should be self-evident: a guide consisting of written information that is used to help the various constituencies of the clinical experience understand the process and procedures. For faculty members who have developed and used one, the value of a guide is accepted. However, some faculty members have not considered using a guide, much less developing one.

The term "clinical education guide" may be self-explanatory, but at the same time, it is not the only usable term. Faculty members may have developed some type of clinical education handout and placed another label on it, such as clinical supervisor's guide, internship experience, instructional guide, or student handbook. The point is not the title, but the substance of the material and its intended and actual use.

In the systems approach to instruction, a basic belief is the required sharing of the intended outcomes of learning with students. No less important is sharing the intended learning outcomes with faculty members. This statement may appear simple-minded at first reading, but in the context of clinical education for a variety of allied health professions the issue is quite serious. In most health professions, the content of the program is ultimately the responsibility of *one* group—the academic faculty. Exceptions to this generality exist. In medical technology, the clinical portion of programs is often the responsibility of another group—the clinical faculty. Even in this case, however, the trend is clearly toward academic and clinic integration and joint planning. In dental hygiene, programs are taught solely by academic faculty members, with the clinical experience existing directly under their control. There is no dichotomy between didactic teaching and clinical experience. In fact, the major portion of the clinical experience most often occurs in a setting operated by the educational institution. Curriculum models in which the academic faculty work directly with the students in the clinical setting also tend to integrate efforts. The nursing education model is the most typical of this type of curriculum design. The fact that the nursing faculty members participate in the delivery of service encourages integration of the didactic and clinical portions of the program. Seaton examines in Chapter 12 the five different models for administration and teaching that are used by educational institutions and health care facilities.

HOW THE GUIDE IS USED

Although this chapter does not directly address integration of clinical and didactic education, the end result of designing and using a clinical education guide is improved integration.

Most programs in the health professions utilize clinical education sites that are external to the academic institution. Most of these sites are in acute care hospitals. (Of course, health care agencies that deliver both direct patient services and public health services are also used.) External clinical sites include both physicians' and dentists' offices. They all depend on health care personnel to serve as clinical instructors unless the health profession programs have *integrated* faculties. Whether the clinical instructors are paid or serve voluntarily may have a bearing on their motivation, but the larger issue is the design of an interrelated clinical experience or, as suggested earlier, the issue of communication. Pascasio emphasizes this point:

> To ensure the success of a clinical affiliation, all concerned must plan and know the curriculum into which the clinical experiences are to fit. The clinical and educational institutions must both know what is being asked *of* the other and *by* the other. Mutual exploration and evaluation based on predetermined criteria are necessary (p. 225).[3]

The clinical education guide cannot replace mutual exploration, but it can help close the gap between what the educational program plans for the students and what the student receives. If the clinical coordinator of a program does little more than arrange for and schedule a student into a clinical site and then periodically visit, the student's clinical experience is bound to be weak. Clinical faculty members will not know what the experience should be, and the student can be of little help.

The first suggestion within a systems approach to clinical instruction is that the teacher know what is to be taught and the student know what is to be learned. Furthermore, if the program is based on behavior, both the teacher and student should know what behaviors are to be exhibited. The clinical education guide can be a bridge to help this occur.[2] If the clinical faculty are separated from the academic faculty, discussion is useful but not sufficient. The substance of the experience must be written and needs to be communicated between the academic faculty and the clinical faculty.

WHAT THE GUIDE CONTAINS

The breadth and depth of the guide can vary from program to program, depending on a number of variables:

1. *Length of the clinical experience.* A four-week experience in a private office as part of a dental assisting or medical assistant program cannot be compared with a respiratory therapy program in which the student spends a full year rotating through five hospitals.
2. *Level of the clinical experience.* The guide should reflect whether the student is at an introductory level, a secondary or reinforcing level, or an intern level with minimal supervision. The length and precision of the guide are directly related to the level of performance required of the student.
3. *Location of the clinical experience.* Sometimes clinical sites are far removed from the academic sites. Students must often locate their own housing and pro-

vide their own transportation. A guide should include information on local conditions of housing and services, particularly as they relate to the responsibilities of the clinical faculty and students.

Like other components that add to a systematic approach to instruction, revisions or additions of the guide are required annually. For this reason, a format that is easily amended is the most economical. Using a loose-leaf binder with pagination by sections is probably the easiest if the guide is of such a length that duplication becomes a major factor. There is no optimal length. However, guides that are too short usually do not answer all the questions pertinent to a clinical experience. Guides that are too long may fail as a communications tool, for they may not be read. The problem of length can be solved by including only the most pertinent items in the body and adding an appendix for incidental, but useful, items.

The following outline is a suggested format to follow. Following it in a cursory form could result in a five-page clinical education guide; following it in detail could result in a fifty-page guide. Faculty, both academic and clinical, must decide how explicit they wish to be.

The descriptive material following the outline explains briefly the content of the outline, as well as the samples taken from various guides, which are included in Appendixes A through E, pp. 177 to 187.

Title page— what, why, where, when, who
- I. Overview—what, why, where, when, who spelled out
  - A. Introduction
  - B. Responsibility of student
  - C. Responsibility of clinical institution
  - D. Responsibility of academic institution
  - E. Responsibility of clinical coordinator
- II. Organizational structure
  - A. Academic
  - B. Clinical
  - C. Personnel
- III. Competency and background of students (didactic)
- IV. Objectives of clinical experience
  - A. Level of difficulty
  - B. Time frames
- V. Evaluation process
- VI. General policies/regulations
  - A. Housing
  - B. Transportation
  - C. Liability coverage
  - D. Absence
  - E. Dress
  - F. Authority chain
  - G. Miscellaneous (library privileges, parking, etc.)
- VII. Special policies/regulations
  - A. Competency waiver
  - B. Long-term illness
- VIII. Appendix
  - A. Agreement forms
  - B. Liability coverage
  - C. Evaluation forms
  - D. Course outlined

I. Overview

The overview explains in detail what the program is, why the clinical site is being used, where the students come from, when the students will be at the clinical site, and the level of the students in the program.

Various subsections should describe the responsibilities of each person or group of persons in the clinical experience. Many problems that arise in the clinical experience are caused by lack of information regarding the various roles and the responsibilities that go with the roles. The overview should be useful in preventing some misunderstandings.

II. Organizational structure

The organizational section addresses the formal relationships that exist within both the educational institution and the clinical setting. An organizational chart *may be* sufficient; the important point is the identification of the chain of command.

III. Competency and background of students (didactic)

Knowledge of the entry level of the students is very important. As indicated in the Prologue, preassessment is an important part of the systems approach to instruction. If this section identifies with some degree of precision the competency level of the student entering the clinical experience, it will save time for the clinical faculty.

Included in this section should be a demographic profile of the students. A description of what positions the average graduate might assume would also help the clinical faculty understand the relationship between where the students are coming from and where they are going.

IV. Objectives of clinical experience

The objectives section is relatively easy to create; it consists of the list of performance objectives for the experience. To help the clinical faculty, the objectives should be divided on the basis of both time and difficulty. The guide may suggest that objectives at the lower taxonomic levels be accomplished in the first third of the experience, while those at the higher levels be reserved for the final portion of the clinical experience. The objectives should be placed in the framework of the whole clinical experience to help the clinical faculty plan a total program.

V. Evaluation process

The evaluation section is important, because clinical supervisors normally are quite concerned with their role in the evaluation process. This section should spell out the *total* process (i.e., who is responsible for what, when it will occur, and how it will be used). Evaluation forms that need explanation should be included in this section; otherwise, they can be placed in an appendix.

VI. General policies/regulations

The general policies section includes answers to all the questions that are raised on a daily basis. This section could be written in a question-and-answer format. It is the catchall that is likely to expand as questions are raised and answered.

VII. Special policies/regulations

The special policies section can be included in the general section, for it, too, deals with policies and regulations. However, policies that may affect only a select number of students may exist within given institutions. Examples in the outline are a competency waiver (when and how it operates) and the policy concerning long-term illness (what procedures are followed for makeup work caused by a long-term illness).

VIII. Appendix

The appendix includes all the information that clinical faculty members may need or want for reference, but does not include information on the day-to-day operation of the clinical experience.

SUMMARY

This chapter provides a simple but effective means to help solve problems that arise from poor communication between the academic institution and the clinical faculty. A clinical education guide cannot supplement personal contact, but it can answer the questions that arise most frequently.

In order to provide the reader with concrete suggestions, several sections from existing guides appear in Appendixes A through E.

REFERENCES

1. Department of Health, Education, and Welfare, Health Resources Administration. *Final Report, National Assessment of Clinical Education of Allied Health Manpower*, Vol. 1. Washington, D.C.: 1974.

    A report on the generic problems that exist in the clinical education of allied health manpower programs.

2. Moore, M. L.; Perry, J. F.; Nourse, E. S.; and Clark, A. W. *Clinical Education in Physical Therapy: Present Status/Future Needs.* Washington, D.C.: American Physical Therapy Association, 1976.

    This work is the most recent major effort by a professional association. Although dealing with the problems of physical therapy, most of the report is quite useful for all allied health professionals.

3. Pascasio, A. Clinical facilities. In C. Ford and M. Morgan (Eds.), *Teaching in the Health Professions.* St. Louis: C. V. Mosby, 1976.

    This chapter focuses on four matters related to clinical facilities: (1) determination of an effective clinical site, (2) decision making in regard to sites, (3) Major concerns, such as contractual agreements, and (4) Accomplishment of objectives.

INTRODUCTION TO APPENDIXES

The set of appendixes is made up of examples from a variety of clinical education guides. For each guide there is a description of the guide and where it is used, a copy of the table of contents, and several sample pages.

APPENDIX A

Guide for Department of Allied Health Education and Research, University of Kentucky*

"This study guide and resource manual has been designed for a number of purposes; among them— (1) a ready source of information to explain what is involved in Kentucky January, (2) a reference document concerning the academic elements of Kentucky January, and (3) a teaching resource for students and faculty" (Foreword).

Table of contents

I. Introduction to the Kentucky January Program
   A. Expectations
   B. Program organization
   C. Program activities
II. Conceptual and academic framework
   A. Learning process for Kentucky January
   B. The team concept
   C. Field models
   D. Team final report
III. The Kentucky January survival guide

Faculty responsibilities

a. Be able to explain objectives and logistics of Kentucky January, and especially of the clinical team component, to students and personnel in the base agency and other field facilities.
b. Be able to explain and interpret the theoretical models of Kentucky January to students and Location Coordinators in the base agency.
c. Arrange for at least four (4) team meetings prior to field experience for coordination of student pre-field tasks.

d. Attend Faculty Sponsor meetings prior to the field experience.
e. Attend the Faculty Sponsor/Location Coordinator Conference held in Lexington and encourage students to participate in the Conference.
f. Make at least one site visit and encourage student participation in the visit.
g. Arrange for appropriate student transportation on the team.
h. Coordinate and gain approval of developed objectives, programs and schedules with Location Coordinator.
i. Be available for inservice sessions, education or consultation at field location as requested by the base institution.
j. While in the field lead daily discussions of team based on day's experiences to develop future plans.
k. Insure that the content of the field experience is consistent with the learning objectives and that such content is integrated by the students.
l. Act as a liaison between student team members and site coordinators (and/or home health service director).
m. Complete evaluation form on each student to be shared with chairman of the student's discipline and Kentucky January Project Director.
n. Write evaluation of team's experience for project director and location coordinator including reactions to current year's experience and suggestions for future years.

Conduct

Students participating in SITE/77 are expected to abide by the "Code of Professional Conduct," College of Allied Health Professions, University of Kentucky:

> The College of Allied Health Professions at the University of Kentucky has the responsibility for insuring that its graduates are properly

---

*From *Study Guide and Resource Manual for AHE 841: Health Systems Clerkship*. Lexington, Ky: Department of Allied Health Education and Research, Center for Interdisciplinary Education in Allied Health, College of Allied Health Professions. University of Kentucky, September 1976. (By permission)

prepared for their role in providing health care for the patient and the community. The obligations assumed by those who are to be entrusted with the care of the sick transcend mere expertise in their chosen field.

Therefore, in addition to academic competence, students in the College of Allied Health Professions are expected to possess and demonstrate those qualities of professional conduct including integrity, morality, discipline, and compassion which in essence reflect their suitability to assume this trust.

In general, you should keep two things in mind regarding professional conduct. First, you are a *guest* in the community you are visiting. This implies basic courtesies with those with whom you are involved (being prompt in meetings and interviews, keeping to the schedule), as well as using a certain degree of tact and good judgment. Second, keep in mind how you would feel if you were in the same place as the person with whom you are in contact. What would *you* expect in terms of preparation and conduct?

There are, however, certain recommendations we would like to make to you so the experience will have as much meaning as possible for you:

1. You are a guest in the community. Your presence in the community is the result of the spirit of professional cooperation that exists between the community and university.
2. Prior to any interview or rotation call the agency and confirm that you are expected.
3. Be sure you understand why you are involved in the observation or participation in the first place. Have a concrete reason for being there. Communicate those reasons to your host.
4. Keep the appointments you have made with the community agency. The agency counts on your presence, so show up on time.
5. If you cannot keep an appointment, call the agency and leave a message to that effect.
6. Ask whatever questions you have to ask, but, if for some reason someone elects not to provide such information, respect their position. Part of their job is making such decisions. Oftentimes the information is available from other sources.
7. If your host asks you for your reactions to what you have seen or participated in, be honest, but use common sense. There is more than one way to respond to such a request if your response is likely to be critical in some respect.
8. Do not ask the agencies or hosts to let you do what they won't even let their own staff members do.
9. Respect confidentiality. With the exception of that portion of your experience which has real meaning for the work of the team, it is assumed that what you may see or hear otherwise will remain a part of the private domain of the agency. To do otherwise is to undermine the entire relationship the agency and university have and the relationships between the agency and the supporting society.
10. Finally, recognize that in order for this placement to have materialized, the Center staff, the faculty sponsor, preceptor, the Location Coordinator, and the agency staff have all been involved. Make the best and maximum use possible from the experience.

APPENDIX B
Guide for Ferris State College*

This clinical education guide is used as a reference for five clinical subrotations that occur during the entire second academic year of a two-year program. It is primarily written for students to use as they develop respiratory therapy skills and a professional attitude and as they prepare for the registry examination.

Table of contents

Section I. Introduction—goals and structures of the clinical year in respiratory therapy
A. Overview
B. Organization chart
C. Code of ethics
D. Therapist instructor roster
E. Clinical subrotations

Section II. Clinical policies
A. General policies
B. Specific policies
    1. Excused absence
    2. Unexcused absence
    3. Late/tardiness
    4. Dress code
    5. Behavior/conduct
C. Grading policy—general
D. Certification of completion
E. Library policy

*From *Respiratory Therapy Clinical Education*, 1975-76. Big Rapids, Mich.: Program in Respiratory Therapy, School of Allied Health. Ferris State College. (By permission)

F. Chain of command
G. Quarter registration
H. Subrotation waiver procedure
Section III. Course outlines and grading
A. Course outlines
B. Grading

Section IV. Objectives for clinical subrotations
A. Oxygen administration and devices
   1. Piping systems
   2. Compressed gases
   3. Pressure regulators
   4. Flowmeters
   5. Oxygen administration
   6. Oxygen administering devices
   7. Oxygen analyzers
B. Aerosol/humidity administration and devices
   1. Principles of humidification
   2. Humidifiers
   3. Principles of nebulization
   4. Nebulizers
   5. Application of aerosol/humidity
C. Basic procedures
D. Basic therapy
   1. IPPB theory
   2. IPPB procedure
   3. Administration of drugs via IPPB

Section V. Objective for clinical subrotation
A. Blodgett Memorial Hospital
   1. Pulmonary function subrotation
   2. Cardiac catheterization/open heart subrotation
   3. Intensive care unit subrotation
B. Butterworth Hospital
   1. Pediatric subrotation
   2. Neonatal intensive care unit subrotation
   3. Surgical intensive care unit subrotaton
   4. Medical intensive care unit subrotation
C. Grand Rapids Osteopathic Hospital
   1. Anesthesia subrotation
   2. EKG subrotation
   3. Departmental therapy subrotation
D. Kent Community Hospital
E. Saint Mary's Hospital
   1. Acute care subrotation
   2. Chronic care subrotation
   3. Pulmonary care subrotation

Blodgett Memorial Hospital clinical performance objectives

Intensive care unit subrotation
I. The student will be able to do the following tasks with the below listed mechanical ventilators:
   A. Classify the ventilator according to its characteristics
   B. Draw a pressure/flow pattern
   C. Set up the ventilator for patient use with all systems operational
   D. Change the ventilator circuit
   E. Trouble shoot any mechanical problem with the ventilator
   F. Explain the function of any dial on the ventilator
   G. Manipulate the machine parameters/dials so as to correct for any blood gas condition
   H. Explain machine limitations with regard to ventilator selection for long term ventilator patient
      1. Ohio CCV
      2. Bourns
      3. Bennett MA-1
      4. Baby Bird
II. The student will be able to demonstrate the following skills and/or explain the basic concepts in the following points about weaning from a mechanical ventilator:
   A. Necessary indications for weaning: VC, TV, inspiratory force, blood gases
   B. Concepts and goals of conventional weaning technique
   C. Rationale behind IMV
   D. Measurement technique of ventilatory parameters to verify potential weaning from mechanical ventilation
   E. Set up and monitor IMV
   F. Management technique in the weaning of the ventilator patient
III. The student will be able to do the following tasks that are related to respiratory care skills:
   A. Describe the characteristics of rales, rhonchi, and wheezing as well as recognize these patterns when listening to patient's chest with stethoscope
   B. Recognize abnormal ventilatory patterns as well as be able to give an explanation as to their predisposing factors
IV. The student will be able to do the following tasks that relate to basic airway and bronchopulmonary care skills:
   A. Set up and assure proper functioning of any humidity/aerosal device
   B. Explain the indications, goals, methods of administration, effects, and hazards when administering aerosol/humidity
   C. Using sterile technique, demonstrate effective suctioning technique
   D. Demonstrate positioning and/or percussion of patient that will best drain any given lobe or segment of the lung

E. Explain the indications and contraindications in performing chest physiotherapy

F. Set up and assure proper function of any oxygen administering device

G. Explain the indications, goals, effects, hazards, flowrates/concentrations, when administering oxygen by any oxygen delivery device

H. Demonstrate effective technique when administering the following modalities of respiratory care: IPPB, coughing, and incentive spirometer

I. Explain the goals, effects, indications, and contraindications for administering IPPB, coughing, and incentive spirometer

V. The students will be able to demonstrate the following tasks with the below listed drugs that relate to respiratory care through the use of drugs:

A. Explain the indications, contraindications, actions, and side effects of each drug

B. Recognize the goals and/or purpose of each drug
1. Muscle relaxants
   a. Succinylcholine chloride (Anectine)
   b. Turbocurare chloride (Curare)
   c. Pancuronium bromide (Pavulon)
2. Narcotics
   a. Meperidine hydrochloride (Demerol)
   b. Morphine sulfate (Morphime)
3. Tranquilizing agents
   a. Diazepam (Valium)
   b. Hydroxyzine hydrochloride (Vistaril)
   c. Chlordiazepoxide chloride (Librium)
4. Barbiturates
   a. Amobarbital sodium (Amytal)
   b. Pentobarbital sodium (Nembutal)
   c. Secobarbital sodium (Seconal)
5. Anticholinesterases
   a. Neostigmine bromide (Prostigmine)
   b. Edrophonium chloride (Tensilon)
6. Xanthine bronchodilators
   a. Tedral (phenobarbital, ephedrine, theophylline)
   b. Aminophylline (theophylline, ethylenediamine)

c. Elixophylline (theophylline, potassium iodide)
7. Adrenal corticosteroids:
   a. Dexamethasone (Decadron)
   b. Methylprednisone (Solu-medrol)

VI. The student will be able to do the following tasks that relate to blood gases and their interpretation:

A. Explain the procedure for performing an arterial puncture

B. Explain what measures are done following the arterial puncture to prevent a hematoma

C. Interpretation of blood gases as to blood's acidic/alkalotic state, bicarbonate, base excess, oxygen and carbon dioxide tensions

D. Causes/etiology of the abnormal blood gas condition

E. Therapy that will improve the abnormal blood gas condition

VII. The student will be able to perform the following tasks that relate to understanding the below listed respiratory diseases/conditions:

A. Explain the definition, etiology, and pathophysiology of the respiratory disease/conditions

B. Explain the diagnosis and treatment for the respiratory disease/conditions
1. COPD: Emphysema, chronic bronchitis, asthma, and bronchiectasis
2. Neuromuscular: Myasthenia gravis, Guillain-Barré
3. Pneumonia
4. Overdose: Barbiturate, and salicylate
5. Adult respiratory distress syndrome
6. Flail chest
7. Carbon monoxide/chlorine poisoning
8. Status asthmaticus
9. Pulmonary edema

VIII. The student will be able to do the following tasks that relate to mechanical ventilator/patient management:

A. Explain the indications for initiation of mechanical ventilation

B. Explain the effects of positive pressure ventilation

C. Explain the psychological factors encountered in the patient such as: fear, anxiety, patient/ventilator conflict that must be overcome

D. Explain the complications of long-term mechanical ventilation such as: O_2 toxicity, pneumothorax, pneumomediastinum, subcutaneous emphysema

E. Demonstrate correct technique for checking tidal volume, oxygen concentration, compliance, correct inflation of endotracheal tube cuff, as well as effective ventilation of patient

F. Demonstrate technique for monitoring total ventilator function as well as bedside and laboratory tests/measurements

G. Demonstrate ability to perform as well as explain the importance of the following bedside formulas:
1. Shunt equation
2. Deadspace/tidal volume ratio
3. Alveolar air equation
4. pH changes per unit change in PCO_2 in both chronic and acute respiratory conditions
5. Change in tidal volume or deadspace and its relationship to changes in PCO_2

APPENDIX C
Guide for College of St. Scholastica*

This manual is intended to assist clinical supervisors and students through the directed-practice clinical experience of a medical records administration program.

Table of contents

Purpose of manual and general instructions to student

The manual is designed to guide both you and your Clinical Supervisor through your directed practice and affiliation clinical experience. You are asked to read it carefully prior to your DAP [Directed Affiliation Practice]. You have the option to either purchase or borrow the manual. If it is borrowed, please do not write in the manual; *it is to be returned to the Clinical Coordinator on completion of the DAP.*

The Intermediate Objectives are designed to assist you in meeting the End-of-Course Competencies. The objectives guide you in acquiring an overall experience in a working environment and assist you to function more effectively within that setting. You will note that the objectives make reference to your being prepared to discuss the contents of them. This you will be doing, not only as you proceed through the clinical experience, but also on your return to the College when you participate in the DAP seminar and during the Post-DAP conference that is held with each student by the Clinical Coordinator.

Specific instructions

A. Written assignments and reports
  1. Student general reports: Separate reports are to be completed for both your directed practice and affiliation experiences. The *student activities* listed under the various Intermediate Objectives will make up the contents of the reports along with a copy of the General Information Sheet on both of the clinical sites. The report may be done by each student individually or by two or more students working together *as long as the author of each section of the report is identified.* (You may want to complete *some* of the student activities individually and others as a group working together.) Complete the reports in duplicate (typewritten). The original of the reports is to be handed in to the Clinical Coordinator at the Department of Health Information Ad-

*From *Manual for Clinical Supervisors*. Duluth, Minn.: Department of Health Information Administration, College of St. Scholastica, 1976. (Prepared through Allied Health Special Improvement, Grant 3 DO1 AH 50724-0151). (By permission)

ministration at the College. The copy of the reports is either mailed by you or given directly by you to your Clinical Supervisor at the health care facilities in which you did your directed practice and affiliation (unless the Clinical Supervisor indicates to you that he/she does not wish to receive a copy).

2. Administrative project report: You will note under the *student activities* for Intermediate Objective C for End-of-Course Competency II—Directed Practice that you are asked to complete an administrative project which calls for problem-solving and creative thinking. You should be spending at least 20 hours of your own time on it. The Administrative Project Report is to be completed in duplicate (typewritten). The original is to be given to your Clinical Supervisor prior to leaving the directed practice site and the copy handed in to the Clinical Coordinator at the College.

3. Student evaluation of clinical experience Part I: Two copies of Part I of the Student's Evaluation Report are completed by you for both the directed practice and the affiliation experiences. Part II: One copy of Part II of the Student's Evaluation Report is completed by you for both the directed practice and the affiliation experiences. *All copies* of the Evaluation Reports I and II are turned in to the Clinical Coordinator at the College.

4. Log sheets: Record your activities as well as your impressions and values of the experience. The originals are handed in to the Clinical Coordinator at the College. No copies are necessary.

If you desire to keep a copy of any of the above, it will be necessary for you to make additional copies.

The above reports, evaluation and log sheets must be completed and turned in by the end of the winter quarter in order for you to receive a grade with the administrative project, which must be completed prior to your leaving the clinical site.

B. Progress and clinical supervisor evaluation of student

Your Clinical Supervisor has been asked to discuss with you periodically where both you and the Clinical Supervisor are at in terms of expectations, needs, and interests. This should help keep both you and the Clinical Supervisor on the right track. Your Clinical Supervisor has also been asked to complete an evaluation on

you (he/she has the option of discussing it with you), and then forward it to the Clinical Coordinator at the College. You will have the opportunity to review and sign this evaluation either at the clinical site or at the College during the Post-DAP conference.

C. Additional information and instructions regarding directed practice and affiliation

1. Report at the directed practice or affiliation site at 9:00 AM the first morning unless otherwise indicated by either the Clinical Coordinator or by the Clinical Supervisor through the schedule. Find out from the Clinical Supervisor what time to report on subsequent mornings. It is important that you report to work on time. You will be working eight-hour days, forty hours per week. The Clinical Supervisor may include an evening, night or weekend shift in your schedule if he/she feels it would be helpful to your learning experience.

2. It would be well for you to write home and to the Clinical Coordinator here at the College when you arrive at both the directed practice and affiliation sites.

3. Take time to review your notes prior to leaving for your clinical experience, particularly if you've never worked in a Medical Record Department before. Take with you to your sites, your notes on Information Systems and Management or any other reference materials that you feel would be helpful to you.

4. While you are at the clinical site, you are directly responsible to the Director of the Medical Record Department or to the Clinical Supervisor if he/she was so delegated. You are asked to abide by the protocol of the clinical site concerning break periods, parking, etc., as well as abide by all departmental and hospital policies and regulations.

5. Problems that may arise should be brought to the attention of your Clinical Supervisor. If you would run into major problems with your project or in any way, also feel free to call the Clinical Coordinator at the College (218) 728-3631 Ext. 441.

6. Remember to wear your student identification insignia on your uniform, lab coat or working apparel.

7. Keep in mind that your Clinical Supervisor may not be familiar with the term "DAP." Some are familiar with the terms "directed practice" and "affiliation."

8. Make every effort to refrain from being absent from work. If you necessarily have to be absent, be sure to inform the Clinical Supervisor as soon as possible. Check with your Clinical Supervisor to see whether you need to make up the time.

9. Keep in mind that you will be sharing your experience with your fellow students during the seminar and that each student will be giving a presentation on some aspect of the DAP during the seminar. Experiences that are unique to your site and may not be available to other students in some way are especially important to share.

10. You will periodically be receiving correspondence and/or memos from the Clinical Coordinator while you are at your clinical site. Included in them will be information regarding the date, time, and place in which the seminar will be held.

11. For directed practice only:
    a. Hand carry a copy of your physical examination to the directed practice site. This is to be given to your Clinical Supervisor the first day.
    b. Keep track of the time spent on your administrative project outside of the time spent at the clinical site.

12. For affiliation only:
    a. A school holiday falls during your affiliation experience. The Clinical Supervisor is aware of it, and has the option of giving you the holiday off, an alternate day off, or no day off.

APPENDIX D
Guide for Department of Physical Therapy, University of Kentucky*

This handbook is used to guide the students and clinical instructors through a 2-week clinical clerkship, a 14-16 week clinical internship consisting of three rotations through three health care facilities, and a student independent study.

Table of contents

---

*From *Student Handbook, 1976-77 (Working Draft)*. Lexington, Ky.: Department of Physical Therapy, Clinical Education Program. College of Allied Health Professions, University of Kentucky. (By permission)

Lexington, Kentucky   Student _____

	Pre-planning task sheet	# 7-75	
Task to be performed	**Sub-task or component parts of the task**	**Knowledge needed to complete the task**	**Result, outcome, behavior expected when task completed satisfactorily**

To be able to evaluate a patient with complaint of a painful shoulder.	I. Patient history, including C/C, description of pain (type, duration), onset, previous history, other medical problems, patient profile
	II. Examination
	  A. Cervical movements Active, passive (including over-pressures), resistive
	  B. Shoulder movements Active, passive (including "locking")
	  C. Elbow movements Active, passive, resistive, joint stressing
	  D. Wrist and hand movements Active, passive, resistive, articulation
	  E. Neurological Dermatome, myotome, reflexes
	  F. Lower extremities Neurological check
	  G. Shoulder-joint play
	  H. Other goniometrics, etc.
	III. Correlation with lab, X-ray, etc.
	IV. Identification of location of pain
		1. Maitland's scheme of eval. (see attached)
		2. Working knowledge of cervical anatomy, functional anatomy, dermatomes, myotomes, and reflexes
		3. Working knowledge of shoulder, functional anatomy
		4. Definition of overpressure, contractile tissue, joint play
		5. Joint play movements of shoulder
		6. Able to test and interpret reflex findings
		7. Able to R/O cervical pathology
			At the completion of 4 weeks, the student should be able to perform Steps 1-3 satisfactorily without assistance. Step 4 should be performed at 75% accuracy (when comparing student's to physical therapist's results).

APPENDIX E
Guide for Chicago Medical School*

These companion guides, compiled by K. A. Shriver and Sister L. Ramaeker, are designed for student teachers in an upper division program of radiological science. One, of course, is directed to the students, the other to the supervising teacher.

Instructional Guide for Supervising Teachers

*From *Instructional Guide for Supervising Teachers* and *Student Teaching Handbook*. Chicago: Department of Radiological Sciences, School of Related Health Sciences, University of Health Sciences, Chicago Medical School. (By permission)

Intent of the manual

We have described our program—singling out the educational courses for specific explanation and we have stated the philosophy of our educational component. It now remains for us to outline what we expect of our student teachers as a result of these courses, during the time they are at your institution.

We have prepared this manual for you for the following reasons:

It will:

1. Provide ease in your assimilation of the material.
2. Provide a reference for you at the time the Student Teacher is at your institution.
3. Enable us to treat only those specific areas in which you would like additional information.
4. Consolidate two seminars into one (thus conserving your time and ours) while still preparing you for having a student teacher.

Student Teaching Handbook

The student teacher wants to know

1. When do I begin actual teaching?
   Actual teaching begins at the beginning of the quarter. However, prior to this, a student will spend some time becoming acquainted with the physical environment, schedules, students' names, planning course contents, as well as the general routine of the institution before assuming teaching responsibilities.

2. Who will supervise my teaching?
   The supervising teacher to whom you are assigned and the cooperating program will regularly observe you at work. He or she will do most in helping you evaluate your performance with the class in a follow-up conference. The University supervisor will observe your teaching periodically and discuss the progress with you and the supervising teacher.

3. What is expected with regard to discipline?
   It is your responsibility to acquaint yourself with the policies of the supervising teacher and the college or hospital regarding discipline and control problems. In view of this, if a problem does arise, handle it as best you can. Discuss alternative ways to handle similar situations with supervising teacher in a conference later. Thorough planning will prevent or control most discipline problems.

4. Do I have the same privileges as other college instructors regarding the use of the faculty lounge, smoking, use of telephone, etc.? The use of these privileges and facilities will depend upon the nature of the facilities and the college policy. Use good judgment in the amount of time spent in the enjoyment of any one of these privileges and maintain the highest professional standards in the discussion of the program, students or professional problems at all times.

5. How much detail is expected in written lesson plans?
   The lesson plan is a device to help you do an adequate and successful job. Consequently, the length and detail of them will be determined by your competence. Lesson plans should include behaviorally stated objectives and should be cooperatively developed and evaluated by the student teacher and the supervising teacher.

6. Which school calendar do I follow during the student teaching?
   The University calendar is to be followed.

7. What is my responsibility if I find it necessary to be absent?
   You will be expected to inform both your supervising teacher and the University supervisor.

8. How will I be evaluated?
   The process of evaluation will permeate the entire student teaching period. However, the final evaluation will be done in a conference of the University supervisor and your supervising teacher. Final authority and responsibility in grading rest with the University.

9. For what reasons may I ask to be excused from student teaching duties?
   You may ask to be excused for:
   a. Interviews on placement—you are encouraged to arrange for interviews during nonteaching hours.
   b. A day to visit the hospital, community college, or university for which you have a contract. Do not ask to be excused unless your future employer requests your visit.
   c. Unavoidable illness.

10. Is liability insurance available to student teachers?
    Your liability is covered through the malpractice insurance that you secured through the University at the beginning of the school term. This policy includes coverage during college and clinical affiliation.

11. Will I be expected to serve as a substitute teacher when any of the supervising teachers are absent?

The hospital or college is expected to provide a substitute teacher when the regular teacher is absent. Only in cases of emergency on a short term basis, when no substitute is immediately available, will you be expected to serve in this role. At no time will you be expected to serve as a substitute for teachers in the program other than your assigned supervising teacher.

12. What is the procedure for requesting Letters of Reference?
    a. Prior to listing anyone's name as a reference, first obtain that person's consent and willingness to write the letter.
    b. Ask the individual(s) who best know(s) your qualifications for the position.
    c. Select individuals who can give a *current* report of your abilities.

14
SELF-ASSESSMENT

Harold G. Smith

Recently public and third-party payers for medical expenses have demanded an explanation of the spiraling costs of health care. Within the past ten years, the cost of medical care in the United States has increased dramatically. It has become a major item in the budgets of most families in the United States. The staggering costs are forcing the federal government and health professionals to identify alternative methods of health care designed to reduce the cost. One response at the national level has been the establishment of Health Systems Agencies (HSAs) to oversee health care in local communities.

The federal government has also provided incentives to bring about accountability in publicly financed health care. Its establishment of the Professional Services Review Organizations (PSROs) represents an initial attempt to assess the efficiency of the health care process in Medicare and Medicaid programs. The PSROs will provide a mechanism for review of the health delivery process. The review will be accomplished by peer, self, or external agencies.

The demand for accountability has also found its way into the educational processes. Leon Lessinger[9,10] has long advocated accountability by publicly financed educators. Students are insisting that their educational experiences be made relevant to their personal goals. Consumers are demanding that graduates of educational institutions be able to perform at a satisfactory level. Parents are demanding that the money they spend on providing an education for their children be efficiently spent and that it produce a product (graduate) capable of performing in the present job market.

Accountability demands a formal assessment plan; that is, a plan must be developed to evaluate the final result and/or the process used to achieve the result. Assessment is the process whereby the outcome is compared to certain criteria stated in behaviorial terminology.[6]

ASSESSMENT METHODS

Leaders in the educational fields, including health care programs, have long recognized the need for a systematic plan of evaluation. A systems approach to assessment is composed of a series of steps. The initial step is identification of the final results that are to be achieved. These outcomes must be identified and stated in specific, observable, and measurable terms. Everyone involved in the process—students, faculty, parents, employees, and employers—must understand and agree on the precise outcomes of the total process of the organization or activity.

After the outcomes are identified, the tasks, skills, and concepts necessary to achieve the final product must be listed. These intermediate steps involved in reaching the final outcome must be identified by persons with a thorough understanding of the process, because they must painstakingly analyze the total process and identify, in sequence, the intermediate tasks, concepts, and skills required to satisfactorily achieve the final outcome. This necessitates working from final results backward to component parts.

After the intermediate tasks, skills, and concepts have been identified and stated in behavioral terminology, criteria must be assigned to each intermediate step. The criteria must answer the question, "What level of activity or knowledge is required to achieve the outcome?" For example, how accurately must the range of motion of the knee be measured before a knee dysfunction can be evaluated? How long can a complete blood count take and still be timely? What level of contrast is required for an X-ray to be acceptable? Each criterion must be stated so that it can be observed and measured.

These first three steps are usually accomplished through group process or consensus. A task force of knowledgeable individuals in a field or profession identify the desired outcomes, establish the intermediate steps, and assign criteria to each of the necessary tasks, skills, or concepts. Once these preliminary steps have been performed, an individual or a small group of individuals working with the materials previously prepared by experts can construct the assessment instrument.[5]

RATIONALE FOR SELF-ASSESSMENT

Traditionally, the assessment of an employee's job performance was accomplished by a supervisor telling the employee how well the employee had performed. The process was employer initiated, administered, and delivered. Education used the same process to evaluate student performance, with the instructor initiating and delivering the assessment. Rarely was there any student input or feedback in the process.

Several years ago, industrial organizations began to seek better methods of evaluating job performance. General Electric was one of the first organizations to initiate a process of self-assessment. In its program, the employee initiated the process by writing an evaluation of job performance. The evaluation was discussed with the employee's immediate supervisor. At the completion of that discussion, the employee and supervisor together set goals for the employee. At the end of six months, the employee and supervisor met for a progress report and reevaluation of the goals. Thus the evaluation process became a dialogue between the supervisor and the employee. Before the completion of the evaluation, the supervisor and employee had to agree on the final decisions, and both had to be satisfied with the discussion throughout.

This assessment process initially had certain drawbacks. Supervisors were uneasy in the early months of the program. They were uncomfortable in having the employees prepare the written evaluation on their own job performance. In the beginning of the program, the employees did not know what was expected of them during the evaluation process. Almost universally they were unprepared to realistically assess their own job performance.

A six-month follow-up, however, showed many favorable reactions. Employees and supervisors were not defensive during the evaluation interview. The majority of the employees understood the job requirements better. A feeling of cooperative action had developed between management and labor. Employees were able to develop realistic goals for their immediate future. One of the most important advantages of the self-assessment process was the feeling by the employees that they were an essential part of the organization.[1]

As education faced new student-teacher roles in the 1960s and 1970s, educators looked to the self-assessment process for guidance. The self-assessment process provided an opportunity to improve teacher-student dialogues. It helped the student establish meaningful personal and professional goals, particularly in the evaluation of performance of psychomotor and communication skills.[3,4,7,8,14]

EXAMPLES OF SELF-ASSESSMENT

In education, some of the more outstanding examples of self-assessment are found in accreditation of programs and institutions. Regional accrediting agencies have used self-assessment formats for years. In conducting a self-assessment, the university or college prepares a detailed self-assessment document, following the guidelines usually provided by the accrediting agency. The institution or program answers specific questions that pinpoint the strengths and weaknesses of its program. Before an on-site visit, the completed assessment is forwarded to the accrediting agency. While these procedures are time consuming, the general consensus is that the increased self-awareness within the institution seeking accreditation is worth the time and effort expended in preparing the assessment document.

The best examples of self-assessment within allied health are found in the work of the Council on Medical Education, Committee on Allied Health Education and Accreditation of the American Medical Association. The Committee on Allied Health cooperates with thirty-three professional groups to accredit educational programs. It sets forth the outcomes, guidelines, and criteria for the educational programs. Once the programs complete the self-study and forward the completed document to the Council on Medical Education and the appropriate professional organization, an accrediting team makes an on-site visit.*

Passage of the PSRO legislation has stimulated many allied health professions to become interested in peer evaluation. Peer evaluation is the evaluation of one professional by another professional equally trained and experienced. A variety of allied health programs are being designed to encourage self-assessment prior to evaluation by peers. Federal legislation is putting increasing pressure on allied health professionals to participate in both types of evaluation.

In view of these pressures, the clinical setting becomes an ideal area for encouraging self-assessment by the student. The recent task force studying clinical education in physical therapy developed some models for student self-assessment. It recommended that

---

*Changes in the accreditation process have replaced the Council on Medical Education, Committee on Allied Health and Accreditation with the Committee on Allied Health Evaluation and Accreditation (CAHEA).

"Evaluation programs should include emphasis on self evaluation" (p. X).[12] In addition, the report noted that lifelong habits of personal development are fostered by early use of self-assessment techniques.

Industry has found that one difficulty in utilizing self-assessment is a reluctance by employees to either criticize or praise their own performance.[1] If allied health professionals are going to develop skill in self-assessment, they must begin as students. Clinical education provides the ideal place to initiate the process, because in many cases the first step of the process—identification of the required outcomes—has already been accomplished by experts in the students' professional organization.

A MODEL FOR STUDENT SELF-ASSESSMENT

A systems approach to self-assessment is evident in the following example from physical therapy. The clinical education outcomes were determined by the American Physical Therapy Association and adopted by its House of Delegates in 1974. The following model does not represent any specific tool currently being used by a school of physical therapy but is used as an example of the type of outcome that might be expected of graduates:

The curriculum shall be designed so that upon completion of the physical therapy educational program the student will possess competencies in the following categories:
A. Individual patient services
  1. In the area of physical health:
    a. Performance ability to implement programs of patient evaluation and treatment through:
      (1) Treating patient by:
        (a) Utilizing exercise, physical agents, assistive and supportive devices, and other treatment procedures and equipment designed to promote healing[6]

The statement means that any physical therapy student should be expected to perform this outcome during a clinical affiliation. To make the example more specific, a particular physical agent, such as ultrasound, could be specified. Then, the outcome would be the student's ability to use ultrasound in treatment of a patient in order to promote healing. Stated in behavorial terms, the outcome would be:

At the completion of the educational program the student should be able to apply ultrasound to a patient in a safe and effective manner so as to promote healing.

Once the outcome has been selected and stated in behavorial terms, it is time to move to the second step in the systems approach to assessment. This step consists of analyzing the outcome in order to determine what tasks are essential to achieve that outcome. In the physical therapy example, this step produces the following tasks:

In order to be able to safely and effectively apply ultrasound, the student must perform the following tasks:

1. Position and drape the patient
2. Select and arrange the ultrasound equipment
3. Review the patient's medical chart/history
4. Turn on the ultrasound unit
5. Apply ultrasound energy to the patient
6. Terminate the ultrasound treatment

This list is purposely somewhat general. In some instances, the tasks could be further subdivided.

The next step is to determine the essential concepts that the student must understand in order to be able to apply ultrasound to a patient. A partial list of concepts is as follows:

1. Indications and contraindications of ultrasound
2. Physiological effects of ultrasound
3. Mechanical and physical basis of ultrasound energy
4. Patient's diagnosis and pathological condition
5. Procedure for turning on the ultrasound equipment

The list of concepts should be identified and stated so that every individual involved in the process understands them and agrees to their inclusion.

The final group of items to be identified in this process is the set of skills that must be mastered so that the student can apply ultrasound to a patient. Some of the skills are:

1. Communication skills
2. Patient transfer and draping skills
3. Manipulation of ultrasound transducer head
4. Observation of the patient's reaction to the treatment

All three of these sets—tasks, concepts, and skills—should be stated in behavioral terms. Thus the final listing would be translated to read:

At the completion of the clinical affiliation, the student will:

A. Tasks
   1. Demonstrate the proper positioning and draping of a patient for ultrasound treatment
   2. Select and arrange the ultrasound equipment
   3. Review and select all pertinent information from the patient's medical chart/history
   4. Demonstrate the proper technique for turning on the ultrasound unit
   5. Demonstrate the appropriate technique of applying ultrasound to a variety of selected patients
   6. Terminate the ultrasound treatment
B. Concepts
   1. List the indications and contraindications of ultrasound
   2. Discuss the physiological effects of ultrasound on human beings
   3. Discuss the mechanical and physical basis for the propagation of ultrasound energy
   4. Describe the patient's pathological condition and relate the patient's condition to items B_1 and B_2
   5. Demonstrate the appropriate technique of applying ultrasound to a variety of selected patients
C. Skills (affective and psychomotor)
   1. Demonstrate the ability to communicate both verbally and in writing with a variety of individuals (patients, physicians, nurses, and other allied health personnel)
   2. Safely transfer and drape the patient
   3. Demonstrate skill in moving the ultrasound transducer on the patient during treatment
   4. Observe the patient's reaction to the treatment and alter treatment appropriately

When the essential or required tasks, concepts, and skills have been determined, the next step is to assign criteria to each of the selected tasks, concepts, and skills. The criteria must be met to satisfactorily achieve the outcome. The criteria are normally the minimally acceptable performances.[11] They can be termed the entry-level competencies. In the example that has been given, the criteria would be established as follows:

A. Tasks
  1. Demonstrate the proper positioning and draping of a patient for ultrasound treatment
     Criteria:
     a. The patient will be positioned in a safe and secure manner. The patient will not fall.
     b. The body segment to be treated will be completely exposed, but the patient's modesty will be protected.
     c. The student will treat the patient easily and will utilize appropriate body mechanics.
  2. Select and arrange the ultrasound equipment
     Criteria:
     a. The equipment will be in place before the patient arrives.
     b. All accessory supplies will be within easy reach of the student during the treatment.
  3. Review and select all pertinent information from the patient's medical chart/history
     Criteria:
     a. The student will recite all major categories of information from the chart.
     b. The student will list all secondary diagnoses relating to the patient.
  4. Demonstrate the proper technique for turning on the ultrasound unit
     Criteria:
     a. The transducer will be in contact with the patient when the power is turned on.
     b. The student will manipulate the timer and intensity controls according to the manufacturer's instructions.
  5. Demonstrate the appropriate technique of applying ultrasound to a variety of selected patients
     Criteria:
     a. The student will treat a variety of patients with different diagnoses.
     b. The student will treat the patient in positions other than the prone position.
     c. The student will keep the transducer in contact with the patient's skin throughout the treatment.
     d. The student will move the transducer at a slow, steady rate throughout the treatment.
  6. Terminate the ultrasound treatment
     Criteria:
     a. The student will clean the patient's skin and redrape the patient.
     b. The student will replace and prepare the treatment area for the next patient.
     c. The student will make appropriate notations on the patient's chart.

The same criteria-setting process would be followed for the categories of concepts and skills, each time selecting the minimally acceptable level of performance required to achieve the outcome.

After the criteria have been established, it is necessary to decide how the tasks will be tested or assessed. Many possibilities exist, such as paper-and-pencil tests, simulations, discussions, and observations of student performance. Usually discussion, questioning, or observation of student performance is chosen by clinical personnel to evaluate student performance.

In *stating* tasks, concepts, and skills, it is important to pay attention to the domain of learning. The items and criteria should be stated at the required level of the cognitive, affective, or psychomotor domains. In devising an assessment instrument, it is likewise important to measure at the appropriate taxonomic level.[11] All of the steps become part of the systems approach to instruction that Ford discusses in the Prologue.

When a self-assessment device is used, the student is asked to compare clinical performance with stated criteria and guidelines. The student is encouraged to make decisions regarding personal performance in the clinic. It must be emphasized that this procedure does not relieve the clinical instructor of the responsibility for making decisions about the student's performance in the clinic. In the self-assessment process, the student and clinical instructor must agree on the final evaluation. They both make decisions.[1,13]

To evaluate student performance in administering an ultrasound treatment, the student could be given the form shown as Appendix A (pp. 195 to 197) and asked to compare clinical performance with the stated guidelines.

SUMMARY

As the education of allied health professionals becomes more and more sophisticated, it is reasonable to expect clinical education and evaluation to undergo changes. The self-assessment format is suggested as a reasonable and appropriate change to incorporate into most allied health programs.[12,13] It has several advantages:

1. It helps to develop a life-long pattern of self-evaluation. The true professional is not content to remain static in a chosen profession.
2. The student becomes an active and willing participant in the evaluation process.
3. As an active participant, the student is better able to recognize personal strengths and weaknesses.
4. The evaluation process becomes a positive learning experience. The student approaches evaluation with an open mind instead of a closed, defensive attitude.
5. Mutually developed goals for the student's improvement are identified and readily accepted by the student.

These positive attributes more than offset the disadvantages of the process. Some disadvantages of self-assessment are:

1. Students hesitate to realistically evaluate themselves the first time. They must learn to trust the process.
2. Clinical instructors feel unneeded the first few times they use the self-assessment format; however, once they learn to accept and modify the student's self-assessment, they like the positive, open atmosphere of the evaluation interview.

The second disadvantage is really an advantage. The criteria and guidelines must be prepared, and they must be prepared well in advance of the student's reporting to the clinical facility. This forces the clinical instructor to thoroughly prepare for the student's clinical experience. This prevents the clinical experience from being haphazard.

In this day of accountability (personal, program, and institutional), self-assessment provides a positive, meaningful mechanism for the evaluation of student performance in the clinic. Once developed, the habit of self-assessment is likely to prevail throughout the professional life of the individual.

REFERENCES

1. Bassett, G. A., and Meyer, H. H. Performance appraisal based on self-review. *Personnel Psychology, 21,* 1968, 421-430.

    A study contrasting the effects of traditional, manager-prepared appraisals with self-review appraisals. It specifically describes the implementation of self-review in a General Electric plant.
2. Burton, W. H. *The Guidance of Learning Activities.* New York: Appleton-Century-Crofts, 1962.

    A discussion of ways to make learning experiences meaningful to students. It deals with a variety of different methods other than the traditional lecture.
3. Centra, J. A. Self-ratings of college teachers: A comparison with student ratings. *Journal of Educational Measurement, 10,* 1973, 287-294.

    A study that compares the ratings of students at five colleges with teacher self-reported ratings. The study discloses a modest relationship between student and teacher ratings.
4. Diggory, J. C. *Self-Evaluation: Concepts and Studies.* New York: John Wiley and Sons, 1966.

    A review of a progressive study of self-evaluation. It includes theoretical background and projects results of self-evaluation.
5. Ford, C. W. and Morgan, M. K. (Eds.). *Teaching in the Health Professions.* St. Louis. C. V. Mosby, 1976.

    A book containing a series of contributed chapters on a systems approach to allied health education.
6. *Handbook of information concerning the accreditation process for physical therapy education programs.* Washington, D.C.: American Physical Therapy Association, 1976.

    A description of the accreditation process. It contains self-study guides for educational programs in physical therapy.
7. Irby, D. M., and Morgan, M. K. (Eds.). *Clinical Evaluation: Alternatives for Health Related Educators.* Gainesville, Fla.: University of Florida, The Center for Allied Health Instructional Personnel, 1975.

    Papers presented at a workshop. The authors discuss a variety of methods available for evaluating clinical education and some practical suggestions.
8. Jerseld, A. *When Teachers Face Themselves.* New York: Teachers College Press, 1955.

Results of a study designed to assess the importance of self-understanding in the teaching profession.

9. Lessinger, L. Engineering accountability for results in public education. *Phi Delta Kappan*, 52, 1970, 217-225.
   An argument for systematic accountability.

10. Lessinger, L. What is it all about anyway? In B. S. May (Ed.). *Proceedings of a Training Institute–Performance Evaluation.* HEW Grant No. 1 A13 AH00129-01. Washington, D. C.: Department of Health, Education and Welfare, 1973, pp. 8-17.
    An example for implementing accountability.

11. Mager, R. F. *Measuring Instructional Intent.* Belmont, Calif.: Fearon Publishers, 1973.
    The major thesis is that measurement of instructional success is accomplished through the development of situations that match each objective in scope and intent.

12. Nourse, E. S., and Clark, A. W. *Clinical Education in Physical Therapy: Present Status/Future Needs.* Washington, D.C.: American Physical Therapy Association, 1976.
    Contains the results and recommendations of a two-year DHEW contract. It covers all aspects of clinical education in physical therapy.

13. Palmer, M. E. *Self Evaluation of Nursing Performance Based on Clinical Objectives.* Boston: Boston University Press, 1962.
    A report of a study designed to determine if students can determine their own grades in a clinical situation. It includes a format, objectives, and results of the study.

14. Sullivan, R. F. *Self Study: Measurement Devices in Physical Therapy Education.* Proceedings of 1964 APTA-VRA Institute. Washington, D.C.: American Physical Therapy Association, 1964.

APPENDIX A

Self-assessment on use of ultrasound in treatment of a patient

During your clinical experience at this facility, you will be administering ultrasound to a number of patients. In order to satisfactorily complete this affiliation, you must demonstrate competency in administering ultrasound.

Use this self-assessment guide to determine your competency. When you feel that you have satisfactorily performed all of the items listed, complete this form and make an appointment to discuss your performance with the clinical instructor. It is your responsibility to assess your own performance and make an appointment with your clinical instructor.

I. Checklist

Please make a check mark in the appropriate column for each of the following items:

	Satisfactory	Unsatisfactory	Did not perform
A. Tasks 1. Position and drape the patient a. Patient is safe.			
b. Patient is comfortable.			
c. Body segment to be treated is fully exposed.			
d. Patient remains comfortable during treatment.			
2. Select and arrange the ultrasound equipment a. All equipment is in place before the patient arrives.			
b. All supplies are within easy reach of the student during the treatment.			
3. Review the patient's chart/history a. Student knows the diagnosis for treatment before giving the treatment.			
b. Student lists all secondary diagnoses and compares them to indications and contraindications.			
c. Student notes and considers special precautions.			
4. Turn on the ultrasound unit a. The body segment to be treated is properly prepared with coupling agent.			

Continued.

APPENDIX A— cont'd

Self-assessment on use of ultrasound in treatment of a patient— cont'd

	Satisfactory	Unsatisfactory	Did not perform
b. The transducer is in place before the power is turned on.			
c. The student follows the proper sequence in turning on the equipment.			
5. Apply ultrasound energy to a variety of patients a. The student selects an appropriate position for each patient.			
b. The student selects the correct dosage for each patient.			
c. The student keeps the transducer in contact with the patient's skin during the entire treatment.			
d. The student moves the transducer at the correct speed for the patient and condition.			
6. Terminate the ultrasound treatment a. The student cleans the patient's skin and wipes it dry.			
b. The student replaces the equipment in the normal storage area.			
c. The student observes the patient's skin for any unusual reaction to the treatment.			
d. The student cleans the treatment area and prepares it for the next patient.			

APPENDIX A— cont'd

Self-assessment on use of ultrasound in treatment of a patient— cont'd

    B. Skills
       (completed in the same manner)
    C. Knowledge
       (completed in the same manner)
  II. Strengths and weaknesses
List the strengths and weaknesses you demonstrated in administering ultrasound.

 III. Future goals
List the goals that you have established for yourself during the next *(time period)*. These goals should be designed to improve your proficiency in administering ultrasound.

 IV. Comments by clinical instructor

Student _____ Date _____
Clinical instructor _____ Date _____
Facility _____

15

HIGHER LEVELS OF LEARNING

M. Jeanne Madigan
Anthony LaDuca

The issues posed by use of clinical sites in the education of allied health professionals are best addressed from the standpoint of performance evaluation in these settings. Evaluation involves judgments, decisions, and values about observable performance.[3] The purposes of evaluation may be relatively conventional and individual, such as grading a student in a course; or more extensive and elaborate, as in evaluating an entire program or curriculum. This chapter focuses on the evaluation of performance by students in clinical settings.

GENERAL PRINCIPLES OF CLINICAL EVALUATION

Allied health professionals practice disciplines that involve cognitive, affective, and psychomotor operations at various levels and in various combinations. In virtually every field, problem solving and synthesis of concepts and principles can be observed; hands-on and technical skills are manifested in patient intervention and in use of instruments or equipment; and sensitive and empathic interactions are frequently significant in routine procedures. The allied health educator is confronted with a complex evaluation problem since each student is accountable for such a wide array of competencies in the clinical setting.

The one overriding consideration in clinical evaluation is the acceptability of the student's level of clinical performance. Is the student

safe to practice on the public? To answer this question some fundamental rules are in order:

Essential features of clinical performance must be clearly defined. This point addresses the need to identify objectives in advance. Widespread interest in competency-based education has encouraged systematic studies of competence in the health professions. One result, however, has been the unfortunate practice of merely relabeling *objectives* as *competencies*. But whatever the label and however closely Mager's[13] rules are followed, most clinical educators agree that some description of terminal performance is essential to effective evaluation.

Evaluation of clinical performance must be individual. Since the evaluator must make decisions about the individual student's competence, the *individual's* attainment of objectives must be discerned. Measurement of relative position among classmates is simply not pertinent to the evaluation decision. Whether student A performs better than student B is hardly significant if neither is safe.

The performance evaluated must be unquestionably pertinent to the allied health profession. Educational objectives, especially when related to clinical performance, must be defensibly related to competence in the health professions.[1,18] This fact is frequently overlooked when standards and criteria reflect personal biases or unsupported assertions of importance. At the same time, the difficulty of isolating pertinent aspects of competent performance is probably increased in the clinical setting. The educator increases fidelity to the real world by incorporating clinical settings into the educational program. But a corresponding increase in the difficulty of making sound judgments is the price of this fidelity.[4,19]

DIMENSIONS OF CLINICAL PERFORMANCE

Objectives are the key to evaluation in educational programs, whether learning takes place in the classroom or in the clinic. They specify the behavior to be evaluated, the content to which the behavior is related, and often the level of mastery that is acceptable. Several taxonomies have been developed in an attempt to clarify the language and identify a continuum of educational objectives to promote more effective instruction and evaluation. In the Prologue Ford discusses the use of taxonomic levels as a useful device for specifying learning outcomes.

The taxonomies developed by Bloom,[2] Krathwohl,[10] and Harrow[9] are useful constructs for devising objectives and for analyzing examinations and teaching methods to prevent overemphasis on lower taxonomic levels such as recall and recognition. However, when applying these constructs to competent performance in the allied health fields, educators are hard pressed to make clear distinctions among the various levels within and across domains. Frequently, required performance contains elements of several levels and all three domains. Consider, for example, the task of handling a hyperactive, easily distracted child during a Denver Developmental Screening Test.

Gagné[5] expresses some difficulty in using a taxonomy for planning instruction. He offers a different hierarchy of capabilities, with problem solving as the highest level. He conceptualizes problem solving as self-arousal and selection of previously learned rules to achieve a novel combination.

Glaser[7] recently proposed the need for development of a "psychology of instruction" and the necessity for a "prescriptive science of design" that may be appropriate for professional schools. His discussion of the development of competence is particularly pertinent to the educator's concern for measuring clinical performance and emphasizes the complexity of performance being evaluated:

The changes that take place as an individual progresses from ignorance to increasing competence are of the following kinds: (a) Variable, awkward, and crude performance changes to performance that is consistent, relatively fast, and precise. Unitary acts change into larger response integrations and overall strategies. (b) The contexts of performance change from simple stimulus patterns with a great deal of clarity to complex patterns in which information must be abstracted from a context of events that are not all relevant. (c) Performance becomes increasingly symbolic, covert, and automatic. The learner responds increasingly to internal representations of an event, to internalized standards, and to internalized strategies for thinking and problem solving. (d) The behavior of the competent individual becomes increasingly self-sustaining in terms of skillful employment of the rules when they are applicable and subtle bending of the rules in appropriate situations. Increasing reliance is placed on one's own ability to generate the events by which one learns and the criteria by which one's performance is judged and valued (p. 9).

The complicated task of evaluating the performance of students in the allied health professions thus becomes more evident. Evaluation must include measures that encompass all domains; it must address different levels within those domains; and it must assess complex, interrelated combinations of skills.

METHODS FOR DEFINING CLINICAL EDUCATION OBJECTIVES

Before evaluation can take place, the educator must specify the competencies to be assessed. A number of methods have been used to identify behaviors relevant to particular professions.

1. *Role delineation.* Professional roles are identified through review of the literature and/or consensus by a group of experts in the profession. Appropriate responsibilities for each role are specified.[20]

2. *Task analysis.* Trained observers record step-by-step elements of each task or

unit of work activity professionals perform.[6]

3. *Critical incident survey.* Professionals (and consumers) are asked to describe instances when health care workers have done something that was either particularly effective or ineffective. A list of abilities and criteria is extrapolated from these reports.[14]

4. *Professional situation analysis.* A situation universe is identified by combining variables operating in professional encounters. Sample situations are systematically drawn from the universe, and each situation is analyzed to obtain intrinsic performance requirements.[11,12]

Whichever method is used, once the appropriate behaviors are identified, competencies that will serve as the basis for the evaluative measures must then be specified. Competencies identified as essential to competent performance in a particular allied health profession should in turn dictate the site selection for clinical education and evaluation. The important question to be asked is: Can the site efficiently provide appropriate opportunities? (The use of clinical sites to teach and evaluate lower levels of the cognitive domain, such as recall, is inefficient. Recall is much more appropriately and economically assessed by paper-and-pencil tests in the classroom.)

CLINICAL EVALUATION METHODS

Educators are faced with the problem of designing measures that assess the higher levels of the cognitive domain as well as skills in the psychomotor and affective domains. Carefully constructed paper-and-pencil tests, such as an interpretive exercise or patient management problem, can be used to assess analysis, synthesis, evaluation, and problem solving.[8,15] However, while they offer some situation fidelity and performance similarity, they may oversimplify normally complex situations and measure only cognitive skills.

Other simulation techniques, such as the use of role playing, artificial body parts, computers, or videotapes, add both increased fidelity *and* the opportunity to assess motor skills and attitudes along with cognitive abilities. They are appropriate for classroom learning and evaluation because they offer as much reality as possible, while protecting the client from the hazards of an inexperienced student. They can and should be utilized as a means of determining the student's readiness for experience with actual clients in the clinical setting; their use is less defensible in a real setting because of the time and clinical resources they require.

The procedures most appropriate for and most often used in the clinical setting are (1) direct observation of student performance followed by a description or judging of the behavior and (2) observation and judging of pertinent products resulting from student performance. Observation is subject to incompleteness and bias unless explicit data are systematically obtained. Some of the methods that can be used to record observations systematically and objectively are anecdotal notes, critical incident reports, and rating scales and checklists.

Anecdotal notes

The anecdotal note is a recorded description of the behavior and activities of the student during a particular performance of relatively short duration.[16,17] The note is usually written informally without modifying impressions and contains only data that clarify the image of the event. A good anecdotal note separates objective description of student behavior from any interpretations or inferences. In some instances, the evaluator may decide to provide space for recommendations on ways to improve the student's learning or adjustment as soon as a series of anecdotes is available. The evaluator can also provide space for the student to include an interpretation.

A systematic approach should be developed for collection of notes. The evaluator should select in advance those objectives suited for evaluation by anecdotal notes, as well as the number of notes to be provided for each student performance. After the anecdotes are recorded, the supervisor and student should evaluate the recorded behavior. Following are an example of an objective that can be evaluated with this technique, sample criteria, and an example of a note.

Sample anecdotal note

In working with clients, the allied health professional not only must possess the ability to gather appropriate data and use it properly to plan treatment, but should also demonstrate respect for the dignity of the client and be able to communicate effectively in order to engage the client in what is essentially a cooperative venture.

OBJECTIVE: The student collaborates with the client in establishing goals for treatment.

CRITERIA: The student obtains information regarding values and interests, shares results of evaluations with client, discusses client's assets and deficits, determines client's priorities and expectations, and obtains consensus on goals.

Student: Jane Doe   Date: 12/1/
Observer: Roberta Brown

After greeting R. J. as he entered the clinic for his third visit, Ms. Doe pointed out his areas of weakness on the ROM and MMT forms. She then listed for him two short-term and two long-term goals that she had decided were possible. She asked R. J. if he understood, but without waiting for an answer, she told him he could decide which two activities he would rather do to help accomplish the first two goals. When R. J. indicated his preference, she got out the materials and proceeded to demonstrate the process.

COMMENT: Ms. Doe restricts client's decision making to selection between predetermined activities and offers no opportunity for input on goals or even priorities.

Critical incident reports

The critical incident report is similar to the anecdotal note, but it stresses those aspects of the student's performance that the evaluator feels could make a significant difference in the outcome of an activity.[16,17] As with the anecdotal note, the evaluator must identify specific objectives that are appropriately evaluated by this method. The criteria for analysis of an incident are stated in terms of student behaviors that would influence the outcome of the activity either positively or negatively. The evaluator records the student's performance and evaluates the performance according to the stated criteria. (This technique is similar to, but not identical with the critical incident survey that is used to obtain competency statements for the profession.)

Sample critical incident report

Allied health professionals are frequently involved in situations that have the potential for serious harm to the client, to other staff members, or to themselves. Knowledge of hazards and their consqeuences must be combined with a concern for the safety of others and an ability to carry out procedures properly.

OBJECTIVE: The student takes proper safety precautions when handling specimens of potentially infectious patients.

CRITERIA: The student covers open cuts and abrasions with finger cots or gloves, uses Propipette, washes hands after handling specimens, decontaminates spills immediately, and disposes of materials in designated receptacles.

Student: John Hanson   Date: 12/2/
Observer: Ralph Green

Mr. Hanson was at the chemistry bench, pipetting serum specimens. While measuring an aliquot of serum from a tube marked with a warning label for hepatitis, he allowed the Propipette to slip and spilled serum on the bench top. Mr. Hanson placed the pipette in the receptacle for contaminated glassware, wiped the spilled blood with a paper towel, and threw the towel into the contaminated trash receptacle. He then proceeded to draw another sample, completed the dilution, and went on to the next specimen.

POSITIVE FACTORS	NEGATIVE FACTORS
Used proper equipment	Failed to decontaminate area after spillage
Used proper disposal methods	Failed to wash hands

COMMENT: Mr. Hanson endangers self and others by failure to guard against a source of serious infection.

Rating scales and checklists

The relatively unstructured descriptions of student performance obtained with anecdotal notes and critical incident reports differ from the more standardized descriptions found on rating scales and checklists. The latter are de- vices for recording qualitative and quantitative judgments about observed performance or about a product resulting from the performance.[8]

Rating scales consist of a set of characteristics or qualities to be judged together with an

---

Numerical scale: Circle the number that most closely represents the student's ability (5 = Excellent; 1 = Poor).

1. Participates in discussion   5   4   3   2   1
2. Offers pertinent information   5   4   3   2   1
3. Contributes to problem solving   5   4   3   2   1

Graphic scale: Place a check on the continuum that you feel represents the quality of the student's performance.

1. Participates in discussion

    Freely   Never

2. Offers pertinent information

    Completely and accurately   Incompletely or inaccurately

3. Contributes to problem solving

    Cooperates very well   Does not cooperate

Descriptive-graphic scale: Check the box that most nearly describes the student's behavior.

1. Participates in discussion	Speaks without urging, offers information freely	Only offers information in turn or when urged	Gives brief response to direct question or indicates that there is nothing to add
2. Offers pertinent information	Gives all important facts and supplies accurate information	Gives most significant facts, but some are too sketchy	Gives incomplete facts, stresses insignificant aspects, or misses important facts
3. Contributes to problem solving	Offers suggestions, urges others to express views, and considers others' ideas	Lets others give their views, but always presses for own ideas	Frequently interrupts others, belittles others' ideas, or does not participate

appropriate scale for indicating the degree·to which each attribute is present. Several types of scales can be used: numerical, graphic, or descriptive-graphic.

Sample rating scale

An important activity for allied health professionals is participation in the team conference. Through group process, plans for patient care are developed according to stated patient goals. Student effectiveness on the team can be evaluated in terms of participating, reporting observations, and making proposals for action.

Checklists are similar to rating scales, the difference being the kind of judgments the evaluator is called upon to make. While a rating scale requires the observer to indicate the degree to which a characteristic is present or the frequency with which a behavior occurs, the checklist requires only a simple Yes or No judgment (i.e., if the characteristic is present or absent or if an action is taken or not). Consequently, checklists are most useful in evaluating a performance that can be divided into a series of clearly defined, specific actions.

Sample procedure checklist

Allied health professionals employ numerous data-gathering techniques. Knowledge of the correct procedure to gain the necessary data is a beginning skill and can be effectively measured in the classroom, but to determine if the student is competent, the evaluator must measure the student's ability to carry out the procedure properly and safely on clients with a variety of specified conditions. A procedure checklist is one tool to determine whether data gathering has been handled competently.

If student performance results in a product, it may be more desirable to judge the product than the process. Payne[16] suggests that if the answer to any of the following questions is Yes, product evaluation is appropriate:

1. Are the steps involved in arriving at the product either indeterminate or covert?
2. Are the important characteristics of the product apparent, and can they be measured objectively and accurately?
3. Is the effectiveness of the performance to be discerned in the product itself?
4. Is evaluation of the procedures leading to the product impractical? (p. 408)

Under some circumstances, it is preferable to rate procedures during the early phases of learning and to rate a product *after* basic skills have been mastered. Rating scales or checklists can serve the same purposes in product evaluation as in procedure evaluation. They

---

Passive flexion of forearm

Procedure	Yes	No
1. Position client.	____	____
2. Explain motion to client.	____	____
3. Place axis of goniometer at lateral axis of elbow joint.	____	____
4. Line up stationary bar along lateral side of arm.	____	____
5. Line up movable bar along forearm.	____	____
6. Hold arm securely but gently inferior and superior to joint.	____	____
7. Passively extend arm toward neutral (0-degree) position to limit or point of pain.	____	____
8. Observe/measure starting position.	____	____
9. Passively flex forearm as far as possible.	____	____
10. Follow motion with movable bar.	____	____
11. Observe client for signs of pain.	____	____
12. Carefully return forearm to original position.	____	____
13. Record starting and ending measurements.	____	____

Discharge summary checklist

Routine information	Yes	No
1. Type of note identified	____	____
2. Date stated	____	____
3. Client identified	____	____
4. Signature appended	____	____
5. Reason for discontinuation noted	____	____

Discontinuation summary	Yes	No	NA
6. Total length of treatment stated	____	____	____
7. Treatment goals noted	____	____	____
8. Treatment implementation summarized	____	____	____
9. Results of treatment summarized	____	____	____
10. Follow-up or disposition noted	____	____	____
11. Home program noted	____	____	____
12. Recommendations noted	____	____	____

Written reporting skills rating scale

Procedure	Consistently	Frequently	Occasionally	Never
1. Describes client behavior explicitly	____	____	____	____
2. Describes events accurately	____	____	____	____
3. Uses logical sequence	____	____	____	____
4. Communicates essential information efficiently	____	____	____	____
5. Avoids subjective conclusions	____	____	____	____
6. Uses abbreviations appropriately	____	____	____	____
7. Uses technical vocabulary appropriately	____	____	____	____
8. Uses correct grammatical construction, including third-person style	____	____	____	____
9. Uses correct spelling	____	____	____	____
10. Writes legibly	____	____	____	____

can aid in establishing common standards for student products. They can also identify for the student those qualities desired in an acceptable product.

Sample product checklist and rating scale

The ability to report and record actions is a critical behavior in many allied health professions. Aspects of this competency include both skill in writing accurate reports and skill in communicating the information. The appropriateness and comprehensiveness of facts collected and the interpretation and implications derived from them comprise the criteria for accuracy. Criteria for skill in communication encompass clarity of terminology and composition, as well as conciseness and logic in ordering elements of the message.

Rating scales and checklists can introduce objectivity into measuring performance because they direct observations toward specific and clearly defined aspects of behavior, while providing a common frame of reference for judgments of those behaviors. However, certain limitations that exist, such as those listed below, should be noted and minimized:

1. Lack of uniformity with which terms are interpreted by evaluators. Terms used to designate intervals on the rating continuum are particularly susceptible to this error. An operational definition that includes illustrations of acceptable behaviors for each interval improves reliability among evaluators.
2. Personal bias resulting in a general tendency to rate all students at approximately the same position on the rating continuum. This position may be high, low, or at the mean, depending on the bias of the observer.
3. Halo effect or the evaluator's general impression of the student, which influences the rating of specific characteristics. Both this error and error 2 obscure a student's strengths and weaknesses. Scales that require supportive statements to justify the interval selection and reversal of the direction of the scales help to decrease these two limitations.

4. Logical errors, as when two characteristics are rated as more similar than they actually are, because of the rater's beliefs. A clear definition of terms in addition to careful training of evaluators helps to minimize this problem.

Several other useful techniques for obtaining information about the student's ability to analyze, synthesize, and evaluate are worth mentioning.

Case studies

The case study is a comprehensive, step-by-step report of a particular client's problem. Its steps include data gathering, planning, implementation, and reevaluation proposed and/or carried out for the client. The student's written description of thought processes and rationale for actions in meeting the client's needs enables the evaluator to assess the student's judgment and decision-making abilities in relation to the treatment planning process. A case study calls for interpretive and extrapolative behaviors. It has the advantage over observations because the case study can project beyond the student's overt action to the thought process behind the action.

Client care conferences

In a client care conference the student presents a client situation to a peer group for problem solving and critical analysis. The student presents all available information regarding the client, identifies elements of the problem, and proposes several alternate solutions. After the group weighs alternative solutions, identifying possible positive and negative aspects of each, its members select a course of action and give a rationale for adoption of the solution.

Process recordings

Process recording is the verbatim reproduction of verbal and nonverbal communications between two individuals for the purpose of assessing interactions. Although various formats exist, each usually contains four elements: (1) the client's communication, (2) the allied health student's communication, (3) the student's interpretation of the client's communication, and (4) implications of the communication for student action.

The process recording is best used in conjunction with an individual conference so that the supervisor and student can evaluate the total interaction, as well as each of its components. The recording enables the student to gain skill in analyzing an interaction in terms of its elements. As this skill develops, the student becomes more adept at recognizing inconsistencies and misunderstandings in verbal communication. Process recordings can assist the student to identify patterns of behavior in interactions and thus become self-evaluative about interpersonal relationship skills.

Supervisory conferences

The supervisory conference can be useful after an observation of the student by the supervisor. Discussion of the intervention, the rationale for particular measures taken, and the evaluation of the results will assure the supervisor that the student is doing the correct thing because of what is known and deduced rather than by happenstance. If consequences of the student's actions are less than desirable, the supervisor can determine if the student recognizes the problem and its underlying causes, can suggest alternate solutions, can select the most appropriate from these, and can justify the selection. Consequently, the supervisory conference can give insights into the student's areas of strength and weakness and be a learning situation in spite of apparent student failure.

Summary rating scales

The measures discussed thus far are related to specific performance. As such, they are excellent tools to use for formative evaluation. The specific feedback afforded by these measures describes the student's strengths and weaknesses and thus can aid in identifying areas that need further attention and remediation. Rating scales are also used as a means of summative evaluation to provide description of the student's overall performance for a particular phase of education. Summary rating scales serve as a certifying tool and contribute to the assessment of whether the student is safe to practice as a professional.

Because summary rating scales can touch on all aspects of the student's performance, they are more general than the previously described scales. They are also more prone to limitations, such as the halo effect and the possibility that the evaluator will draw conclusions from an inadequate sample of behavior, fail to consider contradictory data, and give disproportionate weight to incidents that have had a disturbing effect on the evaluator. These limitations can be minimized if behaviors are carefully specified and if the more specific measures used during the clinical experiences are utilized as a basis for the summary evaluation. An example of a summary rating is given in Appendix A, pp. 211 to 213.

STAGES OF CLINICAL EDUCATION

Utilization of clinical settings in the preparation of allied health professionals is essential because clinical situations offer opportunities that are very difficult to duplicate in a classroom. They provide stimuli, demands, and reactions that the student must heed, sort out, and respond to. No simulation, no matter how elaborate, can duplicate these provisions. In these situations the student most closely assumes the role of the allied health professional. The clinical setting requires that students demonstrate higher levels of integration and application of skills they have learned. For this reason, evaluation in the clinical setting is crucial. Without it, one lacks meaningful evidence that students are capable of bringing their abilities to bear on real situations to cause beneficial consequences.

Three stages or levels of clinical education can be identified. They differ in the objectives to be accomplished and, therefore, in the time, resources, and manpower required.

Stage one is the laboratory experience. Coupled with didactic course work it provides the student with the opportunity to learn isolated skills. Because the time is limited (a few hours, one or two visits), the resources and manpower required are minimal. However, it should be noted that the student is a novice and comes to the situation with a specific objective that probably does not conveniently fit into the normal clinical center's day-to-day functioning. Intentionally engineered experiences or simulations are most appropriate for this level of experience. An example of skills to be learned might be use of a piece of equipment or administration of a range of motion test.

Stage two is a limited clinical experience. Also coupled with didactic course work but at a higher order of complexity, it is intended to provide the student with the opportunity to integrate and apply closely related skills over a short period of time (several hours over several weeks). The clinical resources and manpower required are minimal, but they require identifying and making available a limited but appropriate set of experiences. An example of a skill to be learned might be evaluation and planning of treatment goals for a specific category of client.

Stage three is field-work experience. Usually taking place near or after the completion of didactic work, it is intended to provide the student with the opportunity to integrate and practice the full range of skills required of the qualified professional. A full-time experience, it extends over a long period of time (at least several months). Resources and manpower requirements are extensive, but the student generally is able to carry out a portion of the normal operations of the facility under the supervision of a qualified practitioner. For this reason, the experience is not normally disruptive to the functioning of the clinical site. Examples of the skills to be learned are evaluating, planning, and implementing treatment for a caseload of clients; reporting findings; collaborating with other team members; and carrying out a portion of maintenance functions of the department or unit to which the student is assigned.

The clinical experience (1) may be integrated with class work, include all three stages as outlined above, and start on day one of the student's professional preparation or (2) may include only the final stage and take place near the completion of the program. Although the first option is preferred, the clinical experience in both cases should be integral to the total educational preparation of the allied health professional.

If the clinical experience is to be an appropriate part of the student's education and not an ill-defined experience tacked onto the end of the student's academic work, then it must be as carefully designed and monitored as the student's academic work. Objectives must be defined, the on-site supervisor must understand and agree with the objectives as outlined, and appropriate learning experiences must be identified. Consequently, the clinical site must be carefully selected so that the learning experiences it offers match the objectives reasonably well.

This process involves active collaboration between faculty and clinical supervisors. The school faculty should submit the objectives to the clinical center; the clinical supervisor should describe the center's program and outline the learning experiences available; both must examine these experiences to determine if the objectives can be met. A general plan for the experience should be laid out, and follow-up evaluations made to determine if the plan is being followed and if it is accomplishing what was intended. This requires the exchange of materials and several meetings before the student arrives, visits to the center while the student is there, and evaluation during and after the experience is completed. Ford discusses these concepts more completely in Chapter 13.

The process does not imply that the school dictates to the center how it is to treat patients and otherwise carry out its day-to-day business. Rather, it demands that the school and center reach consensus on what is to be accomplished by students while they are at the center. The site is selected only if it is capable of fulfilling the objectives as specified by the school. If it cannot, or will not, the school is obligated to select other sites. If the school is to accomplish its goal of educating students in the full spectrum of professional competencies, it cannot accept any site, merely hoping that the students will acquire the designated competencies.

SUMMARY

The discussion in this chapter ranges over a variety of topics related to higher-order learning in clinical education for health professions. Three points bear repeating:

1. Evaluation of student performance is the most fruitful focus for the design and organization of clinical education. This is because the educator is called upon to make decisions about the student's proficiency as an entry-level professional.

2. Useful and defensible student evaluations depend on clear statements of appropriate performance. Such statements need not be excessively descriptive (as is sometimes the case when Magerian rules are followed), but neither should they be so general as to preclude securing agreement on student performance. This latter aspect of agreement further implies that methods of data gathering should be systematic and reliable, while reflecting unquestioned relationships to the characteristics being evaluated. This relationship can be thought of as one type of validity.

3. Evaluators should utilize a variety of measures in the appraisal of student clinical performance. The justification for this recommendation is two-sided. First, the complexity of higher-order performance demands a multidimensional evaluation. Second, the evaluation is more comprehensive if several methods are used. Examples of instruments and suggestions for their construction and use are provided.

Before drawing to a close, a caveat to the health professions educator about the central theme of this chapter is necessary. The concept of problem-solving ability—a synonym for higher-order learning—has been applied in virtually all educational circumstances, from elementary school mathematics through undergraduate and postgraduate training. Appearing prominently in the rhetoric of educators, curriculum designers, and evaluators, it is evident in descriptions of most professions. And yet it is likely that there is inadequate agreement on the meaning of the concept. Perhaps more importantly, there is a corresponding lack of evidence for the validation of problem solving within these separate applications.

It is agreed among members of the health professions that problem solving is essential to the practice of medicine. Most, if not all, studies of problem solving among health professions has been directed at physicians. However, most efforts to isolate problem-solving ability among physicians and medical students have been unsuccessful. Adequate performance under one set of circumstances, i.e., patient problem, is not consistently correlated with success under others. These findings suggest that situation-specific factors may be operating and not some general, cognitive factor that one can label "problem solving."

The purpose of the cautionary note is not to deny the utility of conceptual frameworks. Their effect on promoting attention to higher-order cognition has been undeniably laudatory, but the educator has a responsibility not shared with either professional practitioners or lay consumers. Educators must apply the most rigorous standards to the validation of the frameworks used in their program designs. Self-serving acceptance of high-sounding professional attributes is no substitute for enlightened and systematic research into the validation of these concepts. Put another way, health professions educators must utilize improved methods of setting objectives, defining and assessing student competence, and evaluating educational programs that do not rely solely on unsystematic consensus of "expert" committees. The advent of broader continuing education requirements, recertification, relicensure, and the like serves to make unavoidable the need for defensible decisions about programs, courses, and graduates.

On a more positive note, student evaluation decisions must be made while the quest continues. Although the picture is not entirely clear or consistent, it does appear that more health professions and other educators are addressing the fundamental unanswered questions. The quality of current decision making leaves much to be desired; however, overall improvement is occurring, and the need for revisions is more widely accepted. This augurs well for the health professions and for the quality of health care.

REFERENCES

1. Berg, I. *Education and Jobs: The Great Training Robbery.* New York: Praeger Publishers, 1970.

   A highly regarded critical examination of conventional assumptions about the relationships between education/training and workers. Data from author's studies of blue and white collar occupations are discussed.

2. Bloom, B. S., et al. *Taxonomy of Educational Objectives. Handbook I: Cognitive Domain.* New York: David McKay Company, 1956.

   An early attempt to establish a common frame of reference to assist in cooperation and communication regarding educational evaluation. This reference is the most widely accepted and used classification of the cognitive domain.

3. Ebel, R. L. *Essentials of Educational Measurement.* Englewood Cliffs, N.J.: Prentice-Hall, 1972.

   A textbook covering the history and philosophy of educational measurement, test development, test score interpretation, test analysis, and evaluation.

4. Fitzpatrick, R.; and Morrison, E. Performance and product evaluation. In R. L. Thorndike (ed.), *Educational Measurement,* 2nd ed. Washington, D.C.: American Council on Education, 1971.

   A scholarly treatise of the rationale for and use of performance evaluation. Characteristics of various types of measurement methodologies are explored and examples are included.

5. Gagne, R. M. *The Conditions of Learning.* 2nd ed. New York: Holt, Rinehart and Winston, 1970.

   This noted educator proposes his theory of the learning process including the eight classes of performance change and corresponding sets of conditions for learning.

6. Gilpatrick, E. *Health Services Mobility Study Technical Report No. 12.* New York: Health Services Mobility Study, 1973.

   One report of a nine-year project intended to promote upward mobility in health fields through design of "job ladders." This report describing an elaborate extension of task analysis procedures should prove interesting to health professions educators. Other project reports relate this work to curriculum design.

7. Glaser, R. Components of a psychology of instruction: Toward a science of design. *Review of Educational Research, 46,* (Winter) 1976, 1-24.

   This article proposes the need for a psychology of instruction as a science of design. The author's analysis of competence and his speculation regarding the components of the instructional process are pertinent to educators of professionals in any field.

8. Gronlund, N. E. *Measurement and Evaluation in Teaching.* 2nd ed. New York: Macmillan Company, 1971.

   An extremely useful basic text for teachers interested in improving evaluation procedures. The writing style and liberal use of sample test items makes this work easy to understand and handy to use.

9. Harrow, A. J. *A Taxonomy of the Psychomotor Domain.* New York: David McKay Company, 1972.

   A taxonomy of the psychomotor domain, classifying observable movement behaviors. Although the author has no connection with the groups who developed the cognitive and affective taxonomies, the book is organized in the same manner.

10. Krathwohl, D. R.; Bloom, B. S.; and Masia, B. B. *Taxonomy of Educational Objectives. Handbook II: The Affective Domain.* New York: David McKay Company, 1964.

    This work describes the nature of the affective domain, proposes a classification structure, and describes the evaluation of each level in the taxonomy.

11. LaDuca, A.; Madigan, M. J.; Grobman, H.; and others. *Professional Performance Situation Model for Health Professions Education: Occupational Therapy.* Chicago: University of Illinois, Center for Educational Development, 1975.

    A technical report describing the framework of professional situation analysis for the identification of elements of competence in allied health fields. Examples focused exclusively on application with occupational therapy.

12. LaDuca, A.; Engel, J. D.; and Risley, M. E. Progress toward development of a general model for competence definition in health professions. *Journal of Allied Health 7* (Spring), 1978, 149-156.

    A description of current refinements in the professional situation analysis methodology as applied to clinical dietetics. Topics include nature of competence in health professions, construction of criterion-referenced tests, implications for curriculum, and validation studies.

13. Mager, R. F. *Preparing Instructional Objectives.* Belmont, Calif.: Fearon Publishers, 1962.

    The classic how-to-do-it book of the behavioral objectives movement.

14. McDermott, J. F., Jr.; McGuire, C.; and Berner, E. S. *Roles and Functions of Child Psychiatrists.* Evanston, Ill.: Committee on Certification in Child Psychiatry, American Board of Psychiatry and Neurology, 1976.

    A report of a recent application of critical incident survey to determine elements of competence in a medical specialty. Presents an interesting methodological refinement.

15. McGuire, C. H.; Solomon, L. M.; and Bashook, P. G.: *Construction and Use of Written Simulations.* New York: Psychological Corporation, 1976.

    A complete exposition of written simulations using the latent image. Contains step-by-step instructions for the construction of this measurement technique.

16. Payne, D. A. *The Assessment of Learning.* Lexington, Mass.: D. C. Heath and Company, 1974.

This text covers the planning, developing, interpreting and refining of test instruments. Examples, suggested readings, and summary preview statements make this a useful reference and aid in evaluating learning outcomes.

17. Reilly, D. E. *Behavioral Objectives in Nursing: Evaluation of Learner Attainment.* New York: Appleton-Century-Crofts, 1975.

    Development of objectives and principals of evaluation is applied to a particular health care profession.

18. Sexton, P. C. Lifelong learning. *The Urban Review, 5,* (6), 1972, 5-11.

    An early argument by an eminent sociologist for recognizing the value of skill and knowledge attained in nontraditional locations.

19. Shulman, L. S. Evaluation of problem solving. *Academic decision-making: Issues and evidence,* Proceedings of Association of American Medical Colleges Council (AAMC) of Deans Spring Meeting, April 26-30, 1975, Key Biscayne, Florida. Washington, D.C.: AAMC, 1976.

    This paper discusses various methods of evaluating clinical problem solving, emphasizing features and characteristics of seven different types of instruments. The list of resources is helpful for those who desire more detailed information.

20. Wilson, M. A. Basic Principles of Credentialing Health Practitioners. *Respiratory Care, 21,* (10), 1976, 954-959.

    This inventory of "principles" includes use of clear role delineations. A useful general discussion of issues in the area by a respected figure.

APPENDIX A

Summary rating scale*

Name: _____ Date: _____

Institution: _____ Absences: _____

Type of field work: Physical dysfunction ___   Psychosocial dysfunction ___

Instructions to the rater

The rating scale consists of the activities subsumed under five main factors that have been identified as important for student performance during Phase III. Please indicate where you think the student's level of performance fits on each continuum, according to the key given below. Record your evaluations by *circling* the appropriate point on the scale following each activity.

You are requested to rate the student twice during the experience: midway through (in pencil) and at the end (in ink) of the experience. Your comments on the last page regarding the student's overall performance will be helpful in counseling the student.

Scale key

5	4	3	2	1	(NA)
Shows unusual accuracy and independent function consistently in all types of situations	Usually shows accuracy and independent function, but requires some guidance in complex or unique situations	Needs moderate guidance to carry out functions in an adequate manner	Requires intensive guidance to carry out functions, but exhibits potential to improve	Requires constant guidance, is unable to carry out functions satisfactorily, and fails to learn, so potential is questionable	Not applicable. Insufficient evidence exists to judge because of extenuating circumstances

*As used by the Curriculum in Occupational Therapy, School of Associated Medical Sciences, University of Illinois at the Medical Center.

Continued.

Factor I: Evaluation
A. History (based on written materials)
    1. Documents past medical history   5 4 3 2 1 NA
    2. Documents family and psychosocial history   5 4 3 2 1 NA
    3. Documents current medical/psychosocial status   5 4 3 2 1 NA
B. Interview (based on observations)
    4. Introduces self and explains role in appropriate manner   5 4 3 2 1 NA
    5. Communicates at client's level of understanding   5 4 3 2 1 NA
    6. Selects appropriate setting   5 4 3 2 1 NA
    7. Asks pertinent questions   5 4 3 2 1 NA
    8. Obtains desired information   5 4 3 2 1 NA
C. Evaluation (based on observations)
    9. Selects appropriate evaluation techniques   5 4 3 2 1 NA
   10. Gathers necessary materials   5 4 3 2 1 NA
   11. Explains procedure to client and answers questions   5 4 3 2 1 NA
   12. Positions client appropriately   5 4 3 2 1 NA
   13. Administers standardized tests in prescribed manner   5 4 3 2 1 NA
   14. Recognizes fatigue or frustration in the client   5 4 3 2 1 NA
   15. Concludes procedure appropriately   5 4 3 2 1 NA
   16. Reevaluates client's status at appropriate intervals   5 4 3 2 1 NA
D. Interpretation (based on written materials)
   17. Uses normative data to interpret evaluation findings   5 4 3 2 1 NA
   18. Indicates synthesis of collected data, interview responses, and evaluation results   5 4 3 2 1 NA
   19. Identifies client's assets and deficits   5 4 3 2 1 NA

Factor II: Treatment planning (based on observations
and written materials)
   20. Uses evaluation data in planning treatment   5 4 3 2 1 NA
   21. Establishes goals appropriate to client's condition and socioeconomic and cultural background   5 4 3 2 1 NA
   22. Establishes priorities that are realistic for client and setting   5 4 3 2 1 NA
   23. Selects methodologies that fulfill goals   5 4 3 2 1 NA
   24. Suggests activities that meet goals and client's interests   5 4 3 2 1 NA
   25. Plans collaboratively with client and other professionals   5 4 3 2 1 NA

Factor III: Treatment implementation (based on observations)
   26. Prepares treatment materials and/or environment   5 4 3 2 1 NA
   27. Positions client comfortably and appropriately   5 4 3 2 1 NA
   28. Explains and instructs client regarding treatment procedures   5 4 3 2 1 NA
   29. Uses processes and techniques appropriately   5 4 3 2 1 NA
   30. Modifies standard procedures or techniques as required by client's disability   5 4 3 2 1 NA
   31. Supervises client's activities   5 4 3 2 1 NA
   32. Uses praise and other reinforcers to encourage appropriate behavior   5 4 3 2 1 NA
   33. Adheres to and alerts client to precautions and safety factors   5 4 3 2 1 NA
   34. Adjusts treatment according to client's response   5 4 3 2 1 NA

Factor IV: Communication skills (based on observations and written materials)

35. Clearly communicates instructions and directions   5 4 3 2 1 NA
36. Oral reports of interviews, observations, and evaluations indicate accurate conveyance of data   5 4 3 2 1 NA
37. Written reports of interviews, observations, and evaluations indicate accurate conveyance of data   5 4 3 2 1 NA
38. Reports meet form and content requirements of facility and school   5 4 3 2 1 NA
39. Reports meet time requirements   5 4 3 2 1 NA
40. Communicates effectively with staff   5 4 3 2 1 NA

Factor V: Professional characteristics (based on observations)

41. Conforms to the regulations of the setting (time, dress, policies, and procedures)   5 4 3 2 1 NA
42. Performs in a fair and unprejudiced manner—not letting personal feelings interfere with professional relationships   5 4 3 2 1 NA
43. Respects confidentiality of client-related information   5 4 3 2 1 NA
44. Accepts feedback and modifies behavior accordingly   5 4 3 2 1 NA
45. Asks pertinent questions at appropriate time and place   5 4 3 2 1 NA
46. Seeks learning experiences to improve current level of skills and knowledge   5 4 3 2 1 NA
47. Uses time effectively   5 4 3 2 1 NA

Comments:

1. Comprehends the role of occupational therapist in this setting:

2. Recognizes own strengths and weaknesses:

3. Demonstrates integration of didactic information with clinical experiences:

4. How do you view this student's overall potential to function as an occupational therapist?

5. Other comments:

_____

Supervisor

_____

Date

epilogue **THE ILLUSION,**
THE REALITY—BUT FIRST A DREAM

Charles W. Ford
Margaret K. Morgan

Nothing happens unless first a dream. . . .
CARL SANDBURG

We have worked as long at perfecting the process of education as at almost any human endeavor, yet we are still far from attaining success. Even after centuries of probing, questioning, experimenting, we still know little of how learning occurs or how to evaluate its occurrence.

This has always been a problem in didactic education, but our lack of knowledge about clinical education is even greater. The melding of the didactic and the clinical followed by an assessment of the combination—the preparation of the practitioner—is often more complex than our tools.

Small wonder we are still unclear as to what constitutes a good, much less excellent, program or institution or graduate. Sometimes the reputation for excellence exists without substance. Sometimes others create illusions about our efforts and the product of those efforts. Or we develop an unreal conception of our own. But programs and institutions are most often assessed by others. Something is labeled good, and it becomes good. Unfortunately, a closer examination may suggest the goodness is but an illusion. The phenomenon can also occur in reverse. A judgment—an illusion—based on a single encounter can mark a program or institution as weak or bad.

Actually, reality is usually somewhere between the good and the bad. What do reality and illusion have to do with a book on clinical education? Probably as much as they have to do with education in general. In business and industry, production can be measured by the number of units or by the ledger. In education, number of graduates may tell us something about size, but nothing about quality.

Living with reality is more difficult than living with illusion. Reality depends on more concrete methods of measuring achievement. It depends on providing sufficient evidence to ourselves and others that we are doing what we say we are doing.

215

In clinical education, in order to implement the ideas expressed in this book, we must be willing to examine our methods and administration. This can be painful. We must ask ourselves if, given our resources, we are producing the best clinicians possible.

If the illusion can be put aside and reality accepted, excellence becomes not a dream but reality. A participant in a faculty workshop asked, "How high should a student goal be?" The reply: "High enough that the student will have to stand on tiptoes to reach it!" By isolating one aspect of clinical education at a time and dealing with it systematically, a breakthrough is possible.

The Prologue of this book suggests that one should begin curriculum design with both a philosophy and a theory of learning. Emphasis is also placed on working toward an ideal. Thus the dream of what could be may provide the opportunity for thinking around or over barriers. Reality is what is, illusion is what appears to be, dream is what could be—thus first the dream.

The many threads of clinical education are interwoven with institutions and persons in those institutions. To modify or change a process, the persons involved must be convinced that a possibility for excellence exists. To implement the ideas posed in this book, participants in the process of change must first dream the dreams, then create the environment, which may be based on illusion, in order to move on to substantive areas of reality, and thence to excellence. An old Sufi story serves to illustrate:

A wise man taught his followers from what appeared to be an inexhaustible store of wisdom. His disciples all dreamed that one day they would have access to his source—a thick tome that he kept to himself, not allowing anyone else to open the volume. Upon his death, his disciples anxiously awaited the moment they could open the book and have their dreams fulfilled. When that important moment arrived, they were surprised, disappointed, confused, and even annoyed, for they found writing on only one page: "When you realize the difference between the container and the content, you will have knowledge."

SELECTED BIBLIOGRAPHY

Charles W. Ford
David M. Irby

Adams, W. R.; Ham, T. H.; Mawardi, B. H.; and others. Research in self-education for clinical teachers. *Journal of Medical Education*, 49 (December) 1974, 1,166-1,173.

Allen, A. S. (Ed.) Introduction to Health Professions. St. Louis: C. V. Mosby, 1976.

Allied Health Professions Project: The Development of Job-Related Curricula Using Task Analysis. Pittsburgh: Educational Projects, 1973.

American Association of Community and Junior Colleges. *A Guide for Health Technology Program Planning*. Washington, D.C.: 1967.

American Hospital Association. *Career Mobility: A Guide for Program Planning in Health Occupations*. Chicago: 1971.

American Hospital Association. *Financial Aid Programs in Support of Health Occupations: A Guide for Auxiliaries*. Chicago: 1971.

American Hospital Association. *Health Manpower: An Annotated Bibliography*. Chicago: 1973. Mimeo.

American Hospital Association. *Statement on Role and Responsibilities of the Hospital in Providing Clinical Facilities for a Collaborative Educational Program in the Health Field*. Chicago: 1967.

American Medical Association, Council on Medical Education. *Instructor Preparation for the Allied Health Professions and Health Occupations*. Task Force on Instructor Preparation, Advisory Committee on Education for the Allied Health Professions and Services, Council on Medical Education, American Medical Association, 1971.

American Medical Association, Council on Medical Education. *Self-Analysis Outline for Allied Health Education Programs*. Chicago: 1973. Mimeo.

Baines, T. R. The faculty supervisor. In J. Duley (Ed.), *Implementing Field Experience Education*. San Francisco: Jossey-Bass, 1974.

Banathy, B. H. *Instructional Systems*. Palo Alto, Calif.: Fearon, 1968.

Bandura, A. *Principles of Behavior Modification*. New York: Holt, Rinehart and Winston, 1969.

Barham, V. Z. Identifying effective behavior of the nursing instructor through critical incidents. *Nursing Research*, 14, (Winter) 1965, 65-69.

Barrows, H. S. *Problem-Based Learning in Medicine: Rationale and Methods*. Education Monograph 4. Ontario, Canada: McMaster University, Faculty of Medicine, 1973.

Block, J. H. (Ed.). *Mastery Learning*. New York: Holt, Rinehart and Winston, 1971.

Bloom, B. S., et al. *A Taxonomy of Educational Objectives: Handbook I: Cognitive Domain*. New York: David McKay, 1964.

Bloom, B. S.; Hastings, S. T.; and Madaus, A. F. *Handbook on Formative and Summative Evaluation of Student Learning*. New York: McGraw-Hill, 1971.

Boyles, M. V.; Morgan, M. K.; and McCaulley, M. H. *The Health Professions*. Philadelphia: W. B. Saunders, 1978.

Brown, C. A. The division of laborers: Allied health professions. *International Journal of Health Services*, 3, (March) 1973, 435-444.

Canfield, A. A. (Ed.) *Competencies for Allied Health Instructors*. Gainesville, Fla.: University of Florida, Center for Allied Health Instructional Personnel, 1972.

Carnegie Commission on Higher Education. *Higher Education and the Nation's Health: Policies for Medical and Dental Education*. New York: McGraw-Hill, 1970.

Clapp, R. W.; Goldman, C.; and Madison, D. L. The federal health agency as preceptor in community medicine. *Public Health Reports*, 85, (February) 1970, 151-154.

Collegiate Programs in Allied Health Occupations. 4 vols. Washington, D.C.: American Society of Allied Health Professions, 1977.

Connelly, T., Jr. Health care process: Teaching models for allied health students. *Journal of Allied Health, 4,* (Winter) 1975, 39-45.

Continuum in Health Occupations Education. Report of a Planning Project for Health Occupations Education. Concord, N.H.: New Hampshire Health Careers Council, 1971.

Cross, K. P. *Accent on Learning.* San Francisco: Jossey-Bass, 1976.

Davis, I. K. *Competency Based Learning: Technology, Management, and Design.* New York: McGraw-Hill, 1973.

Davis, L. E., and Andrews, R. B. The health care system looks at allied health personnel. *Clinical Obstetrics and Gynecology, 15,* (June) 1972, 305-318.

Day, D. J. A systems diagram for teaching treatment planning. *American Journal of Occupational Therapy, 27,* (July-August) 1973, 239-243.

Dixon, J. K., and Koerner, B. Faculty and student perceptions of effective classroom teaching in nursing. *Journal of Nursing Research, 25,* (July-August) 1976, 300-305.

Dressel, P. L. *Evaluation in Higher Education.* Boston: Houghton Mifflin, 1961.

Drumheller, S. J. *Handbook of Curriculum Design for Individualized Instruction: A Systems Approach.* Englewood Cliffs, N.J.: Educational Technology Publications, 1971.

Dunkin, M. J., and Biddle, B. J. *The Study of Teaching.* Washington, D.C.: American Association of University Professors, 1971.

Eble, K. E. *The Recognition and Evaluation of Teaching.* Washington, D.C.; American Association of University Professors, 1971.

Engs, R. C.; Barnes, S. E.; and Wantz, M. *Health Games Students Play.* Dubuque, Iowa: Kendall/Hunt, 1975.

Evans, R. L.; Pittman, J. G.; and Peters, R. C. The community-based medical school—reactions at the interface between medical education and medical care. *New England Journal of Medicine, 288,* (April 5) 1973, 713-719.

Fenderson, D. Health manpower development and rural services. *Journal of the American Medical Association, 225,* (September 24) 1973, 1,627-1,631.

Fine, S. A., and Wiley, W. W. *An introduction to Functional Job Analysis.* Methods for Manpower Analysis, No. 4. Kalamazoo, Mi.: W. E. Upjohn Institute for Employment Research, 1971.

Flanders, N. A. *Analyzing Classroom Behavior.* Reading, Mass.: Addison-Wesley, 1971.

Flanders, N. A. *Analyzing Teaching Behavior.* Reading, Mass.: Addison-Wesley, 1970.

Flanders, N. A. The changing base of performance based teaching. *Phi Delta Kappan, 55,* (January) 1974, 312-315.

Ford, C. W., and Morgan, M. K. Teaching in the Health Professions. St. Louis: C. V. Mosby Company, 1976.

Gaff, J. G. *Toward Faculty Renewal.* San Francisco: Jossey-Bass, 1975.

Gage, N. L. (Ed.). *Handbook of Research on Teaching.* Chicago: Rand McNally, 1973.

Gagné, R. M. *The Conditions of Learning.* 2nd ed. New York: Holt, Rinehart and Winston, 1970.

Gazda, G. M.; Walters, R. P.; and Childers, W. C. *Human Relations Development: A Manual for Health Sciences.* Boston: Allyn and Bacon, 1975.

Gerlach, V. S., and Ely, D. P. *Teaching and Media: A Systematic Approach.* Englewood Cliffs, N.J.: Prentice-Hall, 1971.

Gottman, J. M., and Clasen, R. E. *Evaluation in Education: A Practitioner's Guide.* Itasca, Ill.: Peacock, 1972.

Graham, J. R. Systematic evaluation of clinical competence. *Journal of Medical Education, 46,* (July) 1971, 625-629.

Gromisch, D. S.; Bamford, J. C.; Rous, S. N.; and others. A comparison of student and departmental chairman evaluations of teaching performance. *Journal of Medical Education, 47,* (April) 1972, 281-284.

Gronlund, N. E. *Stating Behavioral Objectives for Classroom Instruction.* New York: Macmillan, 1970.

Harless, W. G.; Drennon, G. G.; Marxer, J. J.; and others. CASE: A computer-aided simulation of the clinical encounter. *Journal of Medical Education, 46,* (May) 1971, 443-448.

Harrow, A. J. *A Taxonomy of the Psychomotor Domain.* New York: David McKay, 1972.

Hawthorne, M. E., and Perry, J. W. *Community Colleges and Primary Health Care: Study of Allied Health Education (SAHE) Report.* Washington, D.C.: American Association of Community and Junior Colleges, 1974.

Hendee, W. R. A collaborative program in allied health training. *Journal of Medical Education, 46,* (August) 1971, 658-665.

Hildebrand, M.; Wilson, R. C.; and Dienst, E. R. *Evaluating University Teaching.* Berkeley: University of California, Berkeley Center for Research and Development in Higher Education, 1971.

Holcomb, J. D., and Garner, A. E. *Improving Teaching in Medical Schools.* Springfield, Ill.: Charles C Thomas, 1973.

Holder, L. Delivery of health care: Implications for allied health educators. *Journal of Allied Health, 2,* (Spring) 1973, 68-75.

Hood, P. D., et al. *Development of Assessment Instruments for Competency Based Education.* San Francisco: Far West Laboratory, 1973.

Hospital Research and Educational Trust. *Training and Continuing Education: A Handbook for Health Care Institutions.* Chicago: 1970.

Howsam, R. B. Performance based instruction. *Today's Education, 61,* (April) 1972, 33-40.

Hubbard, J. P. *Measuring Medical Education.* Philadelphia: Lea and Febiger, 1971.

Husted, F. L., and Perry, J. W. (Eds.). *Manpower Conference on Allied Health Professions Assistants.* Buffalo, N.Y.: State University of New York, School of Health Related Professions, 1970.

Irby, D.; DeMers, J.; Scher, M.; and Matthews, D. A model for the improvement of medical faculty lecturing. *Journal of Medical Education, 51,* (May) 1976, 403-409.

Johnson, C. E. *Competencies for Teachers: A Handbook for Specifying and Organizing Teaching Performances.* Athens, Ga.: University of Georgia, College of Education, 1972.

Johnson, R. B., and Johnson, S. R. *Assuring Learning with Self-Instructional Packages.* Reading, Mass.: Addison-Wesley, 1973.

Johnson, R. B., and Johnson, S. R. *Developing Individualized Instructional Material.* Palo Alto, Calif.: Westinghouse Learning Press, 1970.

Kemp, J. E. *Instructional Design.* Belmont, Calif.: Fearon, 1971.

Kern, B., and Mickelson, J. The development and use of an evaluation instrument for clinical education. *Physical Therapy, 51* (May) 1971, 540-545.

Kiker, M. Characteristics of the effective teacher. *Nursing Outlook, 21* (November) 1973, 721-723.

Krathwohl, D. R., et al. *A Taxonomy of Educational Objectives.* Handbook II: *Affective Domain* New York: David McKay, 1964.

Lessinger, L. M., and Tyler, R. W. (Eds.). *Accountability in Education.* Worthington, Ohio: Charles A. Jones, 1971.

Lewis, J., Jr. *Appraising Teacher Performance.* West Nyack, N.Y.: Parker, 1973.

Light, I., and Frey, D. C. Education and the hospital: Dual responsibility for allied manpower training. *Hospitals, 47* (March) 1973, 85-88.

Mackenzie, R. S. Defining clinical competence in terms of quantity, quality, and need for performance criteria. *Journal of Dental Education, 37* (September) 1973, 37-44.

Mager, R. F. *Developing Attitude toward Learning.* Palo Alto, Calif.: Fearon, 1968.

Mager, R. F., and Pipe, P. *Analyzing Performance Problems or You Really Oughta Wanna.* Palo Alto, Calif.: Fearon, 1971.

Martin, M. C., and Brodt, D. E. Task analysis for training and curriculum design. *Improving Human Performance, 21,* (Summer) 1973, 113-128.

McAshan, H. H. *The Goals Approach to Writing and Using Performance Objectives: Cognitive Domain, Affective Domain, Management by Objectives.* Philadelphia: W. B. Saunders, 1974.

McGuire, C., and Solomon, L. Selected problems in patient management. *Clinical Simulations.* New York: Appleton-Century-Croft, 1971.

McTernan, E. J., and Hawkins, R. O., Jr. (Eds.). *Educating Personnel for the Allied Health Professions and Services.* St. Louis: C. V. Mosby, 1972.

Merritt, D. L. Performance objectives: A beginning, not an end. *Contemporary Education, 43,* (April) 1971, 209-212.

Miller, G. E., et al.: *Teaching and Learning in Medical School.* Cambridge: Harvard University, 1968.

Miller, R. I. *Developing Programs for Faculty Evaluation: A Sourcebook for Higher Education.* San Francisco: Jossey-Bass, 1974.

Miller, R. I. *Evaluating Faculty Performance.* San Francisco: Jossey-Bass, 1972.

Milliken, M. E. (Ed.). *Proceedings: Conference on Teacher Education for Allied Health and Nursing.* Athens, Ga.: University of Georgia, 1974.

Milliken, M. E. (Ed.). *Teacher Education for Allied Health Occupations: Toward Competency-Based Programs.* Athens, Ga.: University of Georgia, 1973.

Moore, M. L.; Parker, M. M.; and Nourse, E. S. *Form and Function of Written Agreements in the Clinical Education of Health Professionals.* Thorofare, N.J.: C. B. Slack, 1972.

Morgan, M. K. (Ed.). *Stretching Resources for Allied Health Faculty Preparation.* Gainesville, Fla.: Center for Allied Health Instructional Personnel, University of Florida, 1977.

Morgan, M. K., and Irby, D. M. *Evaluating Clinical Competence in the Health Professions.* St. Louis: C. V. Mosby, 1978.

Perry, J. W., and Nechasek, J. E. (Eds.). *Health Maintenance: Challenge for the Allied Health Professions.* Buffalo, N.Y.: State University of New York, School of Health Related Professions, 1972.

Phillips, D. F. Laboratory for medical education. *Hospitals, 47,* (March) 1973, 77-82.

Pinkston, D.; Hockhauser, S. L.; and Gardner-O'Laughlin, K. Standards for basic education in physical therapy: A tool for planning clinical education. *Physical Therapy, 55,* (August) 1975, 841-849.

Popham, J. (Ed.). *Criterion-Referenced Measurement: An Introduction.* Englewood Cliffs, N.J.: Educational Technology Publications, 1971.

Popham, W. J. (Ed.). *Evaluation in Education.* Berkeley: McCutchan, 1974.

Popham, W. J., and Baker, E. L. *Systematic Instruction.* Englewood Cliffs, N.J.: Prentice-Hall, 1970.

Proceedings of the National Conference for Evaluating Competence in the Health Professions. New York: Professional Examination Service, 1977.

Purtilo, R. *The Allied Health Professional and the Patient: Techniques of Effective Interaction.* Philadelphia: W. B. Saunders, 1973.

Ramsden, E., and Dervitz, H. L. Clinical education: Interpersonal foundations. *Physical Therapy, 52,* (October) 1972, 1,060-1,066.

Rauen, K. C. The clinical instructor as role model. *Journal of Nursing Education, 13* (August) 1974, 33-40.

Roush, R. E., and Holcomb, J. D. Teaching improvements in higher education: Medical education may be the leader. *Phi Delta Kappan, 55,* (January) 1974, 338-340.

Rovin, S., and Packer, M. W. Evaluation of teaching and teachers at the University of Kentucky College of Dentistry. *Journal of Dental Education, 35,* (August) 1971, 496-502.

Rubin, I., Plovnick, M., and Fry, R. *Improving the Coordination of Care: A Program for Health Team Development.* Cambridge, Mass.: Ballinger, 1977.

Schmieder, A. A. *Competency Based Education. A Pro-file of the States.* Commissioner's Annual Report to the Congress. Washington, D.C.: U.S. Office of Education, 1973.

Shrock, J. G. Evaluation of Clinical instruction and instructors. *Journal of Dental Education, 30,* (March) 1966, 51-53.

Stritter, F. T.; Hain, J. D.; and Grimes, D. A. Clinical teaching reexamined. *Journal of Medical Education, 50,* (September) 1975, 877-882.

Stufflebeam, D. L., et al. *Educational Evaluation and Decision Making.* Itasca, Ill.: Peacock, 1971.

Tichy, M. K. *Health Care Teams: An Annotated Bibliography.* New York: Praeger, 1974.

Travers, R. M. W. (Ed.). *Second Handbook of Research on Teaching.* Chicago: Rand McNally, 1973.

Twelker, P. A. (Ed.). *Instructional Simulation Systems: An Annotated Bibliography.* Corvallis, Ore.: Continuing Education Publications, 1969.

Vanderschmidt, L. Self-instructional materials for health care facilities. In J. Lysaught (Ed.) *Instructional Technology in Medical Education. Proceedings of the Fifth Rochester Conference on Self-Instruction in Medical Education.* Rochester, N.Y.: Rochester Clearinghouse on Self-Instruction for Health Care Facilities, 1974.

Walker, J. D. Favorable and unfavorable behaviors of the dental faculty evaluated by dental students. *Journal of Dental Education, 35,* (October) 1971, 625-631.

Wandelt, M. A., and Stewart, D. S. *Slater Nursing Competencies Rating Scale.* New York: Appleton-Century-Crofts, 1975.

Ware, J. E., and Williams, R. G. The Dr. Fox effect: A study of lecturer effectiveness and ratings of instruction. *Journal of Medical Education, 50,* (February) 1975, 149-156.

Warner, A. NHC's manpower distribution project—finding ways to interest students to practice in shortage areas. *Journal of Allied Health, 4,* (Winter) 1975, 27-34.

Weigand, J. (Ed.). *Developing Teacher Competencies.* Englewood Cliffs, N.J.: Prentice-Hall, 1971.

Wilson, M. A. *Equivalency Evaluation in Development of Health Practitioners.* Thorofare, N.J.: Charles B. Slack, 1976.

Wilson, R.; Gaff, G.; Dienst, E.; and others. *College Professors and Their Impact on Students.* New York: John Wiley, 1975.

Wise, H.; Beckhard, R.; Rubin, I.; and Kyte, A. L. *Making Health Teams Work.* Cambridge, Mass.: Ballinger, 1977.

Wittrock, M. C., and Wiley, D. E. (Eds.). *The Evaluation of Instruction: Issues and Problems.* New York: Holt, 1970.

Wolkon, G. H.; Naftaline, D. H.; Donnelly, F. A.; and Johnson, C. W. Student and faculty evaluation of instructors as measures of teaching effectiveness. *Journal of Medical Education, 49,* (August) 1974, 781-782.

Zuckerman, D. W., and Horn, R. E. *The Guide to Simulations/Games for Education and Training.* Lexington, Mass.: Information Resources, 1973.

INDEX